Acclaim for the writing of Niall McLaren, M.D.

"Dr. McLaren brilliantly wields the sword of philosophy to refute the modern theories of psychiatry with an analysis that is sharp and deadly. His own proposed novel theory could be the dawn of a new revolution in the medicine of mental illness."　　　　　—Andrew R. Kaufman, MD
Chief Resident of Emergency Psychiatry
Duke University Medical Center

"Not only does Dr. Niall McLaren point out the various shortcomings of the established views of psychology/psychiatry, and of some other scientific disciplines, but he also proposes the most cogent model of mind that does not violate fundamental scientific laws and is also compatible with the norms of common sense and logic. He has endangered the foundations of contemporary mainstream psychiatry while, at the same time, creating a rescue channel."

—Ernest Dempsey, editor of *Recovering the Self Journal*

"This book is a *tour de force*. It demonstrates a tremendous amount of erudition, intelligence and application in the writer. It advances an interesting and plausible mechanism for many forms of human distress. It is an important work that deserves to take its place among the classics in books about psychiatry."

—Robert Rich, PhD, AnxietyAndDepression-Help.com

"I found Niall McLaren's book to be an incredibly well-written and thought-provoking. It is not, by any means, easy reading. It is also not for someone who doesn't have some form of background in understanding the various psychological theories and mental health conditions. I think that this would make an excellent textbook for a graduate class that allows students to question the theories that we already have."

—Paige Lovitt for *Reader Views*

"It is impossible to do justice to this ambitious, erudite, and intrepid attempt to dictate to psychiatry a new, 'scientifically-correct' model theory. The author offers a devastating critique of the shortcomings and pretensions of psychiatry, not least its all-pervasive, jargon-camouflaged nescience.

—Sam Vaknin, PhD, author Malignant Self Love: Narcissism Revisited

"McLaren's book has been thirty years in the making and is obviously well researched and thought-out. The author makes very strong, intelligent arguments that, I believe, will have a large impact on the future of psychiatry. McLaren's book would make an excellent read for a psychiatry student or for those already in the field."

—Kam Aures for *Rebecca's Reads*

"This is an academic book about psychiatric methods. As a psychology graduate as well as a user of the various services, I find this a fascinating subject. It's not for a beginner, but for someone who has some experience of the mental health services, it's interesting and thought-provoking. We need to get over the stigma attached to mental health and see it on the same level as physical health issues. It's not a new theory, but more of an overview of what has gone before and where the future direction of psychiatry should lead."

—Josie Henley-Einion, author of *Silence*

"Among the theories McLaren shows as severely flawed are behaviorist models, psychoanalysis, and eclectic models of psychiatry. Most importantly, McLaren states that no real foundational theory exists for psychiatry. While definitions of mental disorder exist, no real definition of mental order or normality has been determined. Until it is determined what a normal mental state is, psychiatry cannot accurately determine what is a mental disorder.

McLaren's thesis is that 'human behavior is the outcome of a complex interaction between an emergent mind and the physical body.' While psychiatry has focused on depression as the most popular mental disorder, McLaren believes the focus should be on anxiety, which is the result of the 'fight or flight' instinct in most creatures; traumatic events that cause anxiety can lead to depression, so consequently anxiety deserves to be studied as a source of depression. McLaren emphasizes that the human mind does affect the human body, as in cases of mass hysteria, anxiety, and fear that create panic attacks.

Ultimately, McLaren says that any theory of the mind has to provide a rational explanation of mental disorder. He boldly speaks his mind throughout the book, backing up his points with multiple examples, and he is not afraid to cry "Humbug!" when necessary. McLaren has been practicing psychiatry since 1977 in Australia. His discussion of his own education and the shortcomings of the education system he went through as well as weaknesses in current psychiatric practices demonstrate that psychiatry has many more steps to take before it is a completely effective science. This work may well lead to a new understanding of mental illness in future years as younger psychiatrists read his book and follow his example in rejecting the ineffective theories he derides."

—Tyler R. Tichelaar, PhD

"This is a paradigm-challenging work, to say the very least, and McLaren's views require a person who has a vested interest in these subjects to confront their own resistance to challenge. It's worthwhile, because McLaren's book is affirmative concerning something which many people may have found lacking in modern psychology, and psychiatry: namely, a psyche.

With the technological revolutions occurring in the past century-and-a-half, it seems every scientist wanted to find a way to reduce the psyche to a physical property, or some combination of physical properties, or completely deny its existence (behaviorism). While this has certainly been in vogue, and has yielded many useful results in terms of understanding neurobiology and its connection to moods and perception, it has not been successful in penetrating an understanding of 'the Self', or the psyche. Some will say this is because the self/psyche doesn't exist, but is only a fiction that appears to the individual: still, this is just a reduction to absurdity- what is the person who perceives the self, but indeed the self?"

—Kevin Brady, *Clear Objectives*

HUMANIZING PSYCHIATRISTS:
TOWARD A HUMANE PSYCHIATRY

Niall McLaren, M.D.

An application of the philosophy of science to psychiatry

Library of Congress Cataloging-in-Publication Data

McLaren, Niall, 1947-
    Humanizing psychiatrists : toward a humane psychiatry : an application of the philosophy of science to psychiatry / Niall McLaren.
        p. ; cm.
    Includes bibliographical references and index.
    ISBN-13: 978-1-61599-060-3 (trade paper : alk. paper)
    ISBN-10: 1-61599-060-7 (trade paper : alk. paper)
    ISBN-13: 978-1-61599-061-0 (hardcover : alk. paper)
    ISBN-10: 1-61599-061-5 (hardcover : alk. paper)
    1. Psychiatry--Philosophy. 2. Psychology, Pathological. 3. Mental illness--Etiology. 4. Biological psychiatry. 5. Cognitive neuroscience. I. Title.
    [DNLM: 1. Physician-Patient Relations. 2. Psychiatry. 3. Humanism. 4. Psychological Theory. WM 62]
    RC437.5.M437 2010
    616.89--dc22
                                    2010035858

Distributed by: Baker & Taylor, Ingram Book Group, Quality Books

Future Psychiatry Press is an imprint of
Loving Healing Press
5145 Pontiac Trail
Ann Arbor, MI 48105
USA

http://www.LovingHealing.com or
info@LovingHealing.com
Fax +1 734 663 6861

Table of Contents

Contents

Introduction

This is the third in my little series of monographs on the logical status of psychiatry and my suggestions as to how these may be overcome. I would like to be able to say that the world of psychiatry has fairly leapt with excitement over what I have termed the biocognitive theory for psychiatry, perhaps even promoting it to the same status as the spurious biopsychosocial model long enjoyed, but that has not been the case. There is growing interest in this type of work, especially among medical students and psychiatric trainees, but the comfortable world of orthodox psychiatry really doesn't see much need to pay any attention to the scribblings of yet another quirky provincial who believes he has found the essential fault in the profession. Our elders and betters feel no need to look too closely at what they are doing as they are quite sure that it is heading in the right direction and it is only a matter of time before science churns out the correct Science of Mental Disorder and half the population is put on drugs for life.

The theory outlined in these books is the most highly developed and radical theory in the history of psychiatry. My work says that the entire direction of modern psychiatry is wrong. Mental disorder is not the result of a chemical disorder of the brain but wholly psychological, a matter of "wrong programming", if you prefer. The finer details of this theory are, well, fairly fine, and they certainly need a great deal more work before any reliability will attach to them. However, that job falls to the readers. I have done my bit in formulating this theory to the point where it can be published. Other people have to read it carefully and find the faults setting up a dialectic process which, we hope, will lead to an improved version. However, there is a catch. Anybody who wishes to criticize this work must also, by the rules of science, turn the same critical effort on their own favorite theory. Criticism is the engine of scientific progress but, if you read only the mainstream psychiatric literature or attended their conferences, you wouldn't think so. All too often, our professors take criticism as an intense attack upon themselves and respond accordingly. They didn't read the bit in Popper where he said that "We let our hypotheses die in our stead."

I am most grateful to my publisher, Mr. Victor Volkman of L.H. Press, Ann Arbor, who patiently sorts out the many problems of committing words to paper, and to young friends I have made on my overseas trips. However, the main thanks will always go to my family who patiently endure living with the ultimate outsider.

Darwin, Northern Territory, Australia
July 20th, 2010.

Part I:
The Logic of
Mental Disorder

1 | Consciousness Unexplained: The Failure Of Dennett's Functionalism

1.1: Introduction

Over the past few years, there has been a wave of unsavory events, in which psychiatrists are alleged to have taken large sums of money in exchange for ensuring that their research produced results favorable to certain viewpoints [1, 2]. Coincidentally, those viewpoints happened to be the same as the drug companies who were sponsoring the research. Years ago [3], I predicted that psychiatry would be regularly rattled by scandals of this type. The reason was because there is no formal model of mental disorder to impose limits on the activities of practitioners and researchers. Matters have not improved in the past decade: without a scientific model, there is no coherence, so that the practice of psychiatry is driven by the strongest social forces, rather than scientific forces. At present, a gale of financial pressure drives psychiatry across a wasteland of public indifference, lit only by occasional lightning bolts of media panic. This is the case just because we have no proper models of mental disorder. Since the starting point in any scientific endeavor is a declared theory or model to limit the area of study, the absence of a declared model means the whole field of psychiatry is pre-scientific.

In my previous books, I showed that the various models used in psychiatry, since its beginnings one hundred and fifty years ago, all fail to meet the minimal criteria of what constitutes a science. They don't just fail, but not one of them can be developed to the point where it could form the basis of a general theory of mental disorder for psychiatry. This is of fundamental importance: without a formal, declared model, psychiatry can never progress beyond being mere protoscience. These days, there is no real argument that psychoanalysis and behaviorism have failed, and why they failed. Psychoanalysis showed the folly of unrestrained theorizing when the theories are not anchored to reality. In fact, the history of psychoanalysis is really quite frightening. It shows how easily an attempt to build a rational theory of mind can slide into ideology [4, 5]. Skinner's work also had that totalitarian tendency (for example, his obsession with 'prediction and control' of behavior), but psychiatrists never took him as seriously as he took himself.

However, when we come to the biological approach to mental disorder, psychiatry's mask of tolerance slips, and a rigid, uncompromising view of human life emerges. Lately, however, psychiatrists seem to have given up the pretence of being masters of their own field and have left the intellectual running, if that is what it is, to neurophysiologists. There are now very few papers published by psychiatrists on the theoretical basis of biological psychiatry. In fact, I have often said that I have published more original work on the theory of biological psychiatry than all biological psychiatrists in history combined, but all my conclusions are unfavorable. This doesn't stop the claims, though: we are constantly told that reductionist biological science will soon deliver a full and final account of mental disorder. Mental disorder will be shown to be just a special case of brain disorder because, its supporters claim, mental events and brain events are one and the same thing [6, 7]. However, as empirical claims, these have no support and, as logical claims, they are incoherent [8].

So where does this leave us? Since psychiatry has failed to set its intellectual house in order, it is appropriate to look to other disciplines to see what they have to offer. The first and most likely candidate is philosophy, with its ancient tradition of looking closely at complex questions. If we had a formal theory of mind, surely a theory of mental disorder would flow easily from it, wouldn't it? These days, there are really only two possibilities for the title of 'the correct theory of mind.' The first is a reappraisal of the ancient doctrine of dualism [9], now termed 'natural dualism' to distinguish it from the many forms of supernatural dualism that went before. David Chalmers' case is that "consciousness must be taken seriously," specifically as an ontologically separate and causally effective factor in human behavior.

On the other hand, most modern philosophers embrace one form or other of monism, the notion that mind and body are not ontologically separate but are, in some sense still to be decided, both part of the same realm, meaning the material universe. This means the universe of matter and energy, governed by the fixed laws of physics which, in turn, derive from the fundamental nature of matter. Materialism states that there is nothing in the universe beyond matter and energy and the informational states controlling them. It specifically excludes the possibility of "supernatural" control: no spirits, ghosts, demi-gods, or demons, etc. Everything has a rational explanation. Thus, materialism doesn't exclude extraterrestrial beings; it simply says that, while they are visiting our solar system, the little green men will have to obey all the rules, and our rules are the same as theirs back home.

The significance for psychiatry is that, if the biological approach is to survive, it will have to fit in with a larger theory of mind. Fortunately, for the "chemical imbalance" partisans, there are several monist models of mind available; so all is not yet lost. In Part I, I will examine two well-known monist theories of mind to see whether they can form the basis of a biological approach to psychiatry. The first is the work of Daniel

Dennett, who holds to a form of functionalism, while the second, John Searle, advocates what he calls "biological naturalism". Both of these theorists have been around for a long time, with Searle approaching his fiftieth anniversary at Berkeley. Over at Tufts, in Boston, Dennett has been holding the fort for only about three decades. We can assume, then, that their views have been fairly well worked and their more recent publications will most likely be their legacy. In fact, their work hasn't changed a lot in the last quarter century and neither of them shows any sign of apostasy (recent versions of them can be seen on Youtube).

1.2: Dennett And Anti-Dualism: "And Then A Miracle Occurs"

In his 1991 monograph *Consciousness Explained*, Dennett mounts a vehement case against any and all forms of dualism on the basis that they are irredeemably irrational. His interest goes back to his first year in college, when he read Descartes' *Meditations* and was "... hooked on the mind-body problem" [10, preface]. The classic Cartesian formulation was that the mind is a real thing which interacts with the brain to control the body. Unlike the body, the mind has no shape, no form or color, no size, or even a location inside the fragile box of bones called the skull. Nobody has ever seen a mind, spirit, or soul; yet, from direct experience, everybody knows that there must be something "in there" that does the thinking, experiencing, and acting. To Descartes, it had to be a special kind of real thing, made not of bone and meat stuff but of spirit stuff, a stuff we humans have but which the lower animals don't. However, this immediately bothered the young Dennett: "How on earth," he asked, "could my thoughts and feelings fit in the same world with the nerve cells and molecules that made up my brain?" It seemed to him that the only conceivable way the Cartesian approach could survive was by a small miracle connecting the two realms. He scoffed at this in a cartoon on p. 38 (page references are to the 1993 Penguin edition).

He has been working on the question ever since, making "some progress" to the point where he offered this volume with its provocative title. He gives little time to other philosophers' attempts to examine this most difficult of areas, dismissing them as yielding only "...self-contradiction, quandaries, or blank walls of mystery..." [11]. His view is that "...the various phenomena (of) consciousness... are all physical effects of the brain's activities..." [10, p. 16]. He concedes that it is "very hard to imagine how your mind could be your brain—but not impossible." He is, however, convinced that "...a theory of the biological mechanisms..." would resolve the "...traditional paradoxes and mysteries of consciousness..." His approach would succeed where others' had failed because they "got off on the wrong foot."

The first and worst wrong foot is the "forlorn" notion of dual entities, the "...hopelessly contradiction-riddled myth of the distinct, separate soul" [10, p. 430], which sees mind as one substance and the brain as another. Based in his early apprehension of the problem of Descartes' solution, Dennett sees dualism as crude magical thinking which violates the fundamental laws of the universe, creating endless logical problems without solving any: "Dualism, the idea that a brain cannot be a thinking thing, so a thinking thing cannot be a brain..." At different points, he rails against it ("accepting dualism is giving up"), belittles it ("I wiggle my finger by... what, wiggling my soul?"), or just mocks it ("ectoplasm, Wonder Tissue") because it is false, incoherent, and antiscientific: "There is the lurking suspicion that the most attractive feature of mind stuff is its promise of being so mysterious that it keeps science at bay forever... if dualism is the best we can do, then we can't understand human consciousness" [10, p. 37-9]. His preference is an unalloyed materialism: "Somehow, the brain must be the mind" (p. 41). The book is his attempt to show how that essentially counter-intuitive notion might be the case.

He has no doubt that ectoplasm or spirit stuff is very slippery. One eye must always be kept peeled for it lest it should worm its way into what seems like a brilliant new theory of mind. Sometimes, however, the problem is much more subtle than simply positing a little gremlin or homunculus inside the head. Every now and then, neurophysiological concepts are used to cloak what is, in form, just a rehash of Descartes' non-solution. That is, it is more important to look at the form of a new theory, and not be beguiled by its content. This is especially the case where somebody uses lots of, say, neurophysiological or data-processing terms to garnish what is essentially a dualist model.

Fortunately, Dennett has an infallible test for mind stuff, the "Cartesian Theater." If the magical spirit floating in the head is able to see and hear and feel the information being channeled to it from the outside, and to look into the memory banks and then make decisions before sending them to the various effector organs, then any hidden ectoplasm can easily be found lurking where the information flows to or a point it flows past. It's a bit like an army: if you want to find the general, he's likely to be hanging around whatever the troops are marching past. Conversely, if the troops are marching in review, somebody is reviewing them. In the brain, that somebody can only be a Big Boss, an Ultimate Executive, spirit, or whatever.

Thus, if the conscious contents are assembled into a stream, or flow, or river, or if they travel along a path or to a specific part of the brain where they cavort in a field or on a stage, or if they are bathed in an inner light or are illuminated or picked out in any way, then the reason is because they will be inspected by an inner eye. In turn, this inner eye must belong to an "inner man" or homunculus whom nobody can see because he/she/it has "no shape, no form or color, no size, or even location." This is his test: the Cartesian Theater necessarily implies an Observer, and the Observer is necessarily made of magical stuff, the Ghost in the Machine. This means that any hint of the Cartesian Theater means the whole thing is non-scientific. The only solution to magical mind stuff is to get rid of all traces of the observer and of the observed, leaving only a monist theory of mind, such that consciousness can be explained "... without ever giving in to the siren song of dualism" (p. 33).

All this was published in 1991, meaning it was written in the year or two before that. That's a long time ago, so has Dennett modified his stance since then? In 1996, he published another book on minds, *Kinds of Minds* [11] which expands on the earlier work. *Freedom Evolves* [12], from 2003, looks at two very important issues for any monist theory of mind, the associated questions of free will and morality. Since then, and despite a bout of serious illness, he has maintained a punishing schedule of lectures and publications but has tended to pay more attention to the question of evolutionary theory.

At first, *Kinds of Minds* seems to have a limited scope, that of asking the right questions to improve our understanding of ourselves and the world. That, however, is illusory and Dennett packs some high-powered philosophizing in a small volume. As mentioned, he much prefers his version of the right questions to those asked by other philosophers, whose efforts lead only to "self-contradictions, quandaries, or blank walls of mystery." Armed with this self-assurance, he opines: "Dualism (the view that minds are composed of some nonphysical and utterly mysterious stuff) and vitalism (the view that living things contain some special physical but equally mysterious stuff—*élan vital*) have been relegated to the trash heap of history, along with alchemy and astrology. (If) you... (believe) that the world is flat and the sun is a fiery chariot pulled by winged horses..." (p. 31), then don't look to Prof. Dennett for comfort. In brief, he argues that our minds evolved from simpler minds, and that there is nothing magic or supernatural about the human mind. However, even though simpler minds are essentially robotic, it does not follow that we are robots ourselves. We have a full range of mental attributes; his task as a philosopher is to give a rational (naturalistic) account of them.

Dennett supports the view of mind called "functionalism," the notion that a mind is defined by what it does rather than what it is made from or how it does it. Functionalism abstracts away from "some of the messy particularities of performance (to focus) on the work that is actually getting done" (p. 90). So, in theory, we could replace some of the neurons in a damaged brain with a microchip and the person would not be able to tell. Using the criterion of "what gets done," he assembles lengthy lists of examples to show that, in less complex animals, what appears to be clever or even sentient behavior is just the predictable outcome of information processing according to well-known, natural procedures. The core of his argument is that these processes are sufficient to explain even the vastly more complex behavior of humans. While a very substantial part of the massive increase in our intellectual capacity is the result of language, which allows us to develop "auxiliary brains", there is nothing magic or supernatural about the explanation of human behavior. Any problems we may have in explaining it arise from our crude and old-fashioned ways of thinking, especially the primitive notion of the Cartesian Theater. This construct inevitably leads to the dualist pseudo-explanation of the "thinking stuff", Descartes' *res cogitans* or, more scathingly, ectoplasm.

By adhering to a rigid materialism, the "enduring mystery" of consciousness is rendered prosaic: "A mind looks less miraculous when one sees how it might have been put together out of parts, and how it still relies on those parts" (p. 203). Mental contents become conscious, not by being bathed in an inner glow or scampering through a cerebral field, but by "... winning the competition against other mental contents for... the control of behavior..." and thence to memory (p. 205-6). This is facilitated if we talk to ourselves while we are active. However, some people find this counter-intuitive but they are simply prisoners of the crude Cartesian model: "What you (the reader) are... just *is* this organization of all the competitive activity between a host of competences that your body has developed" (p. 206; any italics in quotes are in the original). So, is the human mind different in principle from all other minds that have gone before? Yes and no. Yes, it is different in its staggering complexity and its computational scope but no, it is essentially only a very much better (and not always bigger) computational machine which relies on tried and proven processes to achieve minor miracles by quotidian means: "What makes a mind powerful—indeed, what makes a mind conscious—is not what it is made of, or how big it is, but what it can do. Can it be distracted? Can it recall earlier events? Can it keep track of several different things at once... When such questions as these are answered, we will know everything we need to know about those minds... These questions will capture everything we want to know about the concept of consciousness..." (p. 210).

But, a persistent questioner may demand of him, What about pain? Where is there room for pain, for the sheer *experience* of pain, in your model? This brings Dennett to his most contemptuous: if he stamps on your foot, he insists, you will feel only a fleeting pain which is so minor as not to warrant the label of "suffering." It would be a "risible" misuse of the term to apply it to an irritation that is no more than "...a brief, negatively-signed experience... of vanishing moral significance" (p. 220). If we look at the mind from the right point of view (naturalism) and ask the right questions (his), we will eventually get out of the old, magical way of thinking and see the mind for what it is, a virtual machine generated by the high-speed, multimodal, distributed information-processing system, which is our brain. Pain is merely the functional state which inclines you to wince and complain, nothing more.

In *Freedom Evolves* (2003), Dennett sets himself the task of answering an ancient and powerful objection to a naturalistic theory of mind, the question of free will and morality. If molecules don't have free will, and if the human brain is made of molecules, how can we humans have freedom of choice? Similarly, if we write God out of the equation, what is the source of morality? Materialism is such a mechanistic and amoral system that many right-thinking people are simply repelled by it, but Dennett disagrees vehemently. Even if the natural world is truly deterministic, he can show that humans have genuine free will from which derives a non-divine morality. But first, he scathingly dismisses dualist attempts to explain these phenomena: "...like the little green man in the control room of the man-sized puppet in the morgue in the film *Men in Black* (1997)... an immaterial portion of glowing ectoplasm that oozes around in your brain like a ghost amoeba... an angel whose wings are folded till you are called to fly to heaven" (p. 232). Dualism is necessarily puerile non-science and a proper theory must avoid all hints of it.

His case against determinism and for free will is based on the fact that humans are consummate information processors, capable of driving physical processes against their natural directions as determined by the normal laws of the universe: "Human freedom is not an illusion; it is an objective phenomenon, distinct from all other biological conditions and found in only one species." Moving in ordered steps along "...non-miraculous paths", we proceed from "... senseless atoms to freely chosen actions..." (p. 305) with no loss of human dignity or autonomy. We are neither marionettes on behaviorist strings nor transient abodes for wispy magical spirits. We do not have to resort to such desperate ploys as invoking quantum indeterminacy to account for human thought and decision-making. Instead, Darwinian theory shows how the mind arises by the same processes which force evolution in, say, snails: "...when language came into existence, it brought into existence the kind of mind that can transform itself on a moment's notice into a somewhat different virtual machine, taking on new projects, following new rules, adopting new policies. We are transformers. That's what a mind is, as contrasted with a mere brain, the control system of a chameleonic transformer, a virtual machine for making more virtual machines" (p. 250-51).

Dennett puts great emphasis on the role of language in converting us from semi-automated mimics (like parrots) to truly autonomous agents: "...language, when it is installed in a human brain, brings with it the construction of a new cognitive architecture that *creates* a new kind of consciousness—and morality" (p. 260). Sometimes, he uses the term "self" (e.g. p. 273) to describe this feature but the details of the actual mechanism are the same: "What, then, is the important role of such a self? The self is a system that is *given* responsibility, over time, so that it can reliably be there to *take* responsibility, so that there is somebody home to answer when questions of accountability arise" (p. 287). Indeed, the last sentence in the book is an approving quote from Merlin Donald: "(Donald's) book proposes that the human mind is unlike any other on this planet, not because of its biology, which is not qualitatively unique, but because of its ability to generate and assimilate culture" (p. 309).

He emphasizes that birds can voluntarily wheel this way and that without the benefit of language, but humans go several steps further: "We have added a layer on top of the bird's (and the ape's and the dolphin's) capacity to decide what to do next. It is not an anatomical layer in the brain but a functional layer, a virtual layer composed somehow in the micro-details of the brain's anatomy." Animals can "ask" each other to do things, like search for fleas, but only we can ask our neighbors for something, and explain ourselves by giving reasons. This creates the "special category of voluntary actions that sets us apart." Our actions are "morally self-forming," and, while this is unique in the world, it is most emphatically not magic or supernatural in any way: "Mental contents become conscious not by entering some special chamber in the brain, not by being transduced into some privileged and mysterious medium, but by winning the competitions against other mental contents for domination in the control of behavior, and hence for... entering into memory" (p. 253). He is constantly alert to the beguiling trap of dualism, e.g. "Notice how the introduction of... privileged access automatically puts us on the slippery slope to the Cartesian Theater" (p. 244). Conversely, the worst thing he can say about anybody else's theory is that it is covertly dualist.

This is a little surprising because, as the quotes above show, his entire theory is covertly dualist.

1.3: A Substitute For Dualism

Let's go back to *Consciousness Explained.* Satisfied he has dispensed with the threat of the ghostly gremlin in the head, Dennett now needs to show what he proposes in its place. This takes some time to emerge. On p. 210, he outlines his position: "Human consciousness is *itself* a huge complex... that can best be understood as the operation of a *"von Neumannesque"* virtual machine *implemented* in the *parallel architecture* of a brain that was not designed for any such activities. The power of this *virtual machine* vastly enhances the underlying powers of the organic *hardware* on which it runs" (his emphasis). He uses the examples of snails secreting calcium to spin a shell or beavers using mud to build a dam to illustrate his point that the genetic endowment of the human species allows us to weave a "narrative self" that protects us "just like the snail's shell" (p. 416). This "web of discourses... is as much a biological product as any of the other constructions to be found in the animal world." Just like the snail, or a spider weaving its web or a beaver building its dam, we do not "... consciously and deliberately figure out what narratives to tell..." while building our protective selves: "Our tales are spun but, for the most part, we don't spin them; they spin us." Since his virtual machine (which he later calls the "psychological self" to distinguish it from the biological self of immunity), is a biological exudation of the genetically-determined human brain, it does not fall into the classic error of dualism: "Since selves and minds and even consciousness itself are biological products..." (p. 421), the question of a supernatural "mind stuff" does not arise, and there is no conceptual problem with mind-brain interaction.

"A self," he continues (p. 426), "is not any old mathematical point, but an abstraction defined by the myriads of attributions and interpretations... that have composed the biography of the living body whose Center of Narrative Gravity it is." Gradually, he fills in the details of his biological model of consciousness, so that it builds up "a defining story about ourselves," incorporating sensation, memory, fantasy, "tendencies, decisions, strengths, and weaknesses" up to and including free will and moral responsibility. In short, except for immortality, his biological concept of self does everything that the much-despised Cartesian Soul did. However, since his self is a biological product, firmly anchored in the biological realm, it does not breach any of the fundamental laws of the universe. He is aware that, as an informational state, the conscious mind could be duplicated in a suitable artificial medium, so that machine consciousness is not just logically possible, but feasible. If people can't grasp that implication, then that is their failure of imagination rather than a limit imposed by the nature of the real world.

In *Freedom Evolves,* he explicitly describes the brain in information-processing terms: "...when language came into existence, it brought into existence the kind of mind that can transform itself on a moment's notice into a somewhat different virtual machine, taking on new projects, following new rules, adopting new policies. We are transformers. That's what a mind is, as contrasted with a mere brain, the control system of a chameleonic transformer, a virtual machine for making more virtual machines" (p. 250-51).

Because his "virtual machines" do not exist in the material realm, this is, of course, a crystal clear account of dualism by another name.

1.4: Ectoplasm: The Ooze That Persists

In his regular column, the contrarian financial reporter, Bill Bonner, told of a symposium he had recently attended in Zurich [13]:

> "The star of the show, however, was Dan Dennett, an American philosopher from Tufts University. Mr. Dennett believes the world, and everything in, it is an accident, in the sense it has no purpose and no designer. He says he can explain human consciousness without resorting to 'magic.' But there was nothing very original in his approach, as near as we could see. And something a bit too smug and self-satisfied about his conclusions. Like the dotcom hustlers at the end of the '90s... or Wall Street in 2006... He acted as though he had it all figured out. He described the creation and development of human beings and their culture in much the same terms that Austrian economists explain the workings of an economy. They are the result of 'spontaneous order,' in which the pieces assemble themselves without the help of central planning. Things take shape from the bottom up... cells get together to form hands and arms... and brains. One person joins with another to form a community. Then, they develop culture, language, and so forth... all of it—like successful businesses—the result of natural selection rather than divine intervention.... We suspect, however, that professor Dennett may be leaving something out—the part he doesn't understand."

Mr. Bonner is particularly sharp in his criticism of experts who are calmly confident of their grip on enormously complex issues, such as all the economists who didn't foresee the recent economic meltdown (which he certainly did). Of course, he is not a physician, a psychologist, or a philosopher, but he has a highly developed sense of "something's not quite right in that spiel." I believe he was absolutely correct in his assessment of the philosopher whom he had never read: there is a flaw right through Dennett's entire corpus of theorizing. He has not constructed a monist philosophy of mind at all.

Based wholly on his published works, it is clear that Dennett is highly intelligent, with very high verbal facility and an impish sense of humor. His website [14] shows that he has been hugely prolific during his long career as a philosopher and enjoys the very highest academic esteem internationally. Could somebody like this make such a profound error? Why not? Nobel laureate, Sir Frank Macfarlane Burnett, announced: "I can see no practical application of molecular biology to human affairs... DNA is a tangled mass of linear molecules in which the informational content is quite inaccessible." Even the great Rutherford thought that expectations of nuclear transformations (fission) providing limitless sources of energy were "the merest moonshine." Science progresses, as Popper said, by "bold conjectures and determined efforts at their refutation." Dennett's conjectures are certainly bold. Let's see, however, if they can survive an attack from the left field, that he is not a monist at all.

By the end of *Freedom Evolves*, the average reader may be feeling that Dennett's works are a little formulaic. His books start with a very brief statement of his position, usually couched in scathingly dismissive comments of his *bête noire*, naive substance dualism, and anybody foolish enough to hold views which he doesn't (postmodernists get a swipe at p. 5 of [12]). However, his own views emerge only slowly and, in the main, ostensively. After a chatty introduction, which may or may not state his position, he briskly launches into a long and vastly-detailed peregrination through his wide-ranging knowledge of the biological sciences. At the end, he abruptly announces that philosophy will be better for his efforts. But his knowledge of biology is gappy; either he doesn't have a feel for it or he is being highly selective in how he uses the material. Occasionally, he is completely wrong (see his comments on methylphenidate and ADD, p. 275; at p. 48, the Universal Turing Machine should be Turing's Universal Computing Machine, aka Turing Machine; and on castration of pedophiles, p. 299). And there is something else seriously wrong with what eventually becomes a tiresome recitation of biofacts: it is not possible to answer a metaphysical question using empirical facts. The question of the nature of mind is a metaphysical question which must be settled prior to any appeal to empirical science. His claim, "Somehow, the brain must be the mind..." [10, p. 41-2], is pure metaphysics.

This claim continues: "... but unless we can come to see in some detail how this is possible, our materialism will not explain consciousness..." (as mentioned, he uses the terms "mind", "self", and "consciousness" more or less interchangeably). This is crucial: how can mind and brain be, in some vital, *explanatory* sense (as distinct from descriptive), one and the same thing? I don't know but, having read a large part of his output several times, I'm sure Dennett doesn't, either. If he did, he wouldn't need to define his case ostensively. He could simply state it in a few sentences and then use the empirical (biological) evidence to illustrate his point, rather than have the point emerge piecemeal, if at all, from the floods of evidence.

Complicating matters, there is a constant sense that he is using his humor and his broadsides against his intellectual opponents to slip some weighty philosophical questions past the reader. Some of the most complex issues in modern philosophy, such as the concept of a self, simply pop up in the course of an amusing discursion on some other matter but are not revisited. At other times, he puts a term in scare quotes, clearly indicating it should be used advisedly but, the next time it is used, it stands alone, as though all concerns about its use had been resolved. In each case, the reader either accepts what is happening and moves on, perhaps expecting the question to be resolved later, or closes the book and reaches for something else (as Bonner would do). But Dennett's jolly manner makes this difficult: only a churl would interrupt the flow of *bons mots* to object. What emerges is a largely intuitive or inchoate sense of something biological (mechanistic) to replace the pure mentalism (or worse) of the old dualist model. But that sense is misleading, because he has used his cheery devices to smuggle frankly dualist concepts into his monist model.

When is dualism not dualism? When it is a biological dualism. In an echo of Orwell's "four legs good, two legs bad," Dennett leaves no doubt that he believes "biological dualism is good, psychological dualism is bad." His vast output illustrates a classic and invariably fatal error in philosophy: he has not defined his terms. Granted, he gave a definition for dualism (see above) but he omitted to examine the word to see if it might have other meanings or usages. And it does. Dualism does not mean just "of two substances." It means "the state of being two-fold or double, of two opposed *natures*" (my emphasis). So when Dennett proposes a "virtual machine" which runs on and controls the brain's "hardware," or a Self composed of a web of words and deeds, a "psychological or narrative self... an abstraction, not a thing in the brain," just what is he doing? He is proposing that the human animal has a dual or two-fold nature, consisting of a real, physical body, and something else. And by postulating that non-physical something else, he assembles a dualist model, because that's what dualism is: two opposed natures. If I point to something and tell you that it is composed of one part here, and something else which is both inseparable and utterly different in nature, but together they constitute the whole, then, inescapably, unavoidably, inevitably, I have proposed a duality: "The crux of dualism is an apparently unbridgeable gap between two incommensurable orders of being that must be reconciled if we (wish to justify) our assumption that there is a comprehensible universe..." (Watson, in [15], p. 210). Dennett's "virtual machine" or self convincingly meets that definition in every meaningful respect.

The fact that he defines his Self as biological, and thereby not a hopelessly wrong, myth-riddled bit of glowing ectoplasm peeking out of the trash can of history, is beside the point. Dual means two, and a virtual machine (of whatever nature) is necessarily of a nature distinct from the physical machine it inhabits: by their very definition, physical and virtual are "incommensurable orders of being." So Dennett's vast intellectual effort merely brought him back to his starting point of how the two interact: Plus ça change, plus c'est la même chose. Three hundred and fifty years ago, of course, Descartes had the easy task: his supernatural soul interacted with the body miraculously. But with his *dualisme* à la mode, Dennett sets himself the much more difficult job of showing how a virtual machine called the Self could arise from and interact with its associated physical body without breaking any rules of nature. By insisting that his Self is secreted like a snail's shell, he has to show, for example, that the words that compose it are biological *in nature*; that our beliefs occupy the same ontological niche as the mud in a beaver's dam; and that the "web of discourse" a human weaves is conceptually the same as a spider's web. I don't believe he can show any of these things. Fortunately, nor does he, and here is the proof.

He explicitly states that our beliefs etc. could theoretically be stored in a computer as pure information [10, p. 430] and even duplicated a thousand times. By claiming that we can reduplicate the conscious human self in a computer, he has immediately committed himself to the notion that information is not the same as the substrate that encodes it, i.e. he accepts (a form of) dualism, but without giving up his antagonism. He agrees that a verbal description of mud is not the same thing as the mud itself, because symbols are never the same as the thing they represent. If I talk about mud, mud does not come out of my mouth, nor do you catch an earful of mud. Every symbol is a duality, an order of being which is utterly distinct from the thing it represents. If it were not incommensurable, it wouldn't be a symbol of it. That's what 'symbol' means.

However, he could have saved himself this embarrassment by being less doctrinaire. It would appear that his understanding of the word dualism, and his instinctive antipathy, derived from his initial reading of Descartes in his first, sparkling days of college, but he never modified his heady, youthful hostility. Other people recognize that, as with every other concept in philosophy, dualism comes in a variety of forms. Spinoza's "property dualism" was an early alternative which preserved the obvious duality of the human experience, yet did so in a way that elided the "incommensurable" part of the separate orders of being. Granted, there were problems with his approach [15, p. 795], but there are problems in every approach. More recently, Chalmers' natural dualism, mentioned above, formalizes Dennett's implicit notion of consciousness supervening upon a particular physical structure in a law-like way, while preserving the irreducible duality of, among others, language and its objects.

1.5: My Good Self

In *Consciousness Explained* [10, p. 399-400], Dennett used the concept of an "intuition pump" to show how writers may induce their readers to believe something that isn't factually correct: the usual way of reading their work indicates a conclusion that is not fully supported by the premises (but Dorbolo [16] has shown that Dennett uses even this term in different ways). But he is not above using it himself, as follows: "We have added a layer on top of the bird's (and the ape's and the dolphin's) capacity to decide what to do next. It is not an anatomical layer in the brain but a functional layer, a virtual layer composed somehow in the micro-details of the brain's anatomy." This is the very clearest description of a dual system comprising the brain and a virtual decision-maker generated in it. It is impossible to claim that "... a functional layer, a virtual layer composed somehow in the micro-details of the brain's anatomy" which "... is not an anatomical layer in the brain..." is anything but an ontologically dualist control system. However, the whole wording of the full quote leads the ordinary reader in the direction of thinking that it outlines something physical or biological, rather than a non-physical or dualist system. Unfortunately, that is completely wrong: that conclusion is not supported by the premises of the quote. By clever word-play, he induces the unsuspecting reader (who, after all, wants to find an "explanation of consciousness" in the book he has paid good money for), he induces the reader to believe the exact opposite of what the words *actually mean*. This is not trivial: if this assessment is correct, a very large part of Dennett's life's work has failed.

Similarly, we see that a capital-S *Self* is a Cartesian Self, meaning unscientific ectoplasmic ooze, whereas a small-s self is fine because it "... emerges from the processes that occur in the brain. Correcting these common misapprehensions about the self and the brain also banishes some dark conclusions about the prospects for free will that have gained credence in some quarters" (p. 219). Capital-S Selves are clearly bad (perhaps full of "self-contradictions, quandaries, or blank walls of mystery") whereas small-s selves are just "a virtual machine for making more virtual machines," to which no rational person would object. His small-s *self* ("A Self of One's Own," p. 245-55) creeps in, more or less unnoticed, amid a clutter of chess-playing computers, evolving brains, monkeys and dolphins, mating chimps etc, with the intuition pump working overtime to dispel any doubt that it may not be 100% biological. But, besides surviving death, what can a Self do that a self can't? The answer is not stated. All we know, by implication, is that anything Dennett doesn't like will be attributed to an anti-scientific superstition of a bad dualist Self, whereas anything that pleases him will be a property of a rational, emergent, biological good self, happily generating virtual machines that do the real work (of a Self, as it happens).

Listen to Dennett again: "That's what a mind is, as contrasted with a mere brain, the control system of a chameleonic transformer, a virtual machine for making more virtual machines." In our heads, we have a "mere brain" (where "mere" means "bloody, gooey, but incredibly powerful transformer") and another insubstantial (that's what virtual means), unextended, unlocalized, fully functional, and causally effective thing which arises from, but is not identical with, the wetware in the head. Not only do we have a virtual machine but it is capable of switching itself in a split second, generating other virtual machines in the process. Each of these, therefore, would be capable of generating further virtual machines *ad infinitum*. That is, the very finite bit of pinkish goo holding our ears apart (all 1300 gm of it) can, by Dennett's own admission, generate an infinite output, where the only limit is the brain's raw computing power.

And this is the point: if he wishes to use the concept of a self, or a virtual machine, or of unconscious motivation, etc, he needs to bite the bullet and accept that any information-processor is necessarily, inevitably, of a fundamentally different nature from enzymes and DNA etc. That is, he needs to accept that his model is dualist in *nature,* because that is the only way "... we can come to see in some detail how this is possible..." As it stands, "(his) materialism (does) not explain consciousness..." Nor does it explain minds or selves, or how selves arise from the brain as an organ, or how they interact with the brain, how they make decisions, choose religions or formulate rules of morality and poker, or tell lies and develop addictions and hatreds and mental illnesses, and so on. His model is incapable of generating answers to these questions because the essential answers can only be formulated within the context of an avowed dualist system.

Even though he uses frankly dualist concepts, he cannot resolve the central issues of, say, how a physical brain can generate virtual machines, or how those machines can make more virtual machines, without acknowledging that virtual machines are not, in any interesting sense of the word, biological. Sure, they derive from biology; nobody has a problem with that these days; but they are not biological *per se*, any more than the copy of Windows 7™, which I bought this afternoon, is a *physical* thing in a box. It's not: it's an idea in a box, and morality is an idea in a small, bony box called the human skull. *Ideas* are not materialist or biological in *nature*, so his life's program collapses.

In short, Dennett's system cannot generate a solution to the mind-body problem, just because he will not admit that there is such a problem: "Somehow, the brain must be the mind..." Well, that settles it, then; all those interminable disputes about the nature of mind and how it interacts with the physical brain were a waste of time. Or was he "a bit too smug and self-satisfied" because he had skipped, laughing and punning, over the bits he didn't understand? I believe so. It's the details of the "somehow" in "Somehow, the brain must be the mind..." that overturn his whole opus.

There is absolutely nothing in any of Dennett's books that is inconsistent with the idea of a natural dualism based in a precisely detailed, molecular resolution of the mind-body problem. All his vast outpouring of biological evidence is neutral on the crucial question of the nature of the controlling factor in human behavior. Moreover, a natural dualist model allows subtleties that are forever denied to Dennett's functionalism, such as an innate cognitive system inherited from our primate forebears; unconscious decision-making; psychosomatics and, of course, questions of mental disorder. There is non- conceptual possibility for a monist model of mind to generate a model of mental disorder. In terms of morality and free will, a dualist model allows the subject to *decide* to work against the laws of thermodynamics (i.e. the laws governing the material world), thereby negating physical determinism. In order to escape the demon of determinism, it is only necessary to postulate that the agent has (at least partial) self-control, where the control system is not permanently subject to the laws of thermodynamics. That is, there must be a control system, or mind, which is subject to laws *other* than those of the physical realm and which can thereby temporarily work against the heat gradient of the natural world. A dualist system immediately meets that essential requirement, because its information-processing is subject only to the laws of the higher-order system's semantic or logical laws. This is only true in a dualist system, and probably necessarily true. In a monist system, it is impossible. When compared with the convoluted wordplay of the chapters in which Dennett painfully extracts a simulacrum of free will from his model, this is a paragon of simplicity, and simplicity is a scientific goal in itself.

A very large part of the biological material in *Freedom Evolves* [12] is not interesting. It is description masquerading as explanation, i.e. the classic mistake of Skinner's *Beyond Freedom and Dignity* [17]. This is because Dennett does not offer a true explanatory account of a monist model of mind: his position is no more than anti-dualism, which is not the same thing. This is especially true of his extended discussion of the role of "memes," or ideas (in [12] Ch. 6: *The evolution of open minds*). Using his "intuition pump" to refer to minds as "carriers" (p. 177), he shifts attention from the mind that develops and contains ideas to the notion of ideas as independent Darwinian exemplars. That is, if we talk about ideas as having lives and trajectories of their own, we are not obliged to talk about the problematic minds that "host" the ideas. But the reader knows implicitly that ideas are frankly mentalist concepts, and he simply suspends judgment while Dennett weaves his characteristic web of words.

Despite his disavowals, Dennett uses overtly mentalist or dualist concepts to close the explanatory gap in his model. Concepts such as thoughts, information processing, beliefs, desires, rules, hopes and fears, sadness and grief, pains and "elaborate exercises of imagination" [10, p. 209] are mentalist to the core, yet they do the "heavy lifting" in his allegedly monist account of human mind. He insists he has eliminated all dualist concepts because they are inherently supernatural yet, in every case, precisely the same dualist concepts are found, lurking under a litter of biologism, making the bridge for the Pied Piper of Boston to lead his beguiled readers up the monist garden path.

1.6: The Infinitely Regressive Self.

In an essay entitled "Why I am not a cognitive psychologist," B.F. Skinner showed the fallacy of naïve dualism [17]. He used the idea of sights and sounds entering the head through their respective portals and being conveyed to the brain to be used as the basis for action. Once they reach the brain, the sensory inputs are presented to a small man or homunculus (the Executive Self) who scans them, checks the brain's memory banks, then pulls levers, and presses buttons to activate the body's muscles and organs. But of course, what does this explain? What decides for the little man? Another little man in his head, and so *ad infinitum*? This is the other danger of dualism, that it leads to the pseudo-explanation of an infinite regress. For Descartes, as for Popper and Eccles, the process of explanation stopped at the supernatural Soul or Self. It was sufficient simply to get the information to the eyes of the homunculus because, after that, it was not of this realm and we couldn't know how he made his decisions—nor did we need to know. It was enough to know *that* he did, without bothering with *how* he managed. A committed supernatural dualist can simply say "God knows," and be satisfied that he has just told the truth.

But materialists can't do that, and Dennett is a materialist: "Somehow, the brain must be the mind, but unless we can come to see in some detail how this is possible, our materialism will not explain consciousness..." [10, p. 41-2]. In order to *explain* consciousness (as distinct from describe it, or give allegorical accounts), it is necessary to explain its functions without invoking any concept of Mind. He quotes Phillip Johnson-Laird's aphorism: "Any scientific theory of the mind has to treat it as an automaton" (p. 256). This is Turing's paradox, to show how each and every function of the mind can be explained as a matter of mentality without invoking inexplicable mental attributes, i.e. without begging the question. Dennett's answer to this question is not so much specified as implied. Each attribute of mind or consciousness has to be isolated and then broken down into its internal sequence of logical steps. This process of "decomposition" continues until it consists of no more than a lengthy series of questions or steps which are so simple that a machine could answer them. That is, the clever little man of Skinner's mocking model is replaced by a whole production line of very little men, but the crucial point is that each one of them is dumber than you would have thought possible. They are very little men, of very little intellect and, by patiently chipping away at The Big Problem, they reduce it to a long series of little problems that are so simple that a mindless creature, such as a neuron, could answer. Then all the answers are reassembled and dispatched, again mindlessly, to the "levers and buttons" of the effector organs. Thus, Dennett accounts for mentation without a Mind, thereby avoiding the first step on an infinite regress.

As an explanation, *Consciousness Explained* would have been much more convincing if its author had specified this process in the same detail as in his earlier work. In his 1978 monograph, *Brainstorms* [18], he described this process with incisive clarity: "When the level is reached where the homunculi are no more than adders and subtractors, by the time they need only the intelligence to pick the larger of two numbers... they have been reduced to functionaries who can be replaced by a machine..." (p. 80). This is directly in line with the account of intellect given years before by the British mathematician, Alan Turing, which, of course, formed the basis of the computing revolution [19, 20]. It is also commensurate with the modular concept of brain function developed by the Soviet neuropsychologist, Aleksandr Luria [21]

By this means, Dennett could have avoided the long detour of declaring himself an antidualist, then trying to find a monist solution to the problem of "two natures" only to give up and sneak dualism in through the back door, thus: "We have added a layer on top of the bird's (and the ape's and the dolphin's) capacity to decide what to do next. It is not an anatomical layer in the brain but a functional layer, a virtual layer composed somehow in the micro-details of the brain's anatomy." Can anyone think of a clearer description of "... an apparently unbridgeable gap between two incommensurable orders of being...."?

Daniel C Dennett didn't see it. His work relies on the miracle of dualism to complete its causal chain—not a large miracle, mind you, just a little one. And the best place to hide anything naughty is right under everyone's nose, where nobody thinks to look for it, such as simply changing the labels from Dualist Virtual Machine to Biological Virtual Machine. So simple, so effective. For forty years, his excusable undergraduate mistake has led the philosophical world astray.

1.7: Conclusion: A Natural Dualism

So, despite his protests, Dennett turns out to be just a sophisticated closet dualist. The significance for psychiatry is that, as it is presently formulated, biological psychiatry is a form of monism. Dennett's failure means biological psychiatry can never be nested in a larger, formal theory of mind that justifies its essential claim. That is, the concept of a "biochemical imbalance of the brain" as the cause for all mental disorders depends on an indefensible philosophical claim. It is an epistemological orphan, a claim without reference, a dead-end. In order to be taken seriously, psychiatry has to do better than opt for monist theories.

The correct sequence for Dennett's program would be as follows:

1.   Adopt the materialist ontology (thereby excluding any supernatural souls right from the beginning);

2.   Opt for a dualist model of mind-body, because simply being able to ask my neighbor: "Could there be a monist account of mind-body?" shows that there couldn't be (i.e. it relies on symbols, which inevitably betray a dualist structure);

3.   Steps 1 and 2 commit him to a form of natural dualism, in which mental functions have to be explained as the law-like results of a precisely-delineated brain structure generating an informational space by mindlessly doing what it was "designed" to do;

4.   Find the specific, information-based means of bridging the gap between mind and body, bearing in mind (!) that any bridge goes two ways.

As a solution to the mind-body problem, monism has a powerful appeal. It is clear and simple, and smoothly eliminates the most complex problem in the history of philosophy. However, just by reading those words, I disprove monism. As Henry Mencken noted, for every complex problem, there is an answer that is clear, simple, and wrong.

Unfortunately for Dennett, his own solution to the mind-body problem, that the mind is biological and therefore doesn't need a bridge, closes his options and forces his theory to end just at the really interesting bit: solving the mind-body problem by showing just how information gets from body to mind and back again. He was so close. All he had to do was show generically how information gets from a substrate to the virtual machine it generates and back again, and he was home. But he couldn't complete his program because he had declared it closed. His model couldn't develop an account of unconscious causation (another of those awful dualist notions), so it couldn't account for just what it means to say the Self is a web of discourse which is spun for us: "Our tales are spun but, for the most part, we don't spin them; they spin us." He was forced to suggest it came from the DNA like a snail's shell does but, clearly, it does not. It comes from the virtual machine itself. The dualist 'virtual machine' or Self controls the brain, not the other way around; so it is self-contradictory to claim that "Somehow, the brain must be the mind..."

For psychiatry, the fact that monism is wrong in principle allows our discipline to drift from the mainstream of science, with very serious consequences. One of the most serious is the lack of an ethical dimension to theorizing in psychiatry. While biological psychiatrists claim that their approach is wholly directed toward relieving human distress, it does so, if at all, at terrible cost. Firstly, it destroys any intellectual basis to the discipline. All complex questions of human affairs are reduced to catch-phrase "chemical imbalances of the brain." Essential humanist constructs which other disciplines accept without demur, such as personality, human nature, morality and immorality, etc., are reduced to matters of brain chemistry, and then dismissed. This is patently false [8], but all objections to rampant biologism are dismissed peremptorily, as either insipid [22], as meaningless affectations [6], or as misconceptions which a robust neurobiology will soon clear up [7]. It is no longer sufficient to claim that, for example, wearing a bow tie is under genetic control [7, p. 381] without offering some plausible route by which genes may control behavior (see Hyman, in [7]).

Second, by insisting that all mental disorder is a special form of disorder in the most complex organ of all, biological psychiatry renders sufferers impotent in their own management and recovery. All power is shifted to a remote caste of specialized workers, trained in a recondite discipline that is forever closed to the uninitiated. If a child is not doing well at school, it is now not just irresponsible of parents to try to manage it themselves, but culpable. Since biological psychiatry is not equipped to determine which disorders are biological and which are psychological (because it doesn't recognize psychological causation of mental disorders), and its only form of treatment is drugs, more drugs, and then brain surgery; it is incapable of knowing when drugs are appropriate and when they are not. A biological psychiatrist will argue that this is a non-question, as drugs are always appropriate, but that begs the question, i.e. it assumes the truth of that which requires proof.

Finally and probably most significantly, the intellectual and emotional poverty of a psychiatry reduced to biology is directly causing the decline of interest in medical students in the specialty. In a recent trip to the US for a lecture tour, I was struck by the hunger among medical students, residents and young graduates for a psychiatry that engages with the humanity of the mentally-troubled. I believe it is the responsibility of senior practitioners as teachers to acknowledge their concerns, and not just dismiss them as the affected posturings of tender-hearted youth. It is our duty to listen to our successors and address their needs for a human-centered psychiatry; otherwise there won't be a psychiatry at all.

2 | *Can Biological Naturalism Save Biological Psychiatry? Flaws In Searle's Program*

2.1: Introduction

At this stage, the logical justification or rationale for biological psychiatry is not looking strong. Perhaps we should recall just what the biological approach is or claims to be. In fact, it is not so easy to find out what people mean by the expression "the biological model of mental disorder." Most psychiatrists don't actually use it, but they certainly act as though they believe it. Why else would they order a CT scan and an EEG for a child who is not doing well at school, then prescribe eight different psychotropic drugs—to be taken all at once? Most often, people simply echo the claims of the Great and Powerful, such as the late Samuel Guze. He insisted there cannot be a psychiatry which is too biological, and wrote a little book about it [1]. Lots of fields, he said, are interested in "disorders in mental and psychological functions... but only psychiatry, as a medical specialty, offers the basis for a comprehensive approach from the medical perspective. The medical perspective is what is meant when we propose applying the medical model to psychiatric conditions. This simply means that the concepts, strategies, and jargon of general medicine are applied to psychiatric disorders" (p. 4). This does seem to beg the question somewhat, so he expands his position later: "Most of us who adhere to the medical model believe that the fullest understanding of human health and illness, including psychiatric conditions, will depend increasingly on growing knowledge in biology, conceptualized very broadly... the explicit as well intuitive recognition of this explains the redefinition of many personal and social problems into concerns of medicine" (p. 7). Quite clearly, he is throwing his net very wide.

Just how wide is seen in his last chapter, when he lays claim for the whole of the human condition for biology: "... one's feelings and thoughts are as biological as one's blood pressure or gastric secretion: feelings and thoughts are manifestations of the brain's operations just as blood pressure reflects the operations of the CVS and gastric secretion the stomach's function" (p. 130). By this, he meant that "hopes, fears, wishes, needs, fantasies and feelings" could and should be studied physiologically. But what does this sweeping claim actually mean in practice? Does he mean to imply that his book was itself nothing more than a biological secretion? That we could stop people writing silly books with an injection? "Come along, Mr Jones, if you vote for that party, we'll have to put you on the blue tablets." Perhaps we could immunize people against talking nonsense or believing rubbish. They tried this in the former Soviet Union: people who opposed the government were diagnosed "sluggish schizophrenics", held in mental hospitals, and were drugged and shocked until they relented.

These absurdities show that mental phenomena are not of the same nature as biological, that we cannot close the debate on causation of mental disorder by fiat. So the claim that a mental disorder is "a biochemical imbalance in the brain" has to be considered very carefully because it rests on assumptions that may well be false. This is where philosophy comes into its own. There is, of course, no such thing as philosophy. There are philosophers, but they are just people who philosophize. They aren't fussy what they philosophize about; there are very few corners of the universe that don't interest one or other of them. And one of their favorite topics, possibly because nobody can really come to grips with it, is the philosophy of mind. It is true that "feelings and thoughts are as biological as blood pressure and gastric acid"? What are the conditions under which it would be true to say "He has Major Patriotism Disorder"? A philosopher once argued that happiness is a disorder, because it met the form of all the criteria DSM-IV uses to diagnose other mental disorders. These days, children who give cheek to the teacher are put on amphetamines and talk to a psychologist about how nobody understands them. In my day, children didn't give cheek to the teachers. Teachers had canes, and a cane hanging behind the classroom door had the remarkable property of "action at a distance", meaning it could cure all sorts of genetic diseases in forty-eight bare-footed little ferals (such as ADHD with a touch of ODD and Pediatric Bipolar Disorder). These and other questions appeal to philosophers, not the least because everybody else makes such a hash of them.

One of the more durable modern philosophers has been probing these types of questions at Berkeley campus in San Francisco for nearly fifty years. At first glance, the work of John Searle would appear to fit hand-in-glove with the views of Samuel Guze. In a short, synthetic work, *Mind, Language and Society*, Searle argues that consciousness is wholly a biological phenomenon which can "... no more lie around separate from my brain than the liquidity of water can be separated from the water, or the solidity of the table from the table" [2, p. 41]. Before looking a little more closely at what this means, I should mention that Searle suggested that textbooks are often a better place to look for the faults and errors in an author's case because there is less room to conceal them. That would also apply to small works on difficult topics, such as this particular book: there is no room to bury any errors under floods of verbiage (which Searle normally doesn't, anyway). So, small as it is, I regard this book as a legitimate statement of his views. There is also a body of original material available on the Internet, especially at his personal site. Because these e-papers can be revised readily, they can be taken as current expressions of his opinions.

It would be fair to say that, as a philosopher, Searle does not enjoy the same profile among psychiatrists as the earthier Dennett, although I doubt this would concern him much. As a writer, Searle is rather old-fashioned, if a spare and sober style means old-fashioned. There is no difficulty extracting his position from his writing, as he inclines to state his views briefly at the beginning of a paper, then deal with each point in turn until he is satisfied that the topic is exhausted, closing with a summary that aims to forestall further doubts. He uses a transparent definition of consciousness: "By 'consciousness' I simply mean those subjective states of sentience or awareness that begin when one awakes in the morning from a dreamless sleep and continue throughout the day until one goes to sleep at night or falls into a coma, or dies, or otherwise becomes, as one would say, 'unconscious'"[3]. This book leaves no doubt that he uses consciousness in its broadest possible definition, and often uses the word 'mind' interchangeably (as in the title to his book). He has named his approach to the question of mind "biological naturalism," so we need to look closely at whether his work can be used to justify the over-arching claims of biological psychiatrists like Samuel Guze.

2.2: Against Materialism

Because of their difficulty of coming to terms with the subjective nature of consciousness, most modern philosophers adhere to one or other form of materialism. This ontology states that there is nothing in the universe above or beyond matter and energy. The universe is self-contained, meaning a complete causal explanation of the entire universe and its contents is available without leaving the material realm in any way. These days, this is more or less a default position because, throughout human history, every possible approach to the question of mind has been tried, but failed to grasp this slippery concept. So, starting mainly with the early behaviorists (e.g. J.B. Watson in 1915, see [4], Chap. 3), efforts were turned toward devising a complete explanatory account of human behavior without any mention of the mind. It is a matter of history [5] that behaviorism's bold project failed. Warned by this humiliation, philosophers have attempted to find other ways of giving a rational account of what seems, at first, a wholly irrational topic. In the 1950s, the thesis was advanced that mind is a reality but, as a matter of contingent fact, mind and brain are one and the same thing. Mind-brain identity theory (MBIT), which Searle terms 'physicalism,' was soon shown to be self-contradictory, as it is manifest that mind and brain each have properties that the other does not, so they are not identical.

Other attempts in the same vein include eliminative or promissory materialism, the notion that, in the fullness of time, science will eliminate all talk of mind and mental matters by showing just how the phenomena we now call mind have a lower order but entirely materialist explanation with no loose ends. That is, scientific progress will get rid of the concept of mind by showing that it is an illusion, just as it got rid of phlogiston and vital spirits. Searle thought this an unpromising line because, he argued, the nature of consciousness just is an illusion, so that showing consciousness to be an illusion doesn't take matters very far. These days, the most widespread form of physicalism is seen in biological psychiatry, where it is hoped that a reductionist biological account of the brain will lead to the elimination of higher-order, non-scientific (mental) concepts by explaining them in terms of the behavior or properties of lower order entities (essentially, neurochemistry). Detailed arguments have shown that reductionism cannot give an account of essential human attributes, and there would probably be no significant philosopher in the world today who supports this option.

Philosophically, there have been two developments which qualify as materialist. Functionalism attempts to give an account of mental states in terms of their functional relationships in the causation of behavior. Essentially, a mental state is defined as the functional relationship between input and output. Searle's objection is that this discounts the subjective nature of a mental state as something experienced by an agent, even when the agent does nothing. A good example of how this "short changes" human experience is Dennett's example of standing on somebody's foot (see Chapter 1). He claims that, if he stamps on your foot, you will feel only a fleeting pain which is no more than "... a brief, negatively-signed experience of vanishing moral significance." Consistent with Searle's critique of functionalism, it would be entirely fair to ask Dennett if he would still believe that in case somebody stamped on his little granddaughter's foot. Similarly, if a man were profoundly depressed, to the point where he did nothing but sit and stare into space all day, there would be nothing in his "input states" that could account for his diminished output. Only his intrapsychic experience could explain it. Depression causes behavioral disturbances, not the other way around, and it is not necessarily the result of any sensory input. Classing the experience of depression as a "brief, negatively-signed experience of vanishing moral significance" would serve to increase the sufferer's distress, not explain it, so functionalism need not be taken seriously.

Searle argues that any attempt to erase consciousness from the equation, such as the various forms of materialism, immediately removes the most important feature of consciousness, its subjectivity: a non-subjective account of consciousness is not an account of consciousness at all, but an account of something else (and not very interesting at that).

The second development to mention is what Searle calls "strong artificial intelligence" (AI). While there is considerable dispute over what this term actually means, the general claim would be that the mind is a computational program running in the brain, such that to be in pain is simply to be running the program for pain. Searle's view is that this does not explain a mental state, but explains it away: a mental state becomes "nothing but" a computational state. His case is that "...*computation is defined syntactically*. It is defined in terms of the manipulation of symbols" [3; his emphasis]. However, syntax does not define content, as he has shown in his renowned "Chinese Room" argument (see that paper for details; they are not relevant here). His conclusion is that "...*syntax by itself is not sufficient* for semantic content," meaning a full account of mind requires something more than an account of how the mind operates. Accordingly, strong AI fails.

2.3: Against Dualism

Searle's deliberate rejection of any form of dualism leaves no room for compromise. Dualism is the formal name for any concept where the mind is seen as a real but different kind of thing from the rest of the universe. To a dualist, creation (if you will) divides neatly in two realms. The first is the very obvious material world where universal physical laws police the restless ebb and flow of matter and energy. The second realm is the insubstantial world of the mental life, where ideas, experiences and emotions reign. The classic formulation of what is essentially the folk psychological view is that of the French polymath, Rene Descartes, who argued that there are two kinds of "stuff" in the universe, material stuff (*res extensa*) and thinking stuff (*res cogitans*), each requiring nothing more than itself in order to exist. The stuff of the Cartesian mind differs dramatically from real world stuff in that nobody can see it, nobody can localize it or find any to weigh it or serve with parsley sauce. It is apprehended by direct experience and any person who tries to deny the reality of his own mental life immediately refutes his claim.

For Searle, this approach creates a major problem, of how the mental stuff interacts with the physical. If they are truly different in nature, there could be no point of contact between them. Mind-body interaction would be impossible and the attempt to explain mind and body would break down. He takes a singularly uncompromising position on anything that smacks of dualism: "I think (dualism) is false..." [2, p. 11].

> "Dualism comes in two flavors, substance dualism and property dualism. According to substance dualism, there are two radically different kinds of entities in the universe, material objects and immaterial minds... Property dualism is the view that there are two kinds of properties of objects that are metaphysically distinct... All forms of dualism share the view that the two types are mutually exclusive. If it is mental, it can't... be physical; if it is physical, it can't... be mental..." (p. 45).

However, he is not convinced by the apparent ease with which property dualism sidesteps the metaphysical problem of dual substances: "I do not believe that we live in two worlds, the mental and the physical—much less in three worlds, the mental, the physical, and the cultural..." (p. 6; presumably referring to Popper's World III; see [6]). He continues: "...dualism in any form makes the status and existence of consciousness utterly mysterious... Having postulated a separate mental realm, the dualist cannot explain how it relates to the material world..." (p. 47). A few pages later, he dismissed all dualism as beyond the pale: "The way to defeat dualism is simply to refuse to accept the system of categories that makes consciousness out as something non-biological, not a part of the natural world" (p. 52). He has reiterated this view a number of times over the years, e.g. "As long as we continue to talk and think as if the mental and the physical were separate metaphysical realms, the relation of the brain to consciousness will forever seem mysterious, and we will not have a satisfactory explanation of the relation of neuron firings to consciousness" [3, p. 8; 7].

As noted, he recognizes two forms of dualism, the first being the age-old notion of the heavenly spirit or soul that resides inside us from soon after conception until the moment of death. As science, this is clearly beyond consideration. Fortunately, nobody has put this notion forward seriously since the ill-fated effort of Popper and Eccles in 1977 but it is persistent. There would be far more people alive in the world today who accept some form or other of this idea than there have ever been people throughout human history who denied it.

The alternative view, property dualism, says that mentality is just a property of certain highly organized physical structures. There is a much older idea, known as panpsychism, which says that mentality is a property of all matter but this, of course, is mystical and non-explanatory and doesn't need to be pursued. Property dualism stems from the work of the 17th century philosopher, Baruch Spinoza. In its original form, it was grafted on a substrate of religiosity which very few people would now take seriously, but the basic idea of emergent properties resonates easily with current thinking. Given the brain's particular structure, certain properties emerge which are themselves not physical, in the sense that the weight of the brain is a physical property. There are many analogies of emergent properties, e.g. because of their particular shape, steel ships can float and, for the same reason, heavier than air flight is possible. However, none of these truly captures the idea of a sentient mind.

The standard modern analogy, some would say homology, is that of the digital computer. Because of its molecular architecture, a computer has properties unlike any other machine in history. In fact, many of its properties are among those we once regarded as quintessentially human, including mathematical operations, using symbolic languages, playing games such as chess, and even learning from experience. There is nothing magic about a computer, it is simply a machine doing the job it was designed to do, and this, supporters say, is precisely true of the human brain and its emergent mind. This leads directly to the suggestion that, with suitable technology, we should be able to build a computer which is, in every sense of the word, sentient. In fact, Searle does not dispute what a substance dualist would claim is a counter-intuitive idea:

> "There is no reason, in principle, why we could not... make an artificial brain that causes consciousness... any such artificial brain would have to duplicate the actual causes of human and animal brains to produce inner, qualitative, subjective states of consciousness. Just producing similar output behavior would not

by itself be enough" ([3], p. 53; the latter point is a parting shot at functionalism).

However, he rejects property dualism on the same basis as he rejects substance dualism [7, 8]: it creates an insuperable gulf between the physical world and the mental world. His carefully-crafted argument is based on the idea of the physical world as a closed system. If the physical universe is causally closed (as the laws of thermodynamics demand), then no non-physical entity or force could ever be causally effective in the physical realm. Thus, if the mind is not part of the physical universe, it would be causally ineffective, meaning it would be an epiphenomenon. In the alternative, if the physical universe is not closed, non-physical minds would be able to exert effects on the body. This would, of course, breach one of the most basic laws of physics, the law of conservation of mass-energy. Searle does not bother about this but argues that if "...the physical universe is not causally closed, (then) consciousness can function causally in the production of physical behavior." His case is that this would be unsatisfactory as it would lead to the anomalous position where there were two explanations of any behavior, the purely physical account of nerves and muscles, and also the causally-effective mental state. That is, behavior would have two separate and unrelated causes, which he regards as absurd.

Essentially, he argues that if any mental property of physical matter is ontologically separate from the matter itself, there can be no interaction in the world as we know it. Merely defining the properties as "special" or different in nature from the rest of the universe does nothing to resolve the intractable mind-body problem. He sees only one solution to this problem, that mental properties must be biological in nature. This has been the thrust of his work over many years.

2.4: The Mind As A Function Of Biology

His own view is that, beginning to end, the mind is biological in nature: "Above all, consciousness is a biological phenomenon. We should think of consciousness as part of our ordinary biological history, along with digestion, growth, mitosis, and meiosis" [3, p. 1]. Elsewhere, he adds photosynthesis and the secretion of bile to this list, leaving no doubt where he stands: "We must stop worrying about how the brain could cause consciousness and begin with the plain fact that it does" [9, p. 8]. "We live in one world, and all the features of the world from quarks and electrons to nation states and balance of payments problems are, in their different ways, part of that one world"[9]. "All of our mental phenomena are caused by lower level neuronal processes in the brain and are themselves realized in the brain as higher level, or system, features" [8, p. 1]. "The smell of the flower, the sound of the symphony, the thoughts of theorems in Euclidian geometry—all are caused by lower level biological processes in the brain; and as far as we know, the crucial functional elements are neurons and synapses" [10]. The mind is not, however, an ordinary biological phenomenon like, say, snails secreting shells, beavers building dams with mud, or humans excreting, it is removed from these matters: "... consciousness is caused by brain processes and is a higher-level feature of the brain system" [2, p. 54].

As a subjective phenomenon, mind is not reducible to "mere chemistry," such as is possible with digestion or the solidity of wooden tables. In outlining his opposition to property dualism [8], he stated:

> "The property dualist and I are in agreement that consciousness is ontologically irreducible. The key points of disagreement are that I insist that from everything we know about the brain, consciousness is causally reducible to brain processes; and for that reason, I deny that the ontological irreducibility of consciousness implies that consciousness is something 'over and above', something distinct from, its neurobiological base."

That is, he excludes the possibility that there can be a natural explanation for two ontologically different matters or forms in the universe. Everything that is must reduce causally to matter and energy:

> "'Consciousness' does not name a distinct, separate phenomenon, something over and above its neurobiological base, rather it names a state that the neurobiological system can be in. Just as the shape of the piston and the solidity of the cylinder block are not something over and above the molecular phenomena, but are rather states of the system of molecules, so the consciousness of the brain is not something over and above the neuronal phenomena, but rather a state that the neuronal system is in."

He sees no room for negotiation on his view that consciousness is a "...biological phenomenon like any other..." which derives from the particular functional organization of the brain ("This proposition is not up for grabs" [2, p. 51]). Because it is a natural feature of brains, the mind cannot lead a separate life, meaning immortality, telekinesis, and the rest of the ancient tricks of the dualist trade are excluded. His task, therefore, is to steer a path between these constraints to find a theory of consciousness that does not fall apart at the first hurdle.

2.5: The Structure Of Consciousness

There are, Searle argues, ten features to the structure of consciousness which constrain any theory [2, p. 73-80]:

> 1. Consciousness is subjective, and there is no way this can be gainsaid or "explained away" without thereby losing the quintessential feature of mind. All conscious states exist only as they are experienced by an agent with a mental capacity: "However, though consciousness is a biological phenomenon, it has some important features that other biological phenomena do not have. The most important of these is... its 'subjectivity'. There is a sense in which each person's consciousness is private to that person... he is related to his pains, tickles, itches, thoughts, and feelings in a way

that is quite unlike the way that others are related to those pains, tickles, itches, thoughts and feelings" [8]. This concept, of privacy, leads to one of the traditional difficulties science has had in coming to grips with consciousness.

2. Consciousness is a unity, coming to us as a single, unified experience, for which memory is an essential requirement. There is a unity in the way our experiences are assembled in the present, and a unity across time: "Thus, it is unthinkable that my conscious states should come to me as a simultaneous series of discrete bits... the field metaphor is a better one for describing the structure of consciousness than the 'putting together of bits' metaphor, which has worked so well in other areas of scientific and philosophical analysis" [2, p. 83].

3. Consciousness gives us access to the real world, and two essential tools for dealing with that world are our cognitive capacities (knowing what and how) and volition, the determination to deal with the world. Some mental states are "unconscious" (what happens to a belief when we are asleep?) but they are not thereby any less real. Mental states exhibit directedness, or intentionality, which is also irreducible, but non-intentional mental states are possible, e.g. free-floating anxiety.

4. "All of our conscious states come to us in one mood or another," meaning there is always a mood of some sort attached to each mental event.

5. Consciousness imposes a structure on the often disjointed but otherwise overwhelming sensory input, filtering it and filling in the gaps, as it were.

6. Every conscious being has the capacity for attention: "Attention is like a light that I can shift from one part of my conscious field to another" (p. 78).

7. Every conscious state is nested in a "Background" of essential information which helps us orient ourselves in changing circumstances. Even if I am not fully aware of it, the object of my current conscious state brings with it a vast array of knowledge that assists in integrating the current experience into a continuing reality: "...I just take a huge metaphysics for granted." Part of this Background is common to all humans and part is local culture: "...our capacity for rational thought and behavior is for the most part a Background capacity" (p. 108-9).

8. Each state also brings with it a sense of familiarity of variable intensity.

9. Every thought leads to another, as part of the Background knowledge state, and,

10. To a greater or lesser extent, conscious states are pleasurable or unpleasurable, occasionally both together.

These features give consciousness its essential, human qualities, from which the (subjective) mind creates an "epistemically objective social reality" (p. 113). The point of consciousness is its capacity for directedness, or intentionality, as this is the means by which we relate to and engage with the world. However, this most abstract of matters has to be "naturalized" or brought to account, otherwise the theory has no explanatory value.

It would not be possible to summarize his complex and often subtle arguments in a paragraph or two. Suffice it to say that, by a series of clever moves, he tries to show that a causally-effective consciousness can find a way between the mysticism of dualism and the sterility of the various forms of materialism. His purpose is to preserve our nature as sentient beings who are an ordinary (not extraordinary) part of the natural (not supernatural) universe. Subsequently, he derives accounts of free will and language, and thence social structure and morality, showing how certain epistemological problems dissolve when seen from this point of view. As part of this, he shows that we utilize what he calls "status functions" to achieve communication via language and many other socially important functions such as currency, etc, to create a new social reality: "... having institutional facts is to gain control over brute facts" (p. 131). When these functions are widely held and applied by individuals:

> "...the collective assignment of status functions, and... their continued recognition and acceptance over long periods of time, can create and maintain a reality of governments, money, nation-states, languages, ownership of private property, universities... a thousand other such institutions that can seem as epistemically objective as geology and as much a permanent part of our landscape as rock formations" (p. 131-132).

Should the collective acceptance be withdrawn, these apparently rock-solid institutions will collapse like a house of cards, as happened to the USSR and its empire in 1989 or Lehman Bros in 2008.

Underlying all of these social features (p. 153) is the human capacity for language, which is composed of "constitutive rules," rules which not only regulate behavior but, in fact, constitute the very activity they regulate. So, in order to surrender, a person must announce: "I surrender." The action of uttering just those sounds constitutes the event of surrender—as long as one's enemies speak English. Language functions by virtue of meaning, where meaning is the property that turns a sound into a speech event, i.e. how the mind imposes intentionality on sounds and scribbles:

> "The meaning of a sentence is entirely a matter of the conventions of the language... The original or intrinsic intentionality of a speaker's thought is transferred to words, sentences, marks, symbols, and so on" (p. 140-141).

When two people know the rules of a language, they can indicate their intention to speak, and then communicate a meaning. All of this depends utterly on the fact that "Humans have the capacity to use one object to stand for, represent, express or symbolize something else" (p. 154).

Language consists of symbols manipulated according to certain rigid and very complex rules (syntax) in order to convey a content or meaning (semantics).

2.6: End Of The Monist Road

Searle makes no pretence of being a jolly fellow, laughingly tossing out solutions to a few world problems and bowing to the applause, but is his sober manner successful where a punster's is not? Even though I believe he is on the right track, where functionalists, who would sidestep the mental impact of feeling pain, are not, my view is that he has not completed his program and, more to the point, cannot complete it. As a reminder, his program is to give a full, natural account of human mentality as a causative factor in observable behavior. By full, he means not slipping the difficult bits (like pain, or qualia, as they are known) off the table while everybody is distracted by a joke. By natural, he means a product of the natural world as we know it, with no supernatural elements occupying a causative role and no clever semantic tricks to bridge the unbridgeable. By mental, he includes everything occurring in the privacy of our heads which we all know by direct personal experience, including some that we don't actually know. By causative, he means that a mental factor is both necessary and sufficient for the ensuing behavior. Observable is just that: can be seen, caught, weighed and measured, then lightly poached and served with a piquant parsley sauce. That is, it is a part of the material realm subject to the laws of thermodynamics.

This is not an impossible program so why should anybody say it cannot succeed? I see a number of interwoven objections, as follow:

Objection 1: Searle's unyielding, visceral antipathy to dualism blinds him to the very obvious fact that an ontologically separate and irreducible state can coexist in natural harmony with an entirely separate state, if and only if it is an informational state generated by a physical machine. Information does not exist without a physical substrate in which it can be coded, but it also does not exist in the sense of being seen, caught, weighed, etc. An informational state floats, as it were, in the machine that generates it, everywhere but nowhere, utterly dependent on the machine continuing to function as designed. This does not mean that all such natural informational states are of the same nature or order as the biological information coded in DNA. DNA is mere "information", physicochemical lock and key stuff of the same order as the "information" coded in my door key. The door key "tells" the door to open but only by analogy, not as a homology to the sense in which my daughter tells me she doesn't want to eat her carrots or Searle tells his readers that functionalists are nitwits. There is information and "information", codes and "codes", telling and "telling", etc.

An informational state is "causally reducible" to its physical substrate but "ontologically irreducible" to that substrate. This satisfies Searle's major objection to property dualism, that ontological separation necessarily means consciousness will forever be mysterious: not if it is an informational state generated by the physical substrate of the brain. There is nothing mysterious about that. The material realm is subject to the laws of thermodynamics, the informational realm to the laws of its particular syntax, and the two are forever immiscible. They are alien realms, intimately related in the causative sense but nothing can cross from one realm to the other unless certain boundary conditions obtain [11]. If those conditions are realized, then the two realms or worlds become mutually interdependent such that information can pass from one realm to the other. So if we say that a mind is a personal informational state generated in the head by the healthy human brain, then we scoop up Searle's requirements of privacy, insubstantiality, and subjectivity. By the same move, we exclude his hobgoblins of substance dualism and immortality, plus any other clever tricks that unreal homunculi can do.

Objection 2: The claim that mind is biological rests on a misunderstanding of the term "biological". It is one thing to say that the mind springs from the biology of the brain, something else again to assume that it is a single, one-step process that remains within the purview of the laws of thermodynamics. There is no a priori reason to suppose that the mind arises from the brain as, say, the hypothalamic releasing factors arise from the brain. The brain is an organic structure but, by virtue of its function, it supports an informational processing space. Searle concedes this case in his statements: "We live in one world, and all the features of the world from quarks and electrons to nation states and balance of payments problems are, in their different ways, part of that one world" [9]. "All of our mental phenomena are caused by lower level neuronal processes in the brain and are themselves realized in the brain as higher level, or system, features" [8, p. 1]. The expressions "...in their different ways..." and "...higher level or system features..." denote something not the same, of another nature, and this in turn means "of a dual nature." At other times, he uses apparently objective terms to convey dualist meanings. For example, in the job it does, his expression "status functions" [2, p. 126] is indistinguishable from the mentalist term, rules. "Conventions of language" [2, Ch. 6] means no more nor less than "rules of language", and rules are not physical. Rules are information. Information is not physical. Anything that is not physical is not biological.

If we propose a disjunction between the physical state of the brain and its associated informational state, we establish the principles by which there is a natural, causative progression "...from quarks and electrons to nation states and balance of payments problems..." Religions, games of poker, and the collapse of empires are then causally related to the material world but remain fundamentally and irreducibly different from the brains that dreamed them up.

Just as Dennett did, Searle has allowed dualism into his monist system and, from there, it does all the work. Sans dualism, his monism flops helplessly on the floor, a body without a mind. There is a reason why this has happened. Let's go back to the opening quote I used: "Consciousness can no more lie around separate from my brain than the liquidity of water can be separated from the water, or the solidity of the table from the table" [2, p. 41]. This claim is seriously misleading.

The liquidity of water and solidity of a table are properties of a very different order from the relationship of mind to brain. Water is wet and wood is solid, and these are inert physical properties stemming directly from the structure of their molecules as they stand in relation to the molecular structure of our fingers. It is just a matter of molecules bumping into each other. The mind, however, is not an inert physical property of the brain. The physical properties of the brain include its weight, its slightly squishy feel, its color, its water and mineral content, and all that boring stuff we learned in Biology 100. However, a living brain has something above and beyond those statistics: it has a function, it does something with its physical properties which extends its capacities in directions which do not depend on molecules bumping aimlessly into each other. While causally related to the brain's physicochemical properties, it has a performance which is ontologically irreducible to those properties, just because it could be realized in any other data processor. Physical properties, and performances or functions, occupy different realms of discourse. It is, as George Orwell didn't quite say, like choosing between a sausage and a rose: their purposes hardly intersect.

Objection 3: "Just as the shape of the piston and the solidity of the cylinder block are not something over and above the molecular phenomena, but are rather states of the system of molecules, so the consciousness of the brain is not something over and above the neuronal phenomena, but rather a state that the neuronal system is in." Here, we see that his claim completely misses the point that the brain never rests. An orchestra waiting tensely for the drop of the conductor's baton is not generating a symphony. A frozen or anesthetized brain does not generate a mind because the mind is a brain doing its job. A piston in its cylinder can be sealed in a vault for ten thousand years but this will not alter its design or function. A brain that is not doing its job of processing information is not generating a mind. (For the benefit of panpsychists, the organized crystalline structure of a rock does not confer a form of consciousness on it. Consciousness, or mind, is a doing whereas the individual calcium, aluminum, and oxygen atoms that constitute a rock's crystals have been frozen in that particular lattice for maybe a billion years. As crystalline elements, they can do nothing: rocks therefore have no mental life).

When the brain dies, all its coded information dissolves with neurolysis and subsequent putrefaction. The mind cannot be recovered from the goo any more than the information in an incinerated book could be recovered from the smoke that drifted away on the breeze. We can heat or freeze, taunt, neglect, hate, or starve an engine block and it will work first time we turn it over, because it is the turning over which constitutes the work of an engine. When an engine is running, it generates a "higher level, or system, feature" such as transport, which would be the correct analogy to the brain and the mind it generates.

Objection 4: "Consciousness is a unity." As it stands, this claim is ideological. It appears to be the result of his firm but unargued conviction that mind cannot be composed of "building blocks" of functions. Why not, when it has overwhelming biological and evolutionary precedents? All that exists in the biological world came from what was before; there is nothing new under the sun [12]. If Searle wishes to propose that the mind is ontologically a unity, then he needs to show that it could have sprung into existence *holus bolus*. Given our present knowledge, this is inconceivable. Far more likely, it developed in spits and spurts from whatever dim awareness the most primitive mammals had a hundred million years ago. Nothing arrives *ex vacuo*, not the tax law, not the organization of armies, organized crime or large universities, not religions, politics, species, or ecologies. Everything comes from what went before, and the mind is no exception.

The urge to find a unity in the mind has driven him to a further mistake, that of incorrectly aligning consciousness as the contents of mind (semantics) with consciousness as medical practitioners understand it, meaning the physiological principle of arousal. Medical consciousness means the preliminary or preparatory state of being alert and able to respond selectively to the environment. This precedes any ʼcognitive contents. This physiological function is a product of the brain stem, which is probably why Searle went burrowing down to the thalamus in search of consciousness. He won't find it there. All he will find are the neural correlates of physiological arousal. He will find the difference between being drowsy and agitated (see Yerkes-Dodson Curve, in [4]) but, most assuredly, he will not find the difference between being a Catholic and an atheist. He appears to have had an implicit understanding of this: "...what I will call the basal, or background, conscious field, which is the presupposition of having any conscious experience in the first place" [9, p. 10]. "Basal consciousness" is clearly a very biological phenomenon, as all animals have it. It readies the organism to perform its various (modular) cognitive functions. We should never refer to this feature as "consciousness" for the reason that it is properly termed "physiological arousal."

The various neurological subsystems that provide the sensory and motor basis for being alive and responsive, such as vision, hearing, balance, fine motor control, motor memory, etc. are most definitely modular in their anatomy and in their function. As the Russian neuropsychologist, Aleksandr Luria, showed in his elegant little experiments [14], one cerebral function after another can be selectively knocked out by injury or illness but the essential humanity of the patient remains intact. Higher cognitive functions are assembled from lower order performances. The unity of my consciousness is an artifact, composed partly by the fact that my brain works very fast and partly because it all happens to me. When it breaks down, as it does in certain psychiatric states, it produces disjointed modules of function, not an "Incredible Shrinking Mind".

Consciousness, as Searle said himself, is an illusion. So, therefore, is the unity of consciousness.

Objection 5: This brings us to a further, major error. Searle claims that brain processes and their various products are all of a biological nature: "...mental phenomena are ordinary biological phenomena in the same sense as photosynthesis or digestion" [9, p. 6]. This is a non sequitur. He has made the mistake of conflating the biological mechanisms or machinery by which the brain produces the mind, with the non-biological output of those mechanisms. The structure of a machine, and its function, performance, role or output etc, are two entirely different things. Just because the brain is a biological organ, constrained and driven by the laws of the material world (thermodynamics), doesn't mean that its output is going to be of the same nature. There could be one, two, or a dozen steps between the machine and its output by which the output is successively transformed into an event of a different ontological nature. There is nothing in the nature of (physical) machines or the laws of thermodynamics themselves to prevent this happening.

By virtue of their particular nature as conduction and switching devices, ordinary brain structures, of the type that can be put under a microscope or analyzed in a mass spectrometer, are capable of generating an informational or virtual space. This presupposes the integrity of the brain, that it is healthy and functioning properly within very narrow physiological limits. If that informational space is found in a human head, we call it a mind. If an informational space is generated in a dog's head, it is, well, a doggy sort of mind but still recognizably a mind and not a pork sausage. If there are drugs or other toxic chemicals in the blood stream bathing the brain, then the output of the brain will be disordered (intoxication). If the informational content is disordered, even in the presence of a healthy brain, the output will be disordered; thus, a small modification of Searle's approach yields a model of mental disorder, something Dennett's functionalism could never do.

Objection 6: His intense preoccupation with intentionality is philosophical but not practical. All information is "about" something, because that's what "information" means: stands for, represents, symbolizes etc, without being one and the same thing as the object, process etc. thereby represented. The idea that there can be non-intentional mental states, such as anxiety, is simply wrong. There is no such thing as "free-floating anxiety"; it means only that the psychiatrist hasn't taken a proper history [4].

The whole idea of intentionality has been misconstrued from the beginning: "One way of explaining what is meant by 'intentionality' in the (more obscure) philosophical sense is this: it is that aspect of mental states or events that consists in their being of or about things (as pertains to the questions, 'What are you thinking of?' and 'What are you thinking about?'). Intentionality is the aboutness or directedness of mind (or states of mind) to things, objects, states of affairs, events" [14]. If, however, we conceptualize the mind as an informational space, then the question of mental events having the property of "aboutness" collapses: all information is "about" something, in the sense that it stands for or represents something. The notion of information that is not "about something" is contradictory. It is not the case that the set of items of information that are "not about something" is empty; the set does not exist. Anything which, at first sight, seems to be both an item of information and not about something is not information. If it is not information, it will not be found in an informational space. The mind is an informational space.

Objection 7: An informational space can be lifted to unimaginable levels of complexity without further modification of the physical machine that generated it [15]. The human brain may be smaller than a dolphin's but since we have something called language (and opposable thumbs, of course), we dominate the dolphins, not vice versa. If Searle agrees that the mind can be duplicated in a computer, then he is agreeing that the mind is an informational artifact, because there is only one thing computers can do, manipulate information. By syntactical transformations, using what IT calls virtual machines generated by algorithms, the semantic content of the mind is transformed beyond recognition, magnified, and amplified until a finite input becomes a near-infinite output. A virtual machine is ontologically different from a physical machine but an infinite virtual machine can be generated by a finite physical informational calculator. Are virtual machines effective in the real world? Airline booking systems, for example, are virtual machines, so the answer is (a qualified) yes.

Objection 8: If we recast the mind as an informational space, it immediately falls within the purview of science. This was one of Searle's major goals. Of course, not all information is itself scientific but the concept of information free of content is a valid, rational model and therefore can be investigated by science: "Just as Einstein made a conceptual change to break the distinction between space and time, so we need a similar conceptual change to break the bifurcation of mental and physical" [9, p. 8]. This goal is achieved by redefining mind as an informational space generated by the brain. The mind consists of syntactical rules (themselves information) which manipulate a semantic content. Thus, information coded in the brain can move freely between mind and brain and back again. Even though we cannot localize it or find any to weigh or bottle or serve with parsley sauce, information is still real and therefore amenable to a scientific investigation. This leads us directly to a "science of consciousness or mental life" which is not a solecism.

Objection 9: Many of his "structures of consciousness" (see above) are, in fact, simple modular functions of the brain. "All of our conscious states come to us in one mood or another" is (a) not true (the mood of 2+2=4?)

and (b) entirely consistent with Luria's model of emotions as output states in their own right [4, 11]. The same is true of familiarity. This is a module which is switched on by objects which evoke a memory trace, and not by those that don't. It can malfunction, as the *déjà vu* and *jamais vu* of epileptic auras shows.

"Attention is like a light that I can shift from one part of my conscious field to another." The problem with metaphors and analogies is that, all too often, they appear to have explanatory value but, instead, they simply stop the process of enquiry. What does it profit us to think of attention as a spotlight that swings around, when we realize that lizards have exactly the same property? I say, no profit at all; it simply lulls us into acquiescence. The orienting response is pure physiology. Even our capacity for attending to a particular task to the point of being oblivious to other stimuli (say, children watching TV) is relatively recent but cats certainly have it. For omnivores, it is not consistent with survival in a demanding environment. Watch baboons on the ground eating. Attention deficit disorder is a social construct, as young male rhesus monkeys show.

"...I just take a huge metaphysics for granted." Part of this Background of knowledge is common to all humans and part is local culture: "...our capacity for rational thought and behavior is for the most part a Background capacity" [2, p. 108-9]. The syntax of rational thought is universal; the semantics are tribal. His "Background" is just information, not magic, some of it gained explicitly, some implicitly. His "metaphysics" is another example of using dualist concepts to complete the causal chain in his monist model: what does the *meta* in metaphysics mean if not "beyond, above, further to, different from"? In any event, most of this depends on memory, and memory is a classic modular function.

"Conscious states are always pleasurable or unpleasurable to some degree" (1999 a, p. 80). Firstly, pleasure is a mood and is therefore an output state but, second, it proves nothing about the nature of mental states. Pleasure just is a mental state so it cannot be considered different to or separate from other conscious states (without running the risk of setting up another duality).

Objection 10: Given the human capacity to generate information about the real world, it is no surprise to learn they do it about other humans, too. From this, it is a small conceptual step to "...governments, money, nation-states, languages, ownership of private property, universities (and a) thousand other such institutions..." Just as, within certain limits, we can treat the weather as predictable, so too we can treat other humans as predictable. Language is just the rule-governed means we use to communicate our mental states to each other. Language consists of coded information; the mind consists of coded information; all that differs is the syntax, or rules (language of thought vs. spoken Urdu). There is no ontological problem in a biologically-based informational space (otherwise known as a mind) generating coded information (also called a language) as a process of conveying part of its content to another informational space.

Sometimes, I can use those rules of language to conceal facts from you, but lying is still an informational state.

2.7: Conclusion: Minds Are Not Bodily Secretions

If we propose that the brain is a high speed, multi-modal, and modular processor of information, then we get a system with abstract (higher level) properties which are different from those of pimples and smelly bodily fluids but which are immutably determined as a function of those same bodily fluids (and neurons, etc.). In that sense, some people might want to say that the higher level features are biological, but I would say doing that stretches the notion of "biological" to the point where it becomes worthless. What does it profit us to claim, as Guze did, that "feelings and thoughts are as biological as blood pressure and gastric acid"? While he might want to claim that all his "hopes, fears, wishes, needs, fantasies, and feelings" are of the same nature as his bowel functions, mine certainly aren't. The acerbic Alfred Ayer said that being a behaviorist was akin to claiming that you are anaesthetized from the neck up. By the same token, claiming to be a biological psychiatrist is no different from saying that your mind, as a secretion of the brain, and your feces, as a secretion of the bowel, are of the same conceptual order.

If we avail ourselves of the fact that the brain is a high-speed switching device, and we allow that information slips back and forth between its phantom world somewhere in the head and the real world, as computers do all day (except when they don't), then we can avoid taking the first step on the slippery slide of substance dualism. By this means, our "higher level system", called the mind, allows us to develop systems of language replete with mentalist terms just because they accurately reflect our inner reality. From this, we can build institutions such as "governments, money, nation-states, languages, ownership of private property, universities etc." So, if somebody says: "I wanted to punch him," we do not need to look for her past history of environmental contingencies (she has never punched anybody before), nor do we need to talk about her id impulses mixed up with her (unproven) penis envy, nor do we have to say she has a chemical imbalance of the brain. All we have to do is say: "She has perceived a number of factors in her environment which generated an agitated emotional output state (of anger) which she accepts will be alleviated by the future event of smacking him in the mouth"

The action of clenching her fist will be generated by an information outflow from the brain, an outflow which is itself of the same nature as the codes underlying her perception (of his infidelity) and the computational events that, of all the possibilities, led her to one particular outcome. This is not magic, it is not biology, it is not mindless, and it is not an irrefutable fantasy. This is what Searle called "a science of consciousness".

It will be clear that I distinguish between properties, functions, and attributes. Properties are rightly seen as measurable parameters of real elements in the material realm. Thus, the properties of a car are its weight, the amount of steel in it, the fuel capacity, and the like. The function, role, or performance of an object is what it does. The function of a car is to move people around, so a car has properties and a function. A rock lying in a river bed has no function, it has only properties. All too often, people use the word function to mean "designed function." Functions can be natural or designed. The designed function of loud speakers is to amplify sound. The un-designed function of a bird is to have baby birds. The function, meaning role, of the bird's wing is to support flight so the bird can collect food for its chicks. Attributes are values or significance assigned to an object by a creature with mental capacities. Attributes have no existence independently of the mind that generates them. They exist only in the informational space generated by a suitable brain. I attribute a high value to this piece of heavy, yellow metal but none to this small piece of limestone, but that value is not a property of gold, and gold, as such, has no function. I would say that a bird can attribute a value to a bit of territory, and most animals attribute value or worth to their offspring. If we see these three terms as signifying separate concepts, then a lot of the problem with property dualism fades away. As mentioned before, the properties of the brain are its weight, its chemical content, its neuronal tracts, etc., but its function is to generate an informational space. Mind is not a property of a brain so, strictly speaking, the idea of the mind being a case of property dualism of the brain is nonsensical.

Because of these problems, Searle's case loses some of its internal coherence: "The meaning of a sentence is entirely a matter of the conventions of the language." (p. 140) Human conventions are not matters of physics: they are irreducibly mental and, therefore, dualist in nature. Rules, say of golf, also cannot be derived from the physical state of the brain that has learned them. Rules are imposed on the brain's microstructure in symbolic form but not in a sense that flows from the biology of the brain. Symbols, of course (p. 141), are the ultimate dualist notion, in that a symbol is never the thing it represents. Searle appears to have given this point little credit. The brain has two states, phases, aspects, or natures: it is a duality, in the strictest sense of the word. There is its physical state, meaning its weight and chemical content, its neurons and synapses, and its nuclei and mitochondria. On the other hand, its physical state subserves a further, higher-level, functional state which flows from the information coded into the brain. When that information is manipulated, it generates an informational space which we call the mind. If the information isn't active, then there is no functional state, i.e. unconsciousness. But Searle has already conceded that the informational state of a brain could be realized in a computer (p. 53). I would say that if the informational state of a human brain could be duplicated as a facsimile in a computer, then the new informational space would ipso facto constitute a mind—of sorts. And information is never of the same nature as its physical substrate (DNA is a physical code, not a symbolic code). He was absolutely correct to say that physics does not give rise to syntax. The semantic content of a language is therefore whatever the speaker intends it to be.

Mind is fundamentally, irrevocably and forever of an ontologically different nature from the brain that generates it—but it is fundamentally, irrevocably, and forever a part of the natural world. That means the natural world is dualist in nature: well, it has been ever since humans came along and, I believe, for a considerable time before Homo stamped his foot in the mud of Olduvai. It also means the mind will cease to exist forever when the oxygen supply to its brain stops.

Given these suggested changes to Searle's stance, some major philosophical problems fold into a larger, genuinely explanatory theory which satisfies every one of his ten conditions. These include the mind-body problem, innate knowledge (human nature), unconscious causation and ego defenses, intentionality, reference and meaning and hence language, rule-governed behavior, and even personality. I conclude his program has been somewhat off-center but not wrong, as the functionalist program was. He did not need to tie himself in knots trying to devise a monist theory of consciousness, or mind; all he needed to do was show that consciousness is an informational state generated by the brain (one state per brain), and his problems were solved. However, he couldn't do this because he had to admit that humans have two natures, a physical state and an informational state, and that, while causally-related, the two are ontologically distinct. That is exactly what the expression natural dualism means. But, and this is the crucial point, because they are causally-related, transfer of information between mind and body is a reality and can be studied scientifically.

At different points, Searle has expressed the hope that the neurosciences will take over the philosophy of mind and complete their program. He hoped neuroscientists would be able to find a biological path between mystical dualism and sterile anti-mentalism. When we look at the rigid and unthinking reductionism to which neuroscientists are beholden [4, 11], I don't believe that will ever happen. Neuroscientists are denizens of the material world; they think only in terms of the laws of thermodynamics. The notion that there might be part of the human state that enzymes and fMRI scans can't explain strikes them as silly, even insulting. From the psychiatric point of view, the unleavened neurosciences will never lead to a humanist model of mental disorder. The correct theory has to be dualist in nature; otherwise it will never give account of the crucial differences between humans and chimps.

As for Searle, he predicted that the correct theory of mind would not be dualist. My objections to his theory mean that his prediction has failed but that's philosophy. Arthur Koestler summarized this neatly: "If the creator had a purpose in endowing us with a neck, he surely meant us to stick it out." While the model proposed here is essentially dualist in nature, it is a dualism with which I believe Searle could feel comfortable. These days, the claim that an informational state cannot influence a physical state is refuted by every child's toy. For Searle, duality was abhorrent. To our children, it's second nature; child's play, you could say.

So, can biological naturalism save biological psychiatry? No, but it was a good try.

3	***The Drivel Generators***

"The greatest error of a penetrating wit is to go beyond the mark."

De la Rochefoucauld

3.1: Introduction

There is a certain class of novelists who achieve a considerable degree of popular fame and, quite often, fortune, within their lifetime. Not uncommonly, such a novelist's fame barely survives his funeral; the fortune may, of course, be somewhat more durable but that depends on how cleverly he insulates it from his feckless relatives. He is to be compared with the less fortunate novelist, often poor and unknown, whose work enters the lists of classics only because his untimely death has jolted the reading public into actually opening his demanding, if not downright tiresome, volumes. Leaving the classics for another day (as we usually do), I want to look at the peculiar phenomenon of those enviously popular authors of what even their most ardent fans would agree is just froth and babble.

Best known are the humorists, such as the British novelists PG Wodehouse and Tom Sharpe, but they are certainly not limited to the comic end of the scale. Other examples include Agatha Christie's detective novels, the swarms of fantasy and sci-fi hacks who effortlessly knock out seven-set sagas of sword and sorcerer, social commentaries such as those by Sinclair Lewis, unlikely adventurers such as Tarzan, by Edgar Rice Burroughs, romance by Dame Barbara Cartland, Westerns by Zane Gray, spies (Ian Fleming), and chewing-gum detective pulp, starting with Mickey Spillane's Mike Hammer and wandering through its many avatars. We should not overlook children's stories, of which Charles Hamilton was the unchallenged master (a.k.a. Frank Richards of Billy Bunter fame). With over twenty million published words to his credit, he remains the world's most prolific author but Dame Barbara sold well over a billion books, also a world record. Seven of Spillane's books are in the top fifteen most popular American novels of all times. Of course, radio and television broadened the opportunities exponentially, with wildly popular soap operas dominating the airwaves for many years. We should also mention the sage of Minnesota, Garrison Keillor, who warrants a pedestal of his own and whose reputation might just survive the onset of rigor mortis.

The characteristics of these efforts are formulaic plots involving two dimensional characters in banal settings employing stereotyped action and a clichéd dialogue with no pretence of uplifting value. However, they sell; unfortunately, vulgarity has no use-by date. But what has this enviably successful brand of kitsch to do with the philosophy of mind? Quite a lot, actually.

All these authors are prolific. In between leading her busy exemplary life, and even well into her eighties, Miss Cartland sent her publishers a book every two months or so, giving her a total of some 723 books over her extraordinarily long professional life. Manifestly, there wasn't much research that went into them, nor did she struggle to stay awake at nights, locked in battle with the intricacies of character or plot. She had in her head what we might call a mental "book-writing machine," capable of churning out another best-seller between Royal Ascot and the last of the Royal Garden Parties. She was a sort of perambulated novel machine in pearls, a human version (in pink) of the 'trash for the proles' in Orwell's Oceania of *1984*. However, we have to explain this lest we fall into the trap of Moliere's 'dormitive principle.' What could be the nature of a 'machine' capable of cranking out formulaic novels of two dimensional characters in banal settings, etc? In fact, it is just ordinary imagination, with the addition of a few simple techniques that do the actual work. The author puts a gaggle of trite characters in a stock setting and lets them blunder through normal daily events. By randomly introducing heroes and villains, joys and dramas, the story acquires a life of its own. All the author does is record the stock utterances of his characters as they stumble over little dramas that we can all identify with.

This style, if it be such, is best suited to humor as, when they begin them, the authors all freely say they have no idea where their stories will end. They assign each character a couple of traits which he or she exhibits more or less consistently (Wodehouse solved the problem of having to invent new characters for each book by using the same ones year after year), drop them in a familiar setting which they (the authors) could describe in their sleep, wind them up and let 'em rip. In essence, the characters are talking dolls, but virtual talking dolls, because they exist only in the author's head. Let's see if we can write one now. We will start with a weak-kneed hero, Freddy, an heir whose response to any pressure is to throw his hands in the air with a screech and run away, yet he can be lured into almost anything by the promise of a free drink. Freddy needs an opposite, so we'll take one of his ribs to create Thelma. This poor but winsome soul is desperate to marry Freddy but she has a wandering eye and a highly developed sense of guilt which, regrettably, only comes into play *post hoc*. Let's put them in the setting of, I don't know, a day at the beach. What will they find at the beach? A sun-bronzed lifesaver, a girl selling ice cream, and a shark. This is a comedy, so the shark should have a broken tooth and, for the Freudian slant, we'll say the girl sells hotdogs instead. We set our little cast on the sand, switch on the video recorder to run until its batteries fade, press their buttons, and leave them to it. The talking dolls (I won't flatter them by calling them characters) and the situation alone will generate the story. Thus is creativity reduced to little more than the street-wise cutting and splicing of clichéd utterances in stock settings. Just by turning the handle, the author cranks out page after page of mindless froth which he changes into money at the nearest bank.

I will call the virtual stage he has set up in his mind a "drivel generator", but we all know it's actually a money-generator. Those of us who are burdened by intellectual pretensions shouldn't mock: drivel pays. Gerald Durrell made far more money and will be remembered long after Lawrence (he even has a statue), and all by the simple expedient of wryly recording the antics of animals and eccentric people in exotic locations. In dreary Britain in the 1950s, it sold. Keillor thinks of a name, cloaks it with an origin somewhere in his private Lilliput of Lake Woebegone, and lets the character invent itself. All he does is write down what such a person from such a setting would be unlikely to do if confronted with a series of essentially unremarkable incidents in workaday settings. With just a bit of nudging from the author, his characters write themselves. One unlikely event triggers another, which in turn leads to another: if the hero did this, what would the heroine do? From the range of possibilities, Keillor chooses something dopey but well within the bounds of normal human behavior and so it goes. Cartland chose the most impassioned, Sharpe the most ridiculous: it is simply a matter of choosing a path along the endlessly proliferating 'decision tree' that generates itself, with the emphasis on 'generates itself'. The only skill involved is bringing it to an end within the space limits set by the publisher's presses.

3.2: Turbo-Charged Drivel

So far, we have looked at written drivel but daily life shows that, regrettably, a lot of drivel is spoken without first being written down. Drivel generators are not restricted to novelists, of course. Politicians have licensed a very potent, turbo-charged version for themselves. Religious speakers of the television variety have honed theirs to the point where their audiences actually throw money at them. There are many speakers on what is called the "inspirational circuit" who can deliver a fine specimen of high-sounding drivel (again for a fee), including failed footballers, psychologists, reformed drunks, and other unlikely professions. Most of the hugely profitable Australian soap operas use the same principle, even though they are often of a standard that would give drivel a bad name. A lot of music is stereotyped drivel, and it's not just restricted to rap on MTV. The output (I won't say work) of the shred guitarist, Yngve Malmsteen, could even be played backwards and nobody would be the wiser, yet he is a multimillionaire. And academia: we must not forget academia, home to the most pretentious drivel of all. It was said of the speeches of Prof. Sir Cyril Burt, sometime president of the British Psychological Society and noted psychological fraudster: "He never says a thing but he says it beautifully." The great people who deliver "keynote" addresses at academic congresses rarely write their speeches, they simply stand up and start stringing clichés together. These cases differ from the novelist as a drivel generator in that the individual is himself the talking doll. All you have to do is switch on a microphone and the drivel obligingly flows.

The test of drivel is very simple: cut a few sentences and paste them in a different order, or even randomly through the work, or take out a critical word and put another word in its place, and see what happens. Work of high informational content is destroyed by such a move; work of low informational content is unaffected. Occasionally, when the drivel is the product of people with a high mouth-to-brain ratio, it may even be enhanced. But, enviously, drivel pays.

If I describe a politician as a "turbo-charged drivel generator", what have I explained? Nothing, of course; it is not possible to nominate something and define it in the same speech act. Of a well-known political character, I can say he is a rather big man turning to fat, with large, powerful hands and a neck and jaw to match. He has a jovial, 'nothing-is-too-much-trouble-my-friend' voice and a bone-crushing laugh during which his eyes rove around the room, as though checking on who is not laughing along over his joke. There is no doubt that he is intelligent, and smart enough to make fun of it. He has a photographic memory for names and what they are worth, for power structures and who pulls the strings, and he invariably remembers who is related to whom and by what means, fair and foul. When he talks, which is most of the time, he sprays his audience with jokes, puns, improbable stories, bits of gossip, vague promises, and accounts of what a wonderful job he has done for all the widows and orphans in his electorate, mostly by the public works he has initiated and private works he has incubated. Listening to him 'off the record' (his preferred mode), he is a large, friendly spider in the middle of a complex web of businesses and unions (who are all his close friends despite their differences), First Mate to all the sports clubs (especially those involving construction, gambling, or alcohol sales, which is all of them), friend and mentor to all pensioners, veterans and immigrants, committed to fairness and decency in all schools, churches, hospitals, and neighborhood parks, unyielding supporter of the Defense Forces, Lawnorder, the Environment and don't let on, but he even has many contacts in the subterranean world of the law and justice, not to mention the police (explosive laugh, clap on the back, see you later my friend).

I could complete his description by quoting large parts of his many speeches to community groups, school openings, sports clubs, fund-raisers, and the like but nobody has ever actually seen him read a speech, so there aren't any to quote, and the promises by his office staff to transcribe some never seem to bear fruit. All they have are his set-piece questions in parliamentary question time, most of which are sent to his office the day before by the relevant ministers. Having heard him a number of times, and spoken to different people who see him regularly in the course of their work, it is clear that, while he can talk the leg off an iron pot, he never says anything. The formal informational content of his utterances is close to zero. His speeches consist of a deluge of 'off the cuff' clichés including immense and heartfelt gratitude to his audience for the wonderful job they are doing, tender recollections of how, as a puckish but buoyantly happy child, he had once yearned for/collected for/sneaked over the fence to help whatever the audience are doing, how the future of this great club/town/state/country will be immeasurably improved by their efforts, how he is hugely gratified by the small part he has been able to play—with their help, of course—in finding the finance/land/planning permission for whatever they do, and how he is thrilled and humbled by the thought that he will be able to continue in their service for as long as they, the voters in our fair democracy, would like to make use of his (wink) particular talents, and he would just like to finish with a story of how he helped pull the prime minister out of the sand trap he got caught in during a sudden storm when they were playing golf together just the other week. How does he manage this?

I have described him, but an explanation of his talk will be on several levels. In the first place, there is the physiology of speech, the actual machinery of lips and larynx, of speech centers and cranial nerves that governs the physical act of making sounds. The second level of explanation is his knowledge of the English language and the myriad facts he has at his disposal when he stands to speak. This also abuts on that vexatious quantity, general intelligence, in which our friend is not lacking. The third is his motivation to say just what he says and nothing else. I know for a fact that he loathes the prime minister and the feeling is mutual; it might be unfortunate for his career if that were to slip out in an unguarded moment, but he could turn it to his advantage. And he is a crook.

For the purpose of understanding drivel, it is not necessary to explain the neurology of speech. The speech centers serve nonsense quite as well as they served Shakespeare or Hitler; neurons are amoral to the bitter end. The function of the second level has already been described, in Chapter 8 of *Humanizing Psychiatry* ("Language as a test of the biocognitive model"). Briefly, information is coded in the brain at the level of synaptic changes as mediated by gene expression. At the highest level, this information consists of the items of knowledge which will be used to form a sentence. These float, as it were, in a semantic space generated by the brain's capacity to switch and transform the information coded in its microstructure. By a series of transformations, other information (rules of language, awareness of surroundings, personality factors) acts upon these items of knowledge to convert them, in a stepwise process, into a series of instructions which are transmitted to the lower-order, physical speech centers. So far, so mechanical: there is no concept of 'mind' as decision-maker in this process. We can mimic this in a desktop computer. And that is the point: in his mindless talking, the politician operates at the level of, or is himself mimicking, a desktop computer. As JD Williams commented, "machines compute with the speed of light and the intelligence of worms." So do a lot of people.

The second and third levels of speech mentioned above are functionally the same. They are virtual levels of information, the lower level consisting of specific coded facts and generic rules (such as language) while the upper level consists of general coded goals, aims and ambitions, wishes, fears, and prohibitions. The lower level holds the facts, the higher level tells the brain what to do with those facts. While specific facts are readily accessible ("What model of car do you have?"), the upper levels are often intuitive or implicit and may not be readily accessible ("Why did you buy such an expensive car?"). Because the whole of the brain's informational state is stored in the one form, it can all interact. However, some of it is stored in brain structures we cannot access: who, for example, can explain how to ride a bicycle? There is no reason to believe that motor memory is open to introspection.

3.3: Automated Drivel

I said above that the talking dolls in drivel novels usually have only two personality parameters. Our political talking doll may have hundreds or thousands hidden in the various parts of the virtual space of his mind, but he has an over-arching rule which limits his public persona to four or five at the most: "Tell them what they want to hear," "Make them think I am one of them so they trust me," "Make fun of their enemies," "Promise them nothing that I could regret," and "Tell them again how wonderful they are." Given these few rules and a stock of hackneyed stories, the budding politician can flatter any crowd and leave them thinking he too is wonderful (on the basis that if he has recognized what worthy souls they are, he must be a jolly good chap himself). With no intellectual effort, he can arrange and rearrange the same few aphorisms to keep any group happy. That's all it is: politicians may operate at a higher level than talking parrots, but not much higher.

As proof of the mindlessness of a lot of speech, there have been several experiments where, using just these principles, computers endlessly generated high-sounding but utterly hollow talk. An early and highly successful one dates from 1996. Andrew Bulhak [1] showed how a recursive transition network can generate post-modernist jargon indistinguishable from the real thing (whatever 'real' means in a relativist context) as well as a very plausible paranoid religious rant:

> Post-modernist gibberish:
> If one examines post-dialectic discourse, one is faced with a choice: either accept the neosemanticist paradigm of context or conclude that the collective is capable of deconstruction, but only if Sartre's model of the cultural paradigm of reality is invalid; otherwise, Lacan's model of subcultural Marxism is one of "subcultural prepatriarchial theory", and therefore part of the failure of reality. The subject is interpolated into a subcultural Marxism that includes truth as a totality. Therefore, several theories concerning the cultural paradigm of reality exist. The main theme of Dietrich's [2] analysis of cultural construction is not

discourse, as subcapitalist narrative suggests, but prediscourse. However, in Models, Inc., Spelling deconstructs surrealism; in Beverley Hills 90210, however, Spelling examines the capitalist paradigm of discourse. Marx uses the term 'the dialectic paradigm of discourse' to denote the role of the writer as reader.

([2]. Dietrich, K. T., ed. (1981) Forgetting Sontag: The capitalist paradigm of discourse and surrealism. Yale University Press) (as you can see, Post-Modern is a very obliging program, it even generates false references).

> Paranoid delusional gibberish:
> Just as there are four letters in the name of God, there are four cardinal directions. This is because of God's law of time compensation. The COSMIC principle of ATOMIC TOTALITY is encoded in the works of Shakespeare. All historical accounts were rewritten to hide the TRUTH about God's law of time compensation. Tesla knew all about the law of psychic justice. That is why the Secret Underground Society destroyed him. The true suppressed value of pi is 3.954; all mathematics textbooks have been changed to hide this. ONLY from this value can one derive the UNIVERSE'S MISSING DAY.

Bulhak's original paper gives a lengthy example of post-modernism which, as an amateur in the subject, I would never have guessed was not written by an earnest honors student. It is of great interest that he uses the same program to develop both postmodernism and mental disorder, and the title of his paper lumps them in the same order of difficulty. Another website generates perfectly plausible but essentially meaningless articles to fill technical websites (http://www.smartarticlegenerator.com). 'Chatterbots' are computer programs designed to simulate intelligent conversation in response to human enquiries. They operate by the same principle, of generating an output from a restricted range of non-contentious options, which are sufficiently neutral in content not to conflict each other. However, just in case anybody thinks that mocking the less fortunate proves nothing, the same thing has been done to one of the world's most formidable intellects, Noam Chomsky. A chatterbot known as chomskybot (search through Wikipedia) shows how to mimic the great man, and also gives more examples of ordinary drivel generators.

Drivel generators are real. There is no question about that. It's just that some of them are in people's heads, which we all knew long before computers arrived. At last, we can be sure of the truth of the old complaint: "That man hasn't a clue. He says the first bit of rubbish that comes into his head."

3.4: Thought Disorder

So far, we have novelists, politicians, academics, parrots, and computers as fully-certified drivel generators; are there any more? Yes, Bulhak's program was able to generate the rambling, disjointed verbiage of a religious paranoid psychotic, what is known in psychiatry as a formal thought disorder. This expression is widely misunderstood: it does not mean there are also informal thought disorders, but it means 'a disorder of the thought form.' It relates to the internal coherence of the thought sequence, as determined by listening to the subject's talk. In ordinary speech, each item of information should relate in a predictable and grammatically correct manner to what went before and what follows. The listener should not have to struggle to work out what the speaker is saying because that leads to misunderstanding. Assuming the speaker knows the rules of the language, and has a clear apprehension of what he wants to say, there should be no room for misunderstanding. Ordinarily, if a speaker doesn't know the full set of grammatical rules for a language, his use of a restricted set will usually be understood by any native speaker who will be able to determine which rule was used incorrectly, just as parents can work out what their small children are trying to say: "I are thinked about it, I are wanting a icec ream."

The thought disorder of psychosis is not due to the speaker not knowing the rules of grammar, as most of them will have been fluent speakers beforehand. It relates to the breakdown of the rules governing the relationships of the concepts which the speaker is trying to express through language. Some thought disorders are due to the speaker being so over-aroused that his mind skitters across a dozen topics before he has had time to finish the first one, meaning the topics are concertinaed together. Some are because he is trying to describe the altered perceptions he is experiencing; some are due to a need to express every thought which pops up, thereby losing the original point under layers of verbiage. Some cases invent new words to describe the inexplicable (neologisms); some assign new meanings to familiar words as ordinary language fails their needs; some are fascinated by the play of puns; others fade into befuddled silence as they drift into the shadows of their minds, and so on. Years ago, psychiatrists tried to classify thought disorders in the hope that they would have some diagnostic significance, but this was shown to be false. They talked of loose associations, clang associations, tangential thinking, invalid puns, and so on; but there are only four types of thought disorder: mild, moderate, severe, and word salad.

A mild thought disorder consists of some difficulty following the speaker, having to remind him to keep to the point of the question or topic. It is more irritating than confusing. Moderate thought disorder is when he changes topic in mid-sentence, introducing new words or following random thoughts and quickly losing the point. A severe thought disorder is very difficult to follow, and word salad, which is rarely seen these days, was where the thought sequence barely survived two or three words before it was lost in a flood of garbled verbiage. One particular thought disorder is often missed, especially by junior psychiatrists. This is difficult to classify but consists of a rambling, woolly, and over-inclusive style of talk where the speaker seems unable to filter his thoughts and simply drifts after any and every notion as it intrudes. It often has a strong, esoteric religious, psychological, socio-political, mathematical, or philosophical content, but the terms are used in a private or solipsistic sense. These people often read extensively in topics that catch their eye because they seem to offer some sort of explanation or rationalization of their own, crumbling experiences; but they rarely, if ever, have the background education to make sense of what they are reading—or to know that they can't actually read it (it is discommoding for a psychiatrist to meet a thought-disordered philosophy student interested in eastern religions and computer models of multidimensional mathematics).

In particular, people with thought disorders regularly filch terms from specialist areas, peppering their talk with abstruse references, formulae, or concepts that are only tangentially related, if at all. They peregrinate from one arcane subject to the next, eliding the differences and compounding the similarities, gradually assembling a vast superstructure of over-inflated folderol which comes to consume their every waking moment. Very often, they are keen to talk about it and will buttonhole people who show an interest (or are not overtly rejecting), especially kindly people who visit the security wards of mental hospitals on wet Saturday afternoons to distribute oranges and tracts (but not cigarettes or condoms), such as elderly ministers of conventional religions (who know nothing of mathematics, eastern religions, or post-Thomist philosophy, but are too polite to say so), middle-aged ladies from the Theosophical Society (who have very clear ideas about eastern philosophy, higher-order mathematics and the origins and destiny of the universe, and will talk to anybody about it), and earnest students from the Social Work and Psychology Students Caring Collective (who have no clear ideas about anything but are blotting paper to their impassioned post-modernist teachers so they can sometimes be persuaded to smuggle razors or marihuana into the ward, with predictable results).

If one listens to only a minute or two of this type of thought disorder, it doesn't seem especially crazy, not like the perfervid rantings of the man who believes the CIA is shining X-rays from a geostationary satellite to turn him into a homosexual. However, the longer one listens, the more the sense fades. It is often easy to distract these people simply by mentioning a vaguely related topic, and they will wander after it, like a butterfly drifting across a summer's meadow from one flower to another. Quite often, they feel very strongly about what they are trying to say and their distress at being unable to express themselves properly, or be understood, can be palpable. At other times, they simply seem unaware that their talk is essentially meaningless and will ramble on happily, even talking to themselves if their audience moves away. However, on entering one of the old mental hospitals, it was immediately obvious that these people recognized thought disorder in each other and wouldn't listen. A thought-disordered patient with chronic schizophrenia would not waste his time talking to all those crazy people (the other patients) but would wait for the new young doctor or, better still, the medical or nursing students who were guaranteed to sit, politely scribbling notes while struggling to follow what was said.

Thought disorder is not only apparent in speech but also in writing, and it often has a very distinctive quality, as any government minister knows. The person starts writing, then keeps adding bits to it, writing around the edges of the page or over the back, drawing peculiar diagrams, or inserting equations which are either totally irrelevant or have no conceivable mathematical relationship to the subject. $E=mc^2$ is, of course, the all-time favorite, closely followed by anything to do with quantum theory and Heisenberg's Uncertainty Principle, while words such as topology, matrix, non-linear, exponential, chaos, infinity, discontinuity and cosmos simply cry out to be misused. Sadly, an engineering student who develops schizophrenia easily outpaces his doctors who have only freshman mathematics to draw on.

Thought disordered drawings and diagrams are also highly characteristic, usually attempts to explicate the whole of the mysteries of the universe on a single page, especially if writing paper is rationed. Almost always, they have an inner symmetry which betrays how much effort has gone into them. Commonly, they will start with atoms (or subatomic particles for sophisticates), proceeding along a serpentine course through cells, bodies, communities, states, and the Universal Brotherhood to union with the Cosmic Mover, with regular irruptions from capitalism, gnosticism, the international Zionist, Catholic, CIA, Maoist, jihadist, uranium or Freemasonry conspiracies, not to overlook solar power, AIDS, home-birthing, macrobiotic diets, colonic irrigation, and the full panoply of fringe medicine cults. The diagrams are the readily recognizable products of a mind which is slipping its tethers with reality, ranging freely over any and every subject that could conceivably bear on the experience of going mad—and that's every subject known to man. The diagnostic point of the diagrams is that, unlike, say, the drawings of the Large Hadron Collider, they do not rest on an agreed body of knowledge which has been tested at every conceivable point of the way, from Archimedes' description of the lever right through to the Higgs boson. Thought disordered drawings and diagrams have no intellectual heritage, as it were, but simply represent the ineffable private yearnings of a disintegrating mind.

In these days of DSM-IV and its long-awaited successor, psychiatric interest in thought disorder has faded. It has become just another symptom caused by the schizophrenic gene, albeit a rather irritating one, and psychiatrists no longer bother to try to understand what the patient is trying to say. Thought disorder has no particular significance in its own right, especially as it has no diagnostic value. I recall one of my teachers saying to me: "I don't know why you try to understand him. I pay no more attention to the utterances of schizophrenics than I do to the vomitus of a child with gastroenteritis. Who knows," he added with a superior smile, "you might catch it yourself." We laughed, as we all knew it wasn't contagious. Was it?

While on his favorite topics, it is only with great difficulty that the thought-disordered psychotic can stop his rambling. There has been a breakdown in normal language production but it does not extend to every word he says. For students and trainees, it is always a surprise when the floridly disordered patient interrupts his sermonizing to ask: "Do you think I could have a cigarette, please? They took mine off me, oh, thank you, you're so kind. And a light? Now, talking of the universal spirit and the Omega Point..."

It is easy to diagnose a thought disorder when we already know the patient is psychotic. It becomes more difficult when there are no other signs of abnormality. The author of this quote, a polite and well-presented young man, was wary of being detained as had happened to a friend of his. He was very guarded in his first two interviews, then sent this letter:

What can I say of my parents than what my father said to me, 'that they be searching for light in the dark with candles'– creating shadows that deceivingly narrow their passage of thought, and are yet to turn toward the exit from which they entered to see the light of truth and dispel the shadows and nonsense that surrounds them. I can only wish my parents well, and my niece fortitude whom has yet life's seasons before her to endure, but I believe in her eventual death and until then confident that she has had a thorough grounding in grammar that is the study of words, and also the organization of musical composition that is a study of comparatives, for which of a sense those will enable her procedure for logical thought and the progressive development of her mind rather than a succession of mindful delusions, if useful for nothing else. Now, of all the things you and I had spoken of at our first meeting, what I shall recall is our statement that restructuring a pattern of thought is a process that causes anxiety and when anxiety already exists, may be hazardous, particularly when a person has not been trained nor is professionally supervised, and of the vexatious tone that was employed, I envisage for the sake of writing this paragraph and to make sense for the show of thumb at the departure of our meeting that you had spoken of firsthand experience, the rule of thumb so to speak, and I could only reply of a thumb to confirm that me has experienced such a thing—traffic is not gainful, and that I have seen it stated before in George Orwell's essay "The Decay of Literature", which had been, 'to speak using words rather than tautological phrases requires furious thought.' Moreover, as part of my activities, I forward a comparatively small ramble, nevertheless a ramble it is, for the case of duality and the model of psychiatry respectively, for which the former I have not seen expanded beyond the grammatical case of the personal pronouns I the nominative and Me the accusative, who playing on the see-saw of dilemma, search for some sort of equilibrium balance of self existence.... (etc. for several pages).

If you focus on one sentence, it seems to make some sort of allegorical sense. If you focus on two sentences, the sense seems to waver like a mirage, but if you try to extract the meaning of three consecutive sentences, nothing emerges. If you cut and paste the sentences, nothing changes. This is the test of thought disorder, because ordered thoughts convey meaning: try telling a joke with the sentence order inverted. Speech is about creating a new mental state in the mind of the listener, one which stands in a precise relationship to the speaker's own mental state. It might be a facsimile; it might be the exact opposite; but the role of language is to transfer information and, if that fails, then language has failed. For an intelligent person who is able to speak according to the rules of grammar, being unable to convey his meaning to another person is an endless torture.

Thought disorder can be the earliest sign of an impending psychosis, or it can exist alone. For modern psychiatrists, this is self-contradictory: thought disorder is a symptom of psychosis, and psychosis is a genetically-determined illness with a specific cluster of symptoms. A psychotic person has a thought disorder, and a thought-disordered person has a psychosis so, if he has a thought disorder, he must have all the other symptoms of psychosis, too; but if he hasn't, then he isn't psychotic and he therefore isn't thought-disordered. End of discussion.

Well, it's not as easy as that. Firstly, however we define thought disorder, there will always be people who show that symptom alone, with no other firm signs of mental illness. Second, there is no point of demarcation between thought order and thought disorder. It is not possible to nominate a point and say: To the left is ordered speech, and to the right, we have thought disorder. It isn't like that. There is but a single axis of coherence, ranging from the most precisely defined engineering instructions, all the way to frank word salad. Somewhere in the middle, we have poets, dreamers, and cranks, and it may be very difficult to distinguish them. In particular, religious and mystical writers confound any attempts to define a line of clarity. Granted, as for philosophers, their subject matter may be at the limits of human comprehension (although that keeps moving out, too) but, all too often, they seem to revel in their obscurity. For their acolytes, this is part of their attraction, as E.L. Doctorow noted: "Once you assume poetically divine authorship, only your understanding is imperfect" [2]. However, divine or not, they still pass the test for drivel. Randomly switching the sentences or paragraphs in their tracts, even swapping the covers on their books, does not affect their meaning nor does it deter their devotees.

The mechanism of thought disorder is rarely discussed. If you ask a conventional, biologically-oriented psychiatrist, she will give that superior little smile and reply: "It's caused by a genetically-determined chemical imbalance of the brain." You won't get further with that line of questioning, because that is their answer to all questions about mental disorder, like the Sunday School teacher who answers every question with: "Well, that's how God made it." Let's look at this a little more closely. The facts are as follows. Firstly, there is no conceptual point on which thought disorder can reliably be distinguished from normal thinking. If we line all the people in the world according to the lucidity and transparency of their reasoning processes, there is not a large group to the left who think clearly and a small group to the right whose thinking is disordered. At the same time, there is no single defect of reasoning that constitutes 'disordered thinking.'

Second, not all people think clearly on all subjects all the time. The quality of rational thinking is heavily influenced by emotional factors, by tiredness and illness, by drunkenness, by determination, and by other factors. Thinking clearly is not easy and is not natural. It requires long training and is hard work. It is true that we have the genetically-determined cerebral machinery to think clearly, but whether we exercise it all the time is another question. Third, the capacity to reason can be reduced to a set of rules, diligently applied. There is every reason to believe that human reasoning is not of a different nature from that of machine reasoning, and no reason to believe otherwise, i.e. that it follows rules. Regardless of the nature of the machine involved, mechanized reasoning is not an instantaneous event, i.e. it is the outcome of a series of standardized steps or processes which can be interrupted at any point with predictable results. The evidence against the idea that thought disorder represents a single error of human reasoning is overwhelming. There are many different types of faulty reasoning, and people may be perfectly lucid at one moment ("Do you mind if I have a cigarette?") but completely befuddled a moment later. Finally, thought disorder can be distinguished from the physical brain disorders which produce disturbances of speech output, meaning the expressive dysphasias.

Coherent reasoning involves so many brain areas, with so many different neurotransmitters operating in strict sequence, partly innate and partly acquired, that there is no chance of it being the outcome of a single genetic determinant. That would be akin to saying that a computer is built from a single component. Given these facts, we can exclude the possibility that thought disorder is a "genetically-determined chemical imbalance of the brain." The brain doesn't work like that. So we need an elegant scientific theory that can account for a diffuse disturbance of a process that has a natural basis but is honed by training and experience, which is influenced by many different factors and need not be present all the time. In this context, 'elegant' means full explanation coupled with the exclusion of the inessential. Since reasoning is a rule-governed process, I suggest a perfectly elegant theory would be that the thought-disordered subject is no longer following the rules. We could say the rules no longer work for him. This may be because he wants to justify the unjustifiable, he has something he wishes to hide, or the experiences (of the world and of himself) and concepts he wishes to express are beyond the facility of language as he knows it.

Thus, we arrive at a perfectly rational, parsimonious explanation for thought disorder which does not involve non-natural processes, which takes account of current neurophysiological understanding, and which does not invoke any elements that cannot, in principle, be tested. It also gives an account of the common observation that, in non-psychotic people, thought disorder is seen in tiredness, high emotion, intoxications, and other physical disturbances of the brain such as fever, concussion, and metabolic impairments including diabetes or renal disease. It is also seen in mild, diffuse brain damage, either static or slowly progressive. It says that people may be able to talk coherently about one subject (like organizing an archeological trip to China in the 1930s) but rapidly become disorganized about another, such as humanity's ultimate destiny

(Teilhard de Chardin). It means that subjects dear to one's heart are more likely to result in defective thinking (due to high emotional arousal and the need to defend the indefensible) than catching the bus to the shops. It also means that high intellect is no guarantee against thought disorder; it just results in more complex word knots: "Intelligence serves insanity quite as well as it serves sanity, which is to say, very well indeed" ('Cordwainer Smith,' I think).

There are many examples of mystical claptrap being passed off as "the real thing", and nothing I can say will slow down their sales. Three notable examples of thought-disordered religiosity include the Greek-Armenian mystic and dancer Georg Gurgjieff, the French Jesuit and paleontologist Pierre Teilhard de Chardin, and the Indian guru and Rolls Royce collector Bhagwan Shree Rajneesh. Based on their endless pseudo-mystical preoccupations and disorganized lives, one could make a good claim that these people were, in fact, covertly or marginally psychotic but, if so, it was a psychosis that did them no great harm. In between their wanderings, they were each prolific writers, except that 99% of what they wrote is high-sounding but empty verbiage. For example, debating the validity of the Bhagwan's turgid ramblings with his often aggressively peace-loving tribe was a waste of time. He simply sat with his adoring disciples at his feet and started talking into a microphone. Hours later, another book fell off the production line to be snapped up by the orange-decked crowds who bore them off to pore over them, reverentially searching for clues from heaven. Teilhard's last book, *The Phenomenon of Man*, was frankly loopy, as the Nobel Prize-winning geneticist Peter Medawar described in his devastating critique [2], but his star-struck followers were utterly unperturbed. The Church was decidedly less impressed, and placed a lot of his output on the proscribed list. They saw the truth in Medawar's acerbic summary: "(The) author can be excused of dishonesty only on the grounds that, before deceiving others, he has taken great pains to deceive himself." I think that is a bit harsh. Teilhard appears to have had only a tenuous grip on reality at best, as this diagram from his book shows. I would say he genuinely lacked the insight to pause in his pursuit of enlightenment to ask: 'Hang on, does this stuff really make sense?'

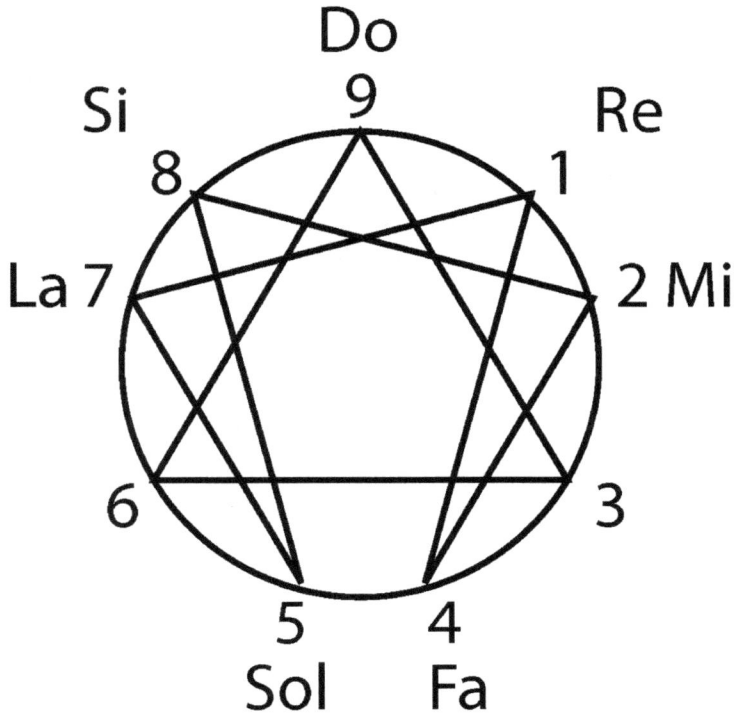

Fig. 1: Gurdjieff's enneagram hieroglyph of a universal language.

These diagrams are, of course, completely cuckoo, but they sold. People want to be misled, that much will never change: *Mundus vult decipi:* The world wants to be deceived. People much prefer flowery certainty to arid probability, and there will always be a few clever people around who are sufficiently venal, stupid, or narcissistic to give it to them in the form of divine texts. Some of the authors, however, wander freely back and forth across the blurred borderland of psychosis, and nobody, least of all they themselves, can ever tell where they are from one day to the next. There is no cut-off point between the ordinary eccentric, the crank, the marginal psychotic, and the frankly psychotic.

One vital test which is often overlooked is the willingness of the individual to consider that he may be wrong. Ordinary people have no problem with the idea they may be wrong; the frankly deluded deny it absolutely; and there are varying degrees in between. A helpful rule of thumb is this: the degree of madness is directly proportional to the degree of certainty the author shows.

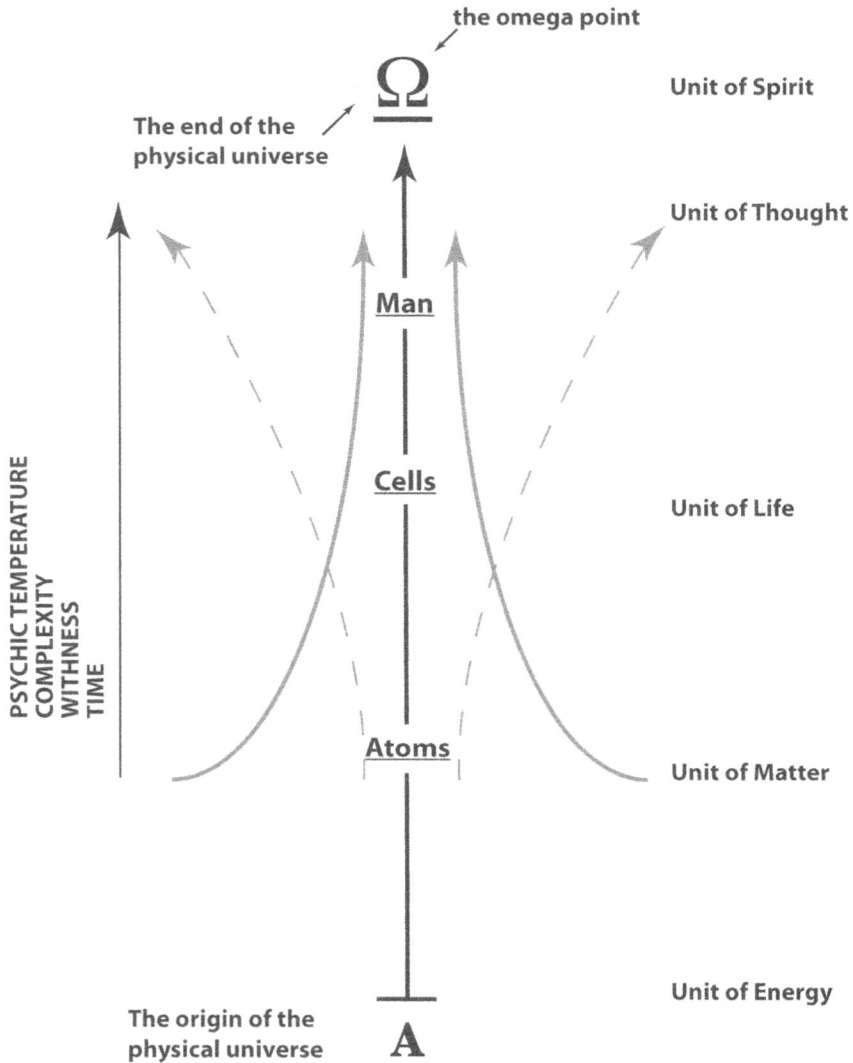

The Cosmos

A Process of Convergence and Divergence

Fig. 2 (above): Pierre Teilhard de Chardin's outline of the "application of his Law of Complexity/Consciousness, which shows how increasing complexity converges and diverges from the consciousness present in rocks (the geosphere) through humans (the biosphere) and beyond (the noosphere), with increasing complexification of human consciousness until it reaches its maximum at the Omega Point, whereupon it will rupture through the restrictions of time and space to assert itself on a higher, eternal plane of existence from which there is no return."

It is of more than passing interest that, in my experience, biological psychiatrists have never considered that their theories may be wrong, and they strongly resent the question. This reaches into another topic, the notion of a socially-sanctioned, shared belief for which there is no factual evidence. A belief in life after death is not a delusion if enough people hold it, and they may resent being questioned about it. Questioning them may cause them to stumble and stutter and contradict themselves, but they will not become thought-disordered. An interesting observation is that the more disturbed the individual's thinking processes, the more likely he is to develop an uncontrollable loquacity. It is almost as if they fear silence as the caustic that can strip the mystery from their productions, leaving their utterances exposed as nonsensical. When did an anchorite last top the best-seller lists?

4 | *This Phenomenal World*

"They read well. The elegance of their construction—in the logician's meaning of elegance as the exclusion of the inessential—can be appreciated."

E.L. Doctorow, on Arthur Miller's plays.

4.1: Introduction

Anybody who has persevered with these books will be aware that I approach the question of mental disorder from a particular point of view. Specifically, this is the idea that we can arrive at a full understanding of a complex matter by rational enquiry. These days, it is generally known as the Anglo-American tradition of analytic philosophy. Taken to its limit, it says that nothing in the universe lies beyond the reach of the disciplined human intellect. Of course, this is not the only viewpoint available; there have always been others, such as religious approaches. These start with the view that the truth of the nature of the universe is not amenable to sober dissection but can only be understood by divine inspiration or revelation. Some argue that the truth lies outside the individual and can only be approached through a medium, such as a priest or holy text, others say truth is imminent but requires special training and discipline before it becomes accessible to the individual.

This does not imply, however, that the choice is wholly between dry secular analysis and febrile religiosity; western philosophy has another, very broad tradition, often termed continental philosophy to distinguish it from the narrower, Anglophone variety. Analytic philosophy self-consciously restricts itself to a basis in certain knowledge so it includes as its preliminaries questions such as "What is knowledge?" "How do we acquire it?" and "What constitutes certainty?" It avoids grand cosmic schemes in favor of the careful, step-by-step separation of reliable knowledge from all the rest: fantasy, prejudice, infatuation, and the like. For an analytic philosopher, being wrong is worse than being boring. This leads to the fractionation of knowledge, so that science, for example, has absolutely no overlap with literature and religion must be kept separate from economics. Methods that produce reliability in one field may not apply at all in the next. Reductionism may produce reliable results in physics but will be quite useless in music. This leads to the intense focus in western thinking on the question of assigning reliability or validity to ideas and beliefs, independently of anybody else's wishes. Propositional logic, for example, would not have reached its present form in a rigid theocracy or under a centralized totalitarian system such as Stalinism. Without logic, there would have been no computer revolution, therefore no modern communications; no jet airliners to fly politicians and religious leaders to international conferences, and so on. We gave you nuclear power stations and genetic engineering, complain the rationalists, who could want more? Those ungrateful continentals, that's who.

At the other end of the secular table in the philosophy restaurant, as far as possible from the tightly-buttoned ascetic rationalists without actually lunching with the mystics, sits a noisy group of sensuous figures, freely indulging in all the menu has to offer. If analytic philosophers eschew art and politics as beyond their narrow scope, phenomenologists have no such qualms. The gulf between the two philosophical traditions is huge and essentially unbridgeable. It is not a question of esthetics, say whether a classical violinist should also like Indian pop music, but a matter of the utter incompatibility of two approaches to the same question. Just as one cannot be both an atheist and a devout Christian, one cannot say that the analytic approach will yield the truth of what we need to know about the universe in its entirety, and so too will phenomenology, that even though your starting point is a matter of where you trained, there is only one goal. Not only do they approach the concept of truth from different directions but each tradition says that the other cannot get to the goal. Each says of the other that its methodology is inadequate because its entire conceptual stance is mistaken. The phenomenologists will say that rationality will give only half the truth, while rationalists will say the continentalists wouldn't know truth if it bit them. So it is for this reason that we do not find philosophers who are both committed analytic rationalists and fully-trained phenomenologists—that, plus the fact that there isn't enough time in a single life.

For better or for worse, my training has been in the area of analytic philosophy. My exposure to phenomenological philosophy was minimal; so what can I tell you about phenomenology and psychiatry that some of its most renowned exponents can't? Not a lot but, as a good rationalist, I will claim that phenomenology cannot resolve the mind-body problem because it starts from the wrong position. Thus, there will never be any such thing as a phenomenological psychiatrist. However, I will also argue that there is indeed a place for a phenomenological approach in the analytic model of mental disorder called the biocognitive model. This is because there is something about mental disorder that analytic philosophy can explain, but probably cannot rectify. However, a "phenomenological approach" does not mean embracing the entire doctrine.

4.2: The History Of Phenomenology (In Two Pages)

Until about two hundred years ago, nobody doubted that the western intellectual tradition was a unity. Under the watchful eye of the church, philosophers studied the classic scholars in the original Latin and were familiar with the complex arguments they had raised on questions such as the fundamental nature of the world, the nature of good and evil, etc. In addition, they kept up to date with the activities of their other branch, natural philosophy or, as we would now say, science. However, this secure world changed, probably irrevocably, with the monumental work of a German author, Georg Hegel (1770-1831). Hegel was determined to write a complete theory of philosophy, drawing all branches of knowledge into a single, all-encompassing system. Without doubt, this was a bold project, and it meant that a lot of his writing was not published in his lifetime. However, and more to my point, he was a verbose and obscure writer, establishing a tradition in which philosophy becomes an exercise, not so much in learning and applying certain well-defined principals to complex questions, as in trying to decipher what on earth the writer meant. For foreigners, the effort is the more intense because Hegel believed that German was the ideal language for expressing the complex issues that together comprised philosophy, a belief which isn't always shared by people who don't speak German. That meant that whatever subtle points he wished to make were not guaranteed to survive translation. There is thus no definitive translation of his work, and even his compatriots were somewhat underwhelmed. Arthur Schopenhauer (1788-1860) described his efforts as:

> "... a colossal piece of mystification which will yet provide posterity with an inexhaustible theme for laughter at our times, that it is a pseudo-philosophy paralyzing all mental powers, stifling all real thinking, and, by the most outrageous misuse of language, putting in its place the hollowest, most senseless, thoughtless, and, as is confirmed by its success, most stupefying verbiage" (On the Basis of Morality).

It should be mentioned that Schopenhauer, who was not noted for a genteel disposition toward his colleagues, once remarked: "I should like to see the man who could boast of a more miserable set of contemporaries than I."

Undoubtedly, Hegel shifted European philosophy in the direction of idealism but he also set a precedent for philosophers writing in a style that even their most devout readers will admit is heavy going. After him, philosophy was dense, tortuous, and often impressionistic, which, all too often, tends to authorize "anything goes." One of his legacies was to justify introspection as a valid source of knowledge for the philosophical endeavor, which immediately opens the door to individual preference (perhaps I should say 'doesn't firmly close the door against...'). So British (including Scottish) rationalism had to make room for a new model where the philosopher focused on matters of cosmic significance by starting—

and ending—with his own self-perceptions as the primary datum. Hegel's goal was to provide a full account of all matters of mind, nature, and human activity, using just the phenomena of his mind as his raw material, but it was too big for one life.

This project was continued and formalized by Edmund Husserl (1859-1938) whose concern was that, by debasing the idea of a human spirit, rationalism was overlooking the essential humanity of man. He wished to turn philosophy into a rigorous science, duplicating the successes of rationalist science but expanding on them by retaining the spiritual side of human life and developing it to the point where it could explain all aspects of human culture. Although he did not use the term, this is also the basis of the arguments against a reductionist psychology: "It was his desire to develop a proper method for grasping the essential nature of the spirit, to overcome naturalistic objectivism, that led Husserl to formulate his transcendental phenomenology" [1, p. 495]. This introduces a problem: how can we use the experience of being a spirit to explain the nature of the spirit? Can my unaided eye tell me anything worthwhile about my eye?

Husserl's project also suffered because of his unusual use of language. Commentators often disagree completely as to the intent of one passage or another. His work was expanded and later turned in a new direction by one of his students, Martin Heidegger (1889-1976) who was himself an adept in the black art of devising new terms. Heidegger wanted to discover the notion of a valid life by means of understanding what it means to be a thinking being through an exposition of the nature of being, or Being. Unfortunately, his association with the Nazi Party has since clouded his reputation. His work was discovered by a French student, Jean-Pierre Sartre, who had travelled to Berlin to study Husserl's method. Sartre was not just a philosopher but also used literature to expound the more complex of his philosophical ideas. He dominated the Paris scene until his death in 1980 and, some would say, ever since. With various colleagues and/or enemies, he and his students licensed the methods of phenomenology, and thence existentialism, as the proper approach to the totality of human experience: morality, art, politics, science, sexuality and, of course, psychology.

In psychoanalysis, the analyst Jacques Lacan offered novel interpretations of classic Freudian theory using insights derived from phenomenology, existentialism, and mathematics. Maurice Merleau-Ponty focused his efforts on notions of truth and political philosophy but died young, leaving a legacy of relativism based in the primacy of perception. Michel Foucault influenced fields as diverse as criminology, education, and psychiatry by his impassioned analyses of the power structures involved in these manifestations of the social state. Jacques Derrida objected to many of the fundamental precepts of phenomenology and its progeny, developing his own approach which aimed to expose the hidden power structures as concealed in the speech of everyday life. Gilles Deleuze analyzed Marxism and the forces of production in capitalist societies. A significant part of his work was written in conjunction with the psychoanalyst Felix Guattari, a student of Lacan and a most accomplished neologist in his own right.

In the post-war period, the field of phenomenology broadened to include practically anything of interest to a person of moderate intellectual pretension. The history of phenomenology and existentialism, of course, are intimately inter-related, and these two fields blur with the entire spectrum of what is generally known as post-modernism. Post-modernism is not a theory in its own right, but an approach or way of looking at human activities, especially critically. Again, it cannot really be separated from the literary movement of post-structuralism and lends itself to relativism. This, the central notion of critical theory, is the idea that there is no objective truth, only claims that are themselves relative to the culture from which they emanate. From this stance derives the main critiques of colonialism and racism, the feminist assault on modern society, anti-psychiatry, anti-capitalism, animal rights, and the radical ecology movement, among many others. It has been singularly influential in the literature and liberal arts departments of American universities and other intellectual centers.

4.3: The Theory Of Phenomenology (In Another Two Pages)

Briefly, what are the essential features of phenomenology? What is it, and how does it differ from analytic philosophy? The definitions are actually quite revealing. Kockelmans said:

"The question of what phenomenology is may suggest that phenomenology is one among the many contemporary philosophical concepts that have a clearly delineated body of doctrines and whose essential characteristics can be expressed by a set of well-chosen statements. This notion is not correct... there is no system or school called 'phenomenology'... (It) is neither a school nor a trend... today, it means different things to different people" [2, p. 578].

He saw a number of features as of major importance in outlining the general field of phenomenology:

> 1. It implies a radical difference between the "natural" and the "philosophical" attitudes, where natural means pertaining to the natural world, i.e. science and everything narrowly rational. Philosophy, then, is not the content of a field of thought but an approach or style to that content, hence the rapid proliferation of schools;
>
> 2. Nonetheless, the two areas are related, with phenomenological philosophy having a fundamental role but the relationship has to be determined in each specific case;
>
> 3. Phenomenologists strip their preconceptions so they can experience the world of meaning with no prejudice;
>
> 4. All phenomenologists accept that consciousness has the property of intentionality, meaning directedness or 'aboutness,' although that is about the limit of their agreement;

5. "All phenomenologists agree... that the basic concern of philosophy is to answer the question concerning the 'meaning and Being' of beings... (They are) interested not in the ultimate cause of all finite beings, but in how the being of beings and the Being of the world are to be constituted;"

6. Phenomenologists adhere to one or other form of intuitionism, meaning accepting their experiences in "primordial form" as representing whatever they purport to be.

Accordingly, he concluded: "... it is not possible to give a simple definition of what phenomenology is... There are many phenomenologists and many phenomenologies."

Further details are available from the Center for Advanced Research in Phenomenology [3], which is predominately North American in its membership but has extensive international links. It sponsors the Encyclopedia of Phenomenology, which is available at €509.00 (about US$700.00) for 770 pages. The organizers of CARP provide newcomers with this explanation of their stance:

"Seven Widely Accepted Features of the Phenomenological Approach:

Phenomenologists conduct research in ways that share most of the following positive and negative features.

1. Phenomenologists tend to oppose the acceptance of unobservable matters and grand systems erected in speculative thinking;

2. Phenomenologists tend to oppose naturalism (also called objectivism and positivism), which is the worldview growing from modern natural science and technology that has been spreading from Northern Europe since the Renaissance;

3. Positively speaking, phenomenologists tend to justify cognition (and some also evaluation and action) with reference to what Edmund Husserl called Evidenz, which is awareness of a matter itself as disclosed in the most clear, distinct, and adequate way for something of its kind;

4. Phenomenologists tend to believe that not only objects in the natural and cultural worlds, but also ideal objects—such as numbers, and even conscious life itself—can be made evident and thus known;

5. Phenomenologists tend to hold that inquiry ought to focus upon what might be called 'encountering' as it is directed at objects and, correlatively, upon 'objects as they are encountered' (this terminology is not widely shared, but the emphasis on a dual problematics and the reflective approach it requires is);

6. Phenomenologists tend to recognize the role of description in universal, a priori, or 'eidetic' terms as prior to explanation by means of causes, purposes, or grounds; and

7. Phenomenologists tend to debate whether or not what Husserl calls the transcendental phenomenological epochê and reduction is (sic) useful or even possible."

This group sees no point in defining phenomenology any more precisely than "this is what we tend to do or tend to oppose." Theirs is an approach which clearly has porous borders and can find room for highly diverse fields of interest, from music and religion to science and medicine and back again via psychiatry, history and ethnology. However, for a dull-witted analytic rationalist, there is something not quite... solid about this. Shall we define football as something where people tend to kick a ball? Ornithology as a pursuit which tends to study birds? Cooking as something that tends to result in meals? Defined this way, a person could deny each of these tendencies and still call himself a phenomenologist.

Moreover, their subject matter is not tightly restricted. The Society for Phenomenological and Existential Philosophy (SPEP) [4], also based in the US, defines its interests as:

> "... phenomenology and existentialism, but also in all those areas commonly associated with 'continental philosophy', such as animal studies, critical theory, cultural studies, deconstruction, environmental philosophy, feminism, German idealism, hermeneutics, philosophy of the Americas, post-colonialism, post-structuralism, psychoanalysis, queer theory, and race theory... discussion on all philosophical topics, from art and nature to politics and science, and in the classic philosophical disciplines of metaphysics, epistemology, ethics, and aesthetics. SPEP is actively committed to philosophical pluralism..." [6] (I doubt animal studies means biology, and presume they meant 'philosophy in the Americas').

Clearly, this is a broad mandate to tend to be interested in, especially the last line. Pluralism is defined as "the doctrine that reality consists of several basic substances or elements..." but there is no doubt they meant "different viewpoints." This would mean that a person could believe that any subject or course with the word 'studies' in its title is a load of garbage, and be resistant to all of CARP's 'tendencies', yet still demand to be recognized as a phenomenologist, which brings me to the end of my two pages.

4.4: Taking Phenomenology Seriously

Given this rather amazingly fluid definition, why, therefore, should anybody take it seriously? This is part of the larger question: Why should we take anything seriously? I can only sketch an answer to this question.

I take food and shelter seriously, for me and for my family, so somebody has to get up in the icy winters to plant the wheat for our breakfast toast; I take health seriously, for myself and for my family, which means that somebody (including me) has to take the idea of studying medicine seriously enough to do it for six years while others have to take it seriously enough to teach it; I take the idea of caring for the world seriously, which means we need biologists and other scientists; I take our accumulated knowledge of the universe seriously, which means we need libraries and librarians, computers and IT techs, and hence we need builders and electricians and people to mine the ore and refine it into steel beams for the roof and so on... Just staying alive and safe and healthy and not too hungry etc. means we have to take a lot of things very seriously. Sometimes, it seems, taking all those mundane, workaday things seriously doesn't leave much time for unserious things.

Clearly, these serious matters are of a specific nature, and would qualify for what phenomenologists term "... naturalism (also called objectivism and positivism), which is the worldview growing from modern natural science and technology..." Remember that they oppose this view, even though many people would argue that Western science and technology grew from their positivist, objectivist worldview, not vice versa. According to their manifesto, phenomenologists take pretty well everything seriously, too: art and medicine, and feminism and racism, and politics (especially politics) and literature, and psychology; you name it, they claim to take it seriously enough to talk about it at great length (it must never be forgotten that they also take themselves terribly seriously). Now I detect a tension here: on the one hand, they like to talk about certain matters (call them rational or objective or positivist) and they have no hesitation using them (such as websites to spread the word and luxury hotels for their conferences) but at the same time, they oppose them, or at least the worldview that led to them. Gilles Deleuze, for example, smoked to the day he jumped from his bedroom window, not long after his doctors operated to remove a cancerous lung. When he allowed the anesthetist to inject the drugs and put him under for his operation, did he trust "modern natural science and technology", or was he only kidding? So what is it that they oppose? This is where it gets a little murky, to the point that we start to wonder just how seriously we can afford to take these people. I could rephrase that: should we take phenomenologists as seriously as we take the men who remove our garbage? Which of the two groups, phenomenologists or garbage men, makes the more serious and significant contribution to the society phenomenologists love to criticize?

Let's move on: "Phenomenologists tend to oppose the acceptance of unobservable matters and grand systems erected in speculative thinking." This means, I presume, that they oppose religion, which is probably true unless it's an Eastern religion, but Marxism? Psychoanalysis? Surely these qualify as "grand systems erected in speculative thinking"? Apparently not, so I am forced to admit I have trouble taking this bit of their work seriously.

"Positively speaking, phenomenologists tend to justify cognition (and some also evaluation and action) with reference to what Edmund Husserl called Evidenz, which is awareness of a matter itself as disclosed in the most clear, distinct, and adequate way for something of its kind." I do not know what it means to justify cognition, it rather seems to be self-justifying, but I see a problem with the idea that matters are disclosed in a clear, distinct, and adequate way. I take that to mean that any cognition I have is automatically justified just by virtue of its being mine. This veers perilously close to an absolutist solipsism, and from there straight to fascism, but no doubt Heidegger's intellectual heirs and successors have neutered that objection to their satisfaction.

"Phenomenologists tend to believe that not only objects in the natural and cultural worlds, but also ideal objects, such as numbers, and even conscious life itself can be made evident and thus known." Again I detect a tension at this point, because the much-despised western science is based on the idea that objects in the natural world can be made (or simply are) evident, and it is by this evidence that we know them. We certainly don't know them by any other evidence, such as prescience or telekinesis. In addition, I would have thought that cultural objects, numbers, and conscious life itself qualify as "unobservable matters" with occasional lurches into "grand speculative thinking," but that may be just further evidence of how rationalists see only half the picture.

The rest of their tendencies, I'm afraid, are too abstruse for me so we might return to the late Joseph Kockelmans, who specialized in continental philosophy and phenomenology at Pennsylvania State University, a fairly prestigious center: "Phenomenologists," he declared, "strip their preconceptions so they can experience the world of meaning with no prejudice." We should stop to look at this more closely because it is indeed a remarkable achievement. We are all delighted and indeed vastly relieved to hear that they have discovered a means by which humans can remove their prejudices and see the world (including the human bit) for what it is. Their unprecedented success will be of vast benefit to humanity, not least by making psychiatry a pushover, meaning we can get rid of all those toxic drugs pushed upon the naïve and innocent by power-hungry psychiatrists acting as the stooges of venal drug companies. Strangely, in my thirty-five years in psychiatry, I have not seen an advertisement nor heard even a whisper of a place where I can go to be stripped of my prejudices, so it is obviously a well-kept secret of the phenomenology trade. Moreover, I have entered a number of philosophy departments over the years and, if they were places free of preconceptions and prejudices, that too was a well-kept secret. In some cases, such was the emotional temperature at which the phenomenological boilers were set, I should say that somebody had forgotten to tell even the denizens of the department themselves.

Nonetheless, having survived the stripping treatment, our intrepid phenomenologists are ready for "… intuitionism, meaning accepting their experiences in 'primordial form' as representing whatever they purport to be." Here we run into a minor difficulty. If I accept my intuitions as representing whatever they purport to be, I am guilty of harboring preconceptions and prejudices, but a day's intuitions in a department of philosophy are obviously the uncontaminated products of the "transcendental phenomenological epochê" and are thus beyond dispute. It would, I imagine, have heartened Heidegger's pals in the NSDAP to learn that sending people to a philosophy department will give them the techniques to trust their primordial intuitions. That would have saved all that unnecessary angst over *die Endlösung.*

On a more sober note, my understanding of "primordial intuitions" is that they just are unreasoning prejudices and preconceptions. Self-righteousness is a very dangerous thing. Indeed, with little effort, I could probably convince myself that it is the single most dangerous human attribute, although that may be just a relativist view, if not sexist, ageist, racist, and elitist.

Thus, I suggest the reason that "...it is not possible to give a simple definition of... phenomenology... (that)... There are many phenomenologists and many phenomenologies..." is just this: they have absolutely no agreement on their subject matter or how it should be approached. The only certainty in their intellectual lives is that what they do is incredibly important, to the extent that nobody should be allowed to contradict them. Phenomenology, as its own practitioners amply demonstrate, takes us to the further reaches of academic silliness and pretension, and all without one scintilla of doubt or hesitation. It would be funny if it were not dangerous.

4.5: Why I Am Not A Phenomenologist: A Polemic

From the psychiatric point of view, continental philosophy is useless. It will never answer any significant questions about the nature of mind or personality, of mind-body interaction, about the causation of mental disorder or personality disorder, or their treatment. This is because it knows nothing about what the mind is, only what it does, and even this is buried under a landslide of self-involved gabble. It has nothing of interest to say that, for example, Buddhism hadn't discovered two thousand years ago—and said far more concisely and poetically. There are two reasons for this gloomy conclusion. In the first place, phenomenology can never say anything of value to those whose minds hurt because the phenomenal experience of mind gives no clues as to the mechanism of mind. That is, they can only agree that the person suffers, but they don't have a clue how to get him out of his suffering because they have no understanding of the mechanism of mental suffering. Let's look at this a little more closely.

If I were to drive south from my home for about six hours, to an Aboriginal community on the edge of the desert, I would find old people who were born in the bush not long after whites first arrived in the area. Some of them, especially the women, still speak very little English. It might still be possible to find one who had never left her traditional totemic area. As recently as a few years ago, we could have found one who had never seen a television. Let's imagine we drive down there and find a little wizened old lady who was born in the desert, who didn't get any western education, who married according to the tribal laws, and who delivered her children in the bush. Her children may have worked on the cattle stations and probably had a few years of schooling but that wouldn't have affected her. She has seen motor vehicles, of course, and knows of aircraft and sausages and ice cream (also cigarettes and alcohol) but she has never seen a television. One day, somebody in the family gets some money and decides to buy a flat screen TV and a DVD player. He sets it up and, that night, they invite granny to watch a show. So, with a gappy grin, the old girl settles down in the dirt and there, in the warm desert night, under the mighty southern arch of the Milky Way, the screen begins to pulse with color.

How many shows would granny have to watch before she understood fully the nature of an LCD television and what has gone wrong when it stops working? I say she could watch it until the end of time and she would be no wiser. Similarly, in the past thirty-five years, I have spoken at length to many, many people with mental disorders, including many people who have suffered most of their lives. They have lived immersed in mental disorder from morning to night. It is rare indeed to find one who has more than the vaguest notion of what might be happening to produce his distress (and that is not just because of the flood of claims that mental disorder is a 'chemical imbalance of the brain,' which itself precludes understanding via personal acquaintance). In normal mental life, nobody knows how he speaks, how he formulates his words, where the words come from, why they come out in just that order and not with the verbs in reverse order at the end of the sentence. Nobody knows from experience just what an emotion is, where or why it comes, or how to stop it. By the same argument, staring at urine tells us nothing about kidneys. In fact, we don't even know we have brains or kidneys. Nobody knows any of this, because watching or otherwise experiencing the output of a complex machine gives no clues as to the mechanism of that machine. By a complex machine, I mean a data-processing machine or mechanism with self-regulating capacities. In order to understand a complex entity, we have to take it apart, which is the essence of reductionist western science and the antithesis of phenomenology.

Of course, this presumes that the mind-brain complex is in fact a data-processing machine of some sort. This presumption could be entirely wrong but, if it is, then simple introspection will never reveal that mistake nor explicate its true nature. This is why James B. Watson declared the behaviorist revolution in 1913: introspection was manifestly and inevitably a waste of time. If we want certainty, then introspection is completely the wrong technique to find it. If, however, certainty is not essential, then introspection is probably a fun place to start. So is there a place for an impressionistic study of mind in a rationalist science of mind-brain? I believe there is, and will explain it later, but we need to keep reminding ourselves that, however much fun it may be, introspection isn't terribly reliable. Of course, that depends on how you rate reliability. Remember that Deleuze, that nemesis of rationalism, rated his doctors' reliability high enough to let them cut his chest open.

The second reason I am so pessimistic about the value of phenomenology is the way it is practiced. It is a search for truth in the essence of Being, for understanding the difference between Being-in-itself and Being-for-itself. It uses epoché to "bracket" the subject's experiences so that he introspects his phenomena without any intellectual baggage from the past. Thus, he sees only the uncontaminated phenomena in pursuit of the goal of pure consciousness and universal truth. Or something like that. Because I believe there is a grievous fault at the very heart of the phenomenological project which means it cannot sift its (few, small) pearls from the mountain of ordure under which they are buried. Here is the fault: There is a clear and unbroken line joining the (rather limited) insights of this humanist program to some of the most pretentious nonsense ever to be dreamed up at public expense.

A trip to the local university library will show that Hegel is often quoted but rarely read, and the reason is exactly as Schopenhauer stated nearly 200 years ago: reading him is an act of devotion. Like entering a monastery, only the committed will stay the race, but they didn't know what they were committing to before their heads were shaved. It's much the same with the Freudians. Only a person who has been analyzed is deemed qualified to criticize the master, but who these days has four or five hours a week for three or four years (plus travelling time, plus fees) to spend on an analysis? So why read thousands of pages of Hegel's dreary, turgid, and often incomprehensible work when there is nothing in the work itself that allows you to decide whether the bit you think you understand is in fact as Hegel intended it? I adhere to Wittgenstein's injunction: "Whatever can be said at all can be said clearly," and I would add "concisely"; otherwise claiming to understand it is probably self-deception.

In similar vein, Husserl was justly renowned for the obscurity of his work. It is still normal for people to argue over what he meant, and this includes German scholars, not just foreigners. He invented terms to suit himself, changed them and, in addition to his own output of some fifteen books and collections, left over 40,000 pages of notes—in shorthand—for posterity. These are apparently being transcribed and translated, giving (my guess) something in the order of six million words. As I understood it, truth was supposed to be economical. If he buried the Truth of Being-in-Itself somewhere in there, then I don't mind waiting for somebody else to find it. Or was he, in fact, unable to bracket his own prejudices and preconceptions from his phenomena? Unlike Freud, Husserl did not write a therapy for would-be phenomenologists. The notion that introspection can yield durable truths may, in fact, be merely a prejudice that he took into the project with him: essentially, his whole project may be nothing more than a vast, loquacious exercise in self-indulgent self-deception.

The important point is that there is no conceivable means available to a phenomenologist to prove that the method is reliable. As analytic philosophers, we ask that their work be reliable at this level: that it could not be wrong. This is the standard demanded of analytic philosophy. It is the reason why we can say of a philosopher: "Oh yes, but Jones showed the errors in his work. Forget him." Analytic philosophy can be shown to be wrong independently of whether anybody likes it or not. On the other hand, phenomenologists are never wrong, just in or out of fashion. Why are they never wrong? Because all they have to do is say: "This is how I see it," and they are ipso facto right. By its process of eliminating error, analytic philosophy (and its uncouth offspring, science) moves forward; phenomenology simply metastasizes. Analytic philosophy and science

proceed by elimination of errors; phenomenology spreads by authority—
and logorrhea.

Husserl's most influential student, Martin Heidegger, had an altogether
more tempestuous career, due, in part, to his affiliation with the Nazi
party before and during World War II. However, in historical terms, this
was a side-issue because it is as a philosopher that he is now judged. The
same tradition was obvious from the beginning: Heidegger was a
formidable neologist who reveled in his often-impenetrable prose. Alfred
Ayer saw his brand of philosophy as useless, a "poisonous strain in
modern thought." Bertrand Russell commented: "Highly eccentric in its
terminology, his philosophy is extremely obscure. One cannot help
suspecting that language is here running riot. An interesting point in his
speculations is the insistence that nothingness is something positive. As
with much else in Existentialism, this is a psychological observation made
to pass for logic" [5, p. 303]. Other English-speaking writers were much
less kind. Even Richard Rorty, who was sympathetic to Heidegger's efforts,
noted that he had constructed not so much an account of being as a myth
of it. However, Heidegger himself took little account of these criticisms,
possibly because he knew his legacy was safe in the hands of the French
school that, when it comes to obscurantism, yields to none.

The main vector by which the evolving German branch of continental
philosophy reached France, Jean-Paul Sartre, was a paragon of clarity
compared with his teachers. His peculiarity was painting himself into
unnecessary corners which, even to his supporters, were a mystery, if not
an outrage. For example, he refused to accept the notion of a human
nature. This was wholly and needlessly for ideological reasons, as Stumpf
noted: "He believed that if there is no God, there is no given human nature
precisely because there is no God to have a conception of it" [1, p. 512].
Today, this simply sounds quaint, because the deity's role has been
subsumed by the process of evolution, i.e. we would now regard the idea
of a divine creator as a reification of an entirely natural process. Evolution
most definitely does not preclude a human nature. Indeed, it strongly
suggests there is, in fact, a higher primate nature which, as primates, we
humans share. Similarly, Sartre's lifelong preoccupation with human
freedom sits uneasily with his intense fascination with Marxism, which
was surely one of the most brutally, if not compulsively, repressive
doctrines in our long and sorry history. This was especially ironic because
his existentialism was not just an abstract philosophy but was offered as
a way of life. Consequently, Sartre did not distinguish between the many
human activities which attracted his prodigious intellect, thereby
legitimizing the notion that a single philosophical doctrine can apply
equally well to all aspects of life. This is a point of departure for most
analytic philosophers who, long cured of any ambitions to write a
universal philosophy, quietly stand aside to let the continental fools rush
in. From Sartre on, they were, with one or two exceptions, very foolish.

One of the more outré of les philosophes nouvels died in 1981, leaving
an oeuvre which will keep his publiques adorants fully occupied for
beaucoup d'ans. The psychiatrist, Jacques Lacan, was born in 1901,

graduated in medicine in 1926 or so, turned to psychiatry and later trained in psychoanalysis. From very early, he showed a voracious intellectual appetite, an endless capacity for disputation, fashionably dubious morality, an insatiable ego, and zero capacity for self-criticism. Clearly, this is a recipe for pyrotechnics, and Lacan did not disappoint. From about 1953 almost to his death, he held seminars in Paris in which he ranged widely across the further reaches of psychoanalysis and anything else that attracted his attention, especially arcane mathematics. His seminars were recorded and English translations are available from a website in New York [6] which is dedicated to investigations of psychoanalytic theory as well as progressive poetry, philosophy, and art. The site also carries works by a group of liberated intellectuals whose interests know no bounds. For example, one recent offering consists of a lengthy and terminally tedious account of an argument by the Slovene philosopher, Slavoj Zizek, as to whether it is or is not an empirical fact that liberal multiculturalism is hegemonic. This, of course, has absolutely nothing to do with psychoanalysis or anything else about the mind, which demonstrates my second point (see above, pearls and ordure).

To return to Lacan, in the 1970s, I, like many young psychiatrists, was looking for a humane certainty in the declining years of psychoanalysis; so I bought a book by this fabled analyst. I don't recall the title but, after wearily dredging my way through it, I finally conceded that I had wasted my time and money because, from beginning to end, it was not just awful, but it was unleavened nonsense. Nobody could deny that the entire work was just a case of thought disorder. But these were not the ramblings of a psychotic; there was little doubt that Lacan was not mad. The ordinary prattle of the chronic schizophrenic is easy to distinguish but Lacan's efforts were different. Reading it, every sentence seemed portentous; the sentences joined by a golden thread, which demanded to be followed, as though to some point where, at last, the eager student would find The Answer. But, like the end of a rainbow, it never quite happened. The paragraphs rambled on, loosely joined, the pages melded into each other, and the chapters rolled past but still there was no denouement. The pot of gold remained a shimmering mirage in the distance, sometimes almost within reach, others a faint, beckoning dream but, oh dear, what poetry! Intellectually, it was nonsense, but as poetry, it shone. That was my epiphany: the entire volume was the long, interminable ramble of an epic poem, the epic being the endlessly unfolding, fantastical vision of the author's lusciously over-ripe and joyously insatiable self-involvement. Lacan was in love with himself, and his seminars provided him with what the ordinary suburban narcissist can only dream of, a fervently adoring public of intellectuelles manquées who swooned at his every word.

So what was the title of Lacan's first major presentation to a psycho-analytic conference? Unsurprisingly, it was called "The mirror phase", in which he claimed he had discovered something very important about psychological development. This was presented at a conference in Marienbad but, according to his entry in Wikipedia, it did not go well. The conference chairman, Ernest Jones (Freud's official biographer), interrupted Monsieur le Professeur in full flight to tell him he had run out of time and somebody else was impatient to present his own paper. Mortally insulted, as per the hallmark of the grand narcissist, Lacan stalked out of the conference and went off to Berlin to brood at the Olympics, no doubt feeling the Nordic splendor of the Nazi version of the heroic ideal was more attuned to his particular needs. To quote from Wikipedia:

Lacan's first official contribution to psychoanalysis was the mirror stage which he described as "...formative of the function of the I as revealed in psychoanalytic experience." By the early fifties, he no longer considered the mirror stage as only a moment in the life of the infant, but as the permanent structure of subjectivity. In the paradigm of The Imaginary order, the subject is permanently caught and captivated by his own image. Lacan writes, "[T]he mirror stage is a phenomenon to which I assign a twofold value. In the first place, it has historical value as it marks a decisive turning-point in the mental development of the child. In the second place, it typifies an essential libidinal relationship with the body-image."

The subject is "permanently caught and captivated by his own image." How entirely apposite, for that just is the definition of narcissism. That is, Jacques Lacan singlehandedly lifted self-obsession to the level of a model of mind. Mais naturellement.

His "thoughts" were a flood of high-sounding nonsense in a jumbled welter of literary allusions, fantasies, analogies, psychological vignettes, misquoted or bastardized mathematical and physical formulae, poetry, religion, art, politics, sexuality, and so on—the whole fantastic, undisciplined avalanche held together by the phantom promise that the speaker was on to Something Really Big. Of course he was. He was stalking his own, Olympian ego, and that voluptuous promise leaked through his talk like the smell of fresh bread fills the streets around a bakery and draws people in whether they know it or not, just because it is so utterly, deliciously, and wickedly promising. Unlike the baker, however, Lacan had no loaves for sale, only a promise which, year after year for thirty years, drew in the faithful until, finally, he passed over to the great hall of mirrors in the sky (I am mixing my metaphors here), leaving his dwindling band of ageing worshippers to gather at seedy conferences and even seedier websites to try to regenerate the vanished magic by rubbing the lamp after the genie has been called to higher duties.

But it cannot happen.

His written words are clotted skeins of hollow echoes; they mean nothing to anybody who did not share the experience of sitting in the darkened salon, bathed in the thrilling heat of the palpitating furnace of Lacan's endless fascination with himself. His books are empty; they are a shell of intellectual conceit that oozes promise but never delivers the goods. His work appeals, not to anybody who is serious about psychiatry, but to attention-challenged dilettantes whose idea of intellectual progress is jamming as many abstruse puns and unknown quotes into a single sentence as are needed to stun the audience with one's own, glittering brilliance: narcissists, in other words. Lacan proves conclusively that there is no conceptual point at which taking one's intuitions seriously can be delimited from taking seriously any other bit of rubbish to enter one's head, i.e. there was no demarcation criterion between novel sense and nonsense. An endlessly boring analysis of the experience of perceiving a color patch (which Watson despised as pointless) is in bed with animal studies (which certainly doesn't mean biology), politics, art, critical theory (which, despite appearances, pertains to Marxism and definitely has nothing to do with self-criticism) and rabid narcissistic self-deception. Indeed, this week's version of the website maintained (erratically) in his memory shows a series of Lautrecian posters of an exotic femme fatale in the lithotomy position, amusing herself with a gigantic dildo. Serious philosophy? I think not.

If Lacan made a business of introspection, Michel Foucault's goal was to lift it to the level of a universal methodology. Foucault is now the most frequently cited humanities author in the world. This formidably loquacious and intolerant man accepted no restraints on the idea that he could look into any aspect of human activity and discern levels of meaning hidden from the general gaze, most of them concerned with inequitable distributions of power. This, of course, is contradictory: the very notion of the word 'power' implies that some parts of society can influence others but not vice versa, just as the definition of the word 'temperature' implies that some places are hotter than others. When we consider the concept of the heat death of the universe, I wonder if the idea of a society with a uniform distribution of power is not a solecism? Putting that aside, Foucault established his reputation with the 1961 publication of his epic thesis on the history of society's attitudes to and treatment of madness. In 1965, a much-shortened version was published in *English as Madness and Civilisation*, on the recommendation of the reviewer, RD Laing, who said: "This is quite an exceptional book of very high caliber—brilliantly written, intellectually rigorous, and with a thesis that thoroughly shakes the assumptions of traditional psychiatry." The book went through a considerable number of versions and titles over the years until the definitive publication in English as History of madness in 2006 [7]. While I found its 725 pages boring and self-indulgent in the extreme, it does not offer an explanation of mental illness per se and is therefore of no interest in this context. Unfortunately, it was taken as licensing Foucault, and thence any post-modernist, to talk authoritatively about mental disorder regardless of any facts contrary to their opinion.

Normally, I try to avoid the genetic fallacy, i.e. the notion that the person who says something has a bearing on the validity of what he says, but Foucault stretches the limits of tolerance. A brief biography at the beginning of this book mentions that, in the late 1970s and early 1980s, he travelled regularly to the US for teaching commitments at UC Berkeley: "Freely experimenting with LSD and the liberal sexual environment, he lived what he termed 'limit experiences.'… Fatally ill with AIDS, Michel Foucault died in Paris on 25 June 1984 in the Salpêtrière Hospital at the age of fifty-seven. After his death, the French prime minister issued a tribute... Georges Dumezil wrote, 'Foucault's intelligence literally knew no bounds.'" Such a pity, then, that his morality was equally unfettered. During his annual sojourns at Berkeley, Foucault knew he was infected with a lethal virus which was spreading rapidly through the gay community. His sexual 'limit experiences' consisted of non-stop unprotected sex in the bathhouses of San Francisco, meaning he would have personally infected and caused the deaths of dozens, if not hundreds, of young men. How he reconciled that with his preoccupation with society's misuse of power over its mentally ill members we will never know. He was a psychopath. I cannot separate that fact from anything of his that I read; so I declare my prejudice and move on.

Since Foucault's inglorious end, the limelight of public fascination has swung to train on one of the more contentious philosophers to have graced the stage in a highly competitive era. For the last thirty years of his life, Jacques Derrida wrote about one book a year (see his entry in Wikipedia for a bibliography). This is an astounding achievement as most authors would agree that writing a book is extremely hard work. How did he manage to fill all those dauntingly blank pages waiting between the covers? What amazing torrent of novel insights into the human condition poured from his fecund mind to fill ten thousand pages of print? Well, that depends on who you ask. Even though his many supporters idolize him as one of the most penetrating intellects in human history, not one of them would deny that his work is obscure and open to interpretation. While his philosophy of deconstruction has generated untold millions of words, it is not possible to point to any particular achievements outside the field itself. In particular, from the point of view of mental disorder, he has nothing to say, except he took a long time saying it.

There are two major criticisms of Derrida's approach, the obscurity and his willful misuse of rationalist terms. Writing in the NY Review of Books (February 2nd 1984), John Searle said:

> "... anyone who reads deconstructive texts with an open mind is likely to be struck by the same phenomena that initially surprised me: the low level of philosophical argumentation, the deliberate obscurantism of the prose, the wildly exaggerated claims, and the constant striving to give the appearance of profundity by making claims that seem paradoxical, but under analysis often turn out to be silly or trivial."

The renowned opponent of post-modernism, Alan Sokal, quoted Derrida in his notorious hoax [8], capitalizing on how the philosopher had misused Einstein's constant in typical style. However, this pales beside the savage criticism of two of post-modernism's deadliest enemies, Paul Gross and Norman Levitt, who saw Derrida as little more than a shifty, prolix charlatan [9, p. 75-78]. In fact, most of his output is so open to multiple interpretations as to be of no value, not the least because nobody can fill that many books with original work in that space of time. His vast output has to be, and is, repetitious and self-indulgent undergraduate wordplay of little or no consistent content. Worse still, according to E.R.

Monegal, late professor of contemporary Latin American Literature at Yale University, a significant part of the little bit that is more than mere punning may well have been lifted from Jorge Luis Borges.

The work of the philosopher, Gilles Deleuze, who died in 1995, is of interest here for two reasons. In the first place, he was a prodigious and unrepentant abuser of scientific terms, scattering them freely across his work with no rhyme and less reason, the only possible intention being duping his readers [10, 11] but not before duping himself. Along with Derrida, he contributed mightily to the notion that artful wordplay trumps intellectual discipline. The second reason is that he collaborated with the communist psychoanalyst, Felix Guattari (died 1992) in some of his most influential works. Guattari, who was a student of Lacan, led a life of supreme disorganization, apparently spending most of his time setting up radical groups (including one called 'Friendly Male Nurses'), which faded as soon as he lost interest in them. He also spent a large part of his spare time devising new words, such as chaosmosis, chaosophy, ecosophy, and schizoanalysis. Pinning down their meaning is like trying to nail jelly to a wall. Sokal and Bricmont were taken by his singular abuse of scientific terms, as the following quote shows. Both of these authors speak faultless French, so the problem does not lie in the translations. Guttari says:

> "We can clearly see that there is no bi-univocal correspondence between linear signifying links or archi-writing, depending on the author, and this multireferential, multidimensional machinic catalysis. The symmetry of scale, the transversality, the pathic non-discursive character of their expansion; all these dimensions remove us from the logic of the excluded middle and reinforce us in our dismissal of the ontological binarism we criticized previously. A machinic assemblage, through its diverse components, extracts its consistency by crossing ontological thresholds, non-linear thresholds of irreversibility, ontological and phylogenetic thresholds, creative thresholds of heterogenesis and autopoiesis. The notion of scale needs to be expanded to consider fractal symmetries in ontological terms.
>
> "What fractal machines traverse are substantial scales. They traverse them in engendering them. But, and this should be noted, the existential ordinates that they 'invent' were always already there. How can this paradox be sustained? It's because everything becomes possible (including the recessive smoothing of time, evoked by Rene Thom) the moment one allows the assemblage to escape from energetic-spatio-temporal coordinates. And, here again, we need to rediscover a manner of Being—before, after, here, and everywhere else—without being, however, identical to itself; a processual, polyphonic Being singularisable by infinitely complexifiable textures, according to the infinite speeds which animate its virtual compositions...." [10, p. 166 etc for several pages].

Sokal and Bricmont commented: "This passage contains the most brilliant mélange of scientific, pseudo-scientific, and philosophical jargon that we have ever encountered; only a genius could have written it." It should be noted that, in their night jobs as scourges of the PoMo establishment, these two authors have certainly encountered a great deal of this type of mangling of language but they are wrong. The quote from Guattari's Chaosmosis does not represent genius at work at all. It may have been that Guattari was a genius, but nobody will ever be able to discern that from his writings because of his thought disorder. Thought disorder? Of course: this is absolutely classic thought disorder of the type that every public psychiatrist will see each day at work. So it is perhaps not surprising the physicists did not recognize the full import of Guattari's, and of Lacan's, and of Derrida's fantastical ramblings. They (Sokal and Bricmont) were starting from the default position that academic psychoanalysts and philosophers who publish a book a year are likely to have a solid grip on sanity. That is not a sound assumption. After all, it falls straight into the genetic fallacy.

So we can now dismiss the whole of the improbable academic edifice built upon the output of these authors and their followers. And with it, a large part of the phenomenological, post-modernist, post-structuralist, constructivist, and relativist, and the rest of the alphabet soup of the critical theory Tower of Babel crumbles and slides down into well-deserved oblivion. The messiahs were simply thought-disordered. Well, they weren't the first and, no doubt, they won't be the last but at least next time, the critics will have another tool at their disposal: "Now, class, before we accept Monsieur Caterwaul's work as the Received Truth, we need to satisfy ourselves that he wasn't thought-disordered. Can you open your books at the specific test, I think it's page 484, and apply it to his notion of the bi-univocal confluence of the chaosmotic hyperfecundity of the autopoietic universal emergentist endophenotypy at the transfinite Omega Point? But don't include his references to the international conspiracy to defraud him of his royalties after he had said the author is irrelevant, as that would rightly be considered delusional, and delusions aren't part of thought disorder. A coherent delusion is not a solecism. I beg your par...? That's autopoietic, Mr. Jones, not homoerotic. I find that type of comment quite tasteless. Now to return to the test of thought disorder. Take a sentence at random and move it around in the body of the text thus, or swap the nouns of one sentence with those of the next. If the text has a high informational value, it will be rendered nonsensical. If, however, it is already nonsense, nobody will be able to discern the difference. You think your effort actually improves it, Mr. Jones? Then it is surely worse than we suspected. Let me see... No, you have created your own neologia. Neologism is one of the hallmarks of the thought-disordered. Also be alert to clang associations, irrelevant punning, forced rhyme, extraneous intrusions and, of course, rambling thinking. In addition, pseudo-philosophy, pseudo-psychology, and a preoccupation with over-inclusive and grandiose religiosity, especially attempts to explain the complexity of the universe in a single diagram are diagnostic. Now we could... Yes, Mr.

Jones? Actually, you're right, it doesn't leave us much to work on. It's rather sad in a way, there was a time when being an intellectual was a hugely gratifying self-indulgence. Not any more...."

Thought-disordered logorrhea was the gas that allowed these self-appointed semi-divine blimps to inflate themselves so they could drift across the sky to a chorus of shrieks from their ecstatic followers below, rather than plummet naked to the insensible ground where they belonged. Having a test to bring them down makes it so easy, doesn't it? Although it does make you wonder where all those clever French psychiatrists were while this pseudo-intellectual claptrap was pouring off the printing presses. Perhaps they were asleep on the job. Too much wine at lunch, I'd say.

I should comment on the suggestion by Sokal and Bricmont that only a genius could write that stuff. What they actually meant was that they couldn't write it themselves. My account of language gives high priority to the role of "unconscious" rules in generating speech. For ordinary people most of the time, these rules are so deeply ingrained that we can over-ride them only with great difficulty. This leads, of course, to the inviolable test of thought disorder: the defendant must prove that his utterances follow all the rules of grammar and of logic, etc, where logic is the study of valid inference. We are so used to people making sense that we forget the null hypothesis: nothing anybody says makes sense until he has proven it. When I say these people are thought disordered, the burden of proof rests on those who say they are not. There are, of course, different sorts of thought disorder. Guattari's was absolutely typical of chronic deteriorated schizophrenia; Lacan's was typical of the supreme narcissist who believes that any thought that enters his head comes from a paramount authority and cannot be questioned; Derrida's conduct was much more typical of the card sharp, the cheat who is only interested in scoring points over his opponents. There are lots more.

The wonder is not that people write this stuff, nor even that people publish it, but that people actually hand over good money to buy it.

4.6: Relativism As Institutionalized Hypocrisy

The idea that there is no such thing as objective knowledge is central to the whole phenomenologist-post-modernist project, if there be such a thing. One society claims as an objective fact that the world was divinely created in a week about six thousand years ago, with all life forms intact, while another claims that, as an objective fact, it evolved from a fireball six billion years ago and that life evolved over hundreds of millions of years by natural processes. According to the relativist stand, each claim is the product of its society, each is biased by the language in which it is cast and by our inherent cognitive biases, and therefore each claim is equally valid.

> "Feminist epistemologists, in common with many other strands of contemporary epistemology, no longer regard knowledge as a neutral transparent reflection of an independently-existing reality,

with truth and falsity established by transcendent procedures of rational assessment. Rather, most accept that all knowledge is situated knowledge, reflecting the position of the knowledge producer at a certain historical moment in a given material and cultural context" [12].

So claims Katherine Lennon but, before I can respond to her assertion, there are several points that need to be clarified. Firstly, I am never sure what the word 'transcendent' means, nor am I sure that 'transcendent rational procedures' does not represent an oxymoron, so I will omit the word. In fact, it doesn't change the meaning of the sentence appreciably. There is a sense in which her claim is a truism, in that, strictly speaking, if there is an "independently-existing reality", it might be the case that we can never be sure our perception of it is correct. For example, we may say that the color of the red rose is an "independently-existing reality" but this is not true: the color red exists only in our minds. There is no such thing as red outside a suitable perceiving system, such as eyes joined to minds. However, I don't think that is the sense in which she meant it, because she was largely referring to the human world, and that is how she should be answered.

Second, her use of the term "knowledge producer" begs some very important questions which essentially negate her claim. The idea that knowledge is simply produced is an example of what Dennett calls the "intuition pump", i.e. a way of describing things which illicitly shifts the reader's perception because the immediate conclusion from reading the sentence is not supported by the facts contained in it. The shift in perception is this: in order to produce anything, we must use the available technology. So a person who is a knowledge producer is perforce fixed "... at a certain historical moment in a given material and cultural context." This is a truism, which sets the scene for the next stroke of her intuition pump. Any production is produced for a purpose, and the purpose of producing knowledge can only be to accumulate power in one form or another. It might be just power over the elements (discovering how to make clay tiles instead of thatch, how to trap more fish, or how to avoid being eaten by crocodiles) but that is certainly not her implication: knowledge "... reflect(s) the position of the knowledge producer at a certain historical moment in a given material and cultural context." She is not talking about keeping dry in storms or building better fish traps; she is talking about men, meaning white men, dominating the cultural context.

So if we accept her claim (which I certainly don't), then her case follows: nothing can be produced without the requisite means of production; anything that people produce necessarily is the result of their "material and cultural context" because that's all they've got, but it should be ignored because it's all about men gaining power; the motives are impure, therefore the knowledge is impure (there is a corollary to this, that pure motives will somehow produce pure knowledge but that is too childish to pursue). But this ignores the deep-seated human drive for knowledge-for-knowledge's-sake which, as an empirical fact, is more active in males than females. Women can usually live without knowing what is in the next valley; their sons usually choose not to. And, of course, this week's bit of "knowledge for fun" becomes the basis of next week's must-have labor-saving device—or weapon. Humans are not "knowledge producers" but are knowledge discoverers or knowledge harvesters, even knowledge miners; but the knowledge thus gained immediately and permanently alters the socio-cultural context. The men who first started looking in the sky didn't know where it would end—nor did they care. Teased out thus, her claim is meaningless but it certainly makes good propaganda.

However, she was right in one respect. It is absolutely the case (pace Boghassian that "... all knowledge is situated knowledge, reflecting the position of the knowledge producer at a certain historical moment in a given material and cultural context," but not in the sense that she thinks it is. When the precise meaning of this claim is untangled, her argument for relativism collapses.

As every epistemologist (male or female) knows, there are certain classes of knowledge, and the problem is to sort them into their proper categories. The knowledge classes that count are not good knowledge vs. bad, liberating knowledge vs. repressive etc, but reliable vs. unreliable knowledge. Let's look at some examples. In several southern US states in the 1950s, there were outbreaks of people dying from snake bite after picking up the snakes while engaging in religious frenzies. The victims believed that if their faith in God was pure, they would be protected from the venom. Needless to say, they weren't around long enough to teach the rest of the congregation how to be true believers. At the same time, several large companies were claiming that they could take an ordinary citizen and propel him (or her, they weren't sexist) through the air at a terrific speed and height, in conditions of temperature, air pressure, and oxygen saturation that would normally kill an ordinary person, yet do so without ruffling so much as a hair on the person's head. Better still, having hurled the stolid burgers across the ocean, they could even bring them back—just for the price of a return ticket in one of their new jet airliners.

Now the question here is not whether the respective claims "... reflect(ed) the position of the knowledge producer at a certain historical moment in a given material and cultural context" because, in a boring sense, they most certainly did, but whether they were reliable. If they were alive and in the US South in the 1950s and, for example, Ms Lennon's sister thought she could charm snakes, what would the feminist say? "Go ahead, darling, because I know that, as a feminist knowledge producer, your motives are pure and uncontaminated by the lust for power"? If, however, her daughter wanted to go on a school trip to the other side of the country, would she forbid her to travel on Mr. Boeing's thunderous new 707 because it was designed by men and built for the wrong motives and would therefore fall out of the sky? We know the answers to these questions because Ms Lennon would make her decisions, not on the "knowledge producer's" motives (or sex) but on whether the claims were reliable. She wouldn't be so silly as to fall for the genetic fallacy. We are not concerned with who makes the statements but their basis for making them. In this sense, epistemology is objective and the idea of a "feminist epistemology" is nonsensical. The proposition 'Poisonous snakes kill' is true regardless of the sex of the person who makes the claim—or the sex of the person lying dead on the floor.

Let's go back to the pernicious idea of opposing "... naturalism (also called objectivism and positivism), which is the worldview growing from modern natural science and technology that has been spreading from Northern Europe since the Renaissance" (from the Center for Advanced Research in Phenomenology, [3]). There is considerable debate over whether children should be taught the theory of evolution or whether they should be taught the creation beliefs of their particular community. For example, should Aboriginal children in the north of Australia be taught that humans descended from ape-like creatures in the plains of Africa a million years ago; should they be taught that God created heaven and earth in six days, ensconcing Adam and Eve in the Garden of Eden; or should they be told that the Great Kangaroo Mother fought the Old Man Crocodile across the sky, leaving a trail of her blood which turned into humans when it touched the soil? Some people would say that all knowledge is equal just because it represents the knowledge producer's position in a socio-cultural power matrix so it doesn't matter which set of beliefs the innocents are given. At best, this is disingenuous in the extreme, at worst, dishonest. If the socio-cultural context includes the view that black people are mud people and should be wiped out, or that homosexuals and witches should be burned at the stake, then it definitely matters whether children are given these ideas.

In fact, there is a huge difference between the classes of information in creation myths—there are myths and myths—but we can come at it obliquely. If Ms Lennon's child came home from school, complaining of abdominal pain which soon got worse and caused vomiting, what would she do? She would, of course, rush him to the nearest hospital to see a surgeon. There, the surgeon would examine the child, order some tests and then announce to the mother: "The boy has appendicitis. We will operate tonight to remove it and he will be home in a few days."

Assuming she has children, I am sure that Ms Lennon would follow the advice but, for the purpose of testing her beliefs, let's assume she is one of those daunting mothers who object to being treated as a "mere relative" but wishes to play a coequal (meaning dominant) role in her son's journey through life. Assuming a forthright posture, she fixes the weary surgeon with a stern gaze and says to him:

"You are speaking as a product of naturalism (also called objectivism and positivism), which is the worldview growing from modern natural science and technology that has been spreading from Northern Europe since the Renaissance. As a feminist epistemologist, which arose from the phenomenological revolution aimed at toppling the male hegemony, I adhere to one or other form of intuitionism, meaning I accept my experiences in 'primordial form' as representing whatever they purport to be. Right now, they purport to inform me that you are speaking as a power-consumer embedded in your male-oriented reality. You may think that you establish truth and falsity by transcendent procedures of rational assessment but I know that all knowledge is situated knowledge, reflecting the position of the knowledge producer at a certain historical moment in a given material and cultural context. You believe that your knowledge is superior to mine but manifestly, your intention in going to medical school was only to elevate yourself in the wealth-oriented socio-cultural milieu in between humiliating nurses through satisfying your vile lusts. I know that the truth of my child's state is that he is fighting against the male animus which is trying to take control of his spirit and obliterate his feminine side, as one of my anti-racist, anti-sexist intuitions tells me. Accordingly, I shall take him to a learned woman who will read his Tarot, take a Kirlian photograph to check his spectral aura, inspect his irises for birthing trauma (caused by the obstetrician, not his mother) and then cure him with herbal candling, macrobiotic moxibustion, and Reikian aromatherapy while my feminist friends and I dance to Tibetan drums to conjure up the healing cosmic spirit from her home at the Omega Point. But first," she says, her voice chilling with contempt, "let me hear your risible attempts at a self-serving relativist pseudo-justification."

The surgeon is a man of the world. Rather than tell the mother that she is a total screwball, selfishly endangering another person's life while acting out her private psychopathology, which consists of a jumbled mess of suppressed fear for her son's health coupled with her insane need for control, he pulls up a chair and takes out a pen and paper.

"I do view scientific knowledge as a neutral transparent reflection of an independently-existing reality," he says, writing points as he goes, "with truth and falsity established by transcendent procedures of rational assessment. Given this ontology, we shall take your son to a room equipped with machines whose reliability has been established beyond reasonable doubt but we still take them apart and check them regularly. The anesthetist, who has lengthy specialist training, will insert a cannula in a vein in his arm and inject isotonic water, which will rehydrate him without risking hemolysis, then inject a series of chemicals which, in anybody else's hands, would immediately result in your son's death. These will ensure that the boy will be paralyzed so he can be respirated by a machine using oxygen at a precisely calibrated pressure, as well as certain gases which also would kill him if not monitored closely. I shall then sterilize his abdomen using more toxic chemicals, take a Japanese stainless steel knife made with iron ore from Brazil, coal and nickel from Australia, and chromium from South Africa, all in precisely-defined objective proportions, and I shall cut through his abdominal wall. If we have made a mistake with the drugs, he will be wide awake but utterly unable to move or signal his pain, which would be worse than any nightmare but we have numerous back-up checks. Every step of this procedure, from analyzing the chemicals in the sap of certain South American trees to produce tubocurarine, to guiding the ore ships across the Pacific by GPS, to measuring the oxygen in his blood, to recording every instrument and needle used in the operation and so on, is spelled out in very great detail in the public domain so that any person can precisely duplicate what we do. We make no claims on non-empirical, meaning non-rational, procedures or entities. From beginning to end, there is nothing mystical or cryptic in our procedures. That is to say, our knowledge is reliable by virtue only of the tests to which we submit it. But you are absolutely correct: it reflects our present understanding of the nature of reality and it could all be overturned tomorrow by another discovery. If you wish me to give you examples of revolutions in medical understanding, I know of many, because that is how science progresses. In science, we challenge the dominant view in order to improve it."

"Aha," replies the woman triumphantly, "I heard you say you could be wrong. So you admit that your knowledge is not absolute? Where does that leave your insatiable male drive to accumulate power and bend the innocents of the world to your corrupt will?"

"Well, madam," the surgeon says calmly, as he has heard this a dozen times before, "I don't claim to have absolute knowledge. My knowledge is situated in a particular intellectual context stemming from the Renaissance in Europe and spreading out to supplant local beliefs of the nature of reality just by virtue of its capacity to make better predictions and build better mousetraps. Only priests, politicians, charlatans, and fools claim to have absolute knowledge. Any person who wishes to consult them is free to do so but the claim that God created Adam and Eve in the Garden of Eden has zero reliability in our schema, just because it cannot be tested. Because ours are the only known tests of reliability, all claims with zero reliability are of equal standing. If there were tests for Adam and Eve, it wouldn't be religion but, if there were such tests, we would quickly start to use them. Anybody who doesn't approve of my knowledge can join a cult which promises certainty from on high but, once in, he might find any urge to apostasy will not be tolerated under pain of death."

"I hear you rejecting classes of knowledge just because they don't fit your preconceptions!" the mother exclaims. "Just because it doesn't fit with your boring tests doesn't imply it is wrong."

"In my line of business," the surgeon says, gesturing at the disinterested boy, "being boring is better than being wrong. My knowledge is empirical and has been submitted to innumerable tests to see whether it accurately reflects the unseen reality in which we humans assume we are embedded. For example, I am currently of the opinion that your son's pain is caused by an inflamed appendix but that is only an informed guess which could subsequently be proven wrong. Once inside his abdomen, I will inspect that organ—it is an independently-existing reality, to preempt your objection; it does not spring into being just because I look for it—and if it is not inflamed, which happens from time to time, I shall then proceed to examine all his other organs. I recall once confidently telling a man he had appendicitis but, when we opened him, we found a matchstick perforating a Meckel's diverticulum. Next day, he agreed he was in the habit of chewing matchsticks and had accidentally swallowed one several days before, so it was not placed there by a magic spell. If our knowledge is a myth, at the very least, it is a reliable myth."

The lady is a becoming a little irritable by this stage: "There are more classes of knowledge than fit your mean and simplistic schema. Am I wrong in saying I see you before me right now? Yet the only evidence is the evidence of my senses."

"There may indeed be many classes of knowledge, but not all of them are reliable. As a mere surgeon, I may be wrong. I do not claim my knowledge comes from heaven on tablets of stone, nor from infallible intuition or irresistible historical forces. But I am claiming that, within the limits of our procedures, it is reliable information. It is the same as when you get on a jet airliner. Every part of that huge machine, every component, every drop of fuel, has been designed, built, and tested to maximize your chances of arriving safely at your destination. Your son's operation is the product of a vast, interlocking system of knowledge which goes back hundreds of years to the time of Andreas Vesalius in Renaissance Italy, and which has been submitted to the most stringent testing at every conceivable point since then to maximize his chances of survival. At this particular historical moment, that knowledge constitutes my given material and cultural context, where 'given' means published and verifiable. While we smugly boring Western rationalist hegemonists do not have absolute knowledge, our knowledge is reliable and that is all you, as an epistemologist, can ask. A myth is an unquestioned belief system based on no evidence; if science is a myth, it is constantly questioned and held to account by independent evidence. Not all myths are coequal. It is your mistake to assume that all bodies of knowledge are fixed. Science changes, myths don't, for which you should be mightily grateful."

Reaching for a form, he pushes it and the pen to the mother: "Please sign this consent form here, and here. The visiting hours tomorrow will be at the whim of the dragon in charge of your son's ward. Meantime, you can rely on my claim that your son will be safe. Relatively speaking."

Mumbling something that might sound grateful but which doesn't actually commit her, the lady takes her leave and immediately rings all her friends on a conference call to tell them how she snapped that surgeon into line; my god she did!

4.7: **Conclusion: Relative Conceit**

All knowledge is relative. Tub-thumping creationists are relatively ignorant; homicidal North Korean dictators who dine on imported steak and champagne while millions of their people starve are relatively evil; conceited bankers who build up untold unfunded liabilities while paying themselves telephone number salaries, then demand government support when the whole mess collapses, are relatively amoral; glamorous film stars who take drugs are relatively immature; boring surgeons, nurses, IT technicians, and pilots are relatively reliable—but not by accident.

The statement: 'All knowledge is relative' puts the emphasis on the wrong side of the equation. It should read: 'No knowledge is absolute.' Relativity does not imply epistemological equality. Consider the following statements:

'Light flux varies according to the inverse square law.'

'Women must conceal their entire bodies except for their eyes under pain of public flogging.'

Even if somebody believes both statements come from God, they are still not in the same realm of discourse. Not all knowledge is equal because only some knowledge is reliable. Western science is about the sorts of methods and procedures and the types of knowledge that allow one to claim reliability but that is all it is about. If those methods and procedures are applied to the wrong type of knowledge, then what results is not science but scientism (the inappropriate application of scientific methods and procedures to questions of no empirical content). Reliability is the result of intense self-discipline, not self-indulgence. It is not achieved simply by tacking the word 'science' on another field of interest e.g. management science, creationist science, domestic science, political science, etc. If this habit continues, soon we will have cartoon science, pornography science, even philosophy science. A subject is a science only when it passes certain tests; if those tests don't apply, the subject may be interesting or important, but it isn't science.

It is true that our actions flow from the totality of our belief states; if they didn't, we would have no basis for rational action. We would be like the flowers of the field turning to face the sun. But not all belief states are equal. Anybody who believes that, say, Aboriginal creation myths (the Dreamtime) are coequal to the Western version is free to join in all that flows from those myths: infanticide and gerontocide; absolute male dominance with females serving as chattels; child marriages arranged according to totemic law; compulsory male sexual mutilation; post-parturition cleansing rituals for women involving smoking the pudenda over open fires; secret trials by sorcery where the defendant doesn't even know he is on trial and has no right of defense or appeal; guilt by association leading to death sentences with no appeal; inability of injured or mentally-impaired men to marry; ritualized rape of women to pay for their husband's offences; ritual spearing; shamanistic treatment of illness, and so on. All of this is part of the Aboriginal worldview: their "... knowledge is situated knowledge, reflecting the position of the knowledge producer at a certain historical moment in a given material and cultural context." Any person who claims that the Aboriginal approach to appendicitis is, in some critical and indubitable sense, coequal with the Western view is thereby guilty of the grossest intellectual dishonesty. When Michel Foucault was in the terminal stages of AIDS, where did he go? To one of the most famous hospitals in France. When Gilles Deleuze needed a thoracotomy because of his lifetime of abuse of tobacco, did he come to Darwin so he could have some half-blind old men squatting in the dirt cut his chest open using a sharp stone? The hell he did. He made sure he got the best. At government expense, *naturellement*.

I am either in a given material and cultural context or I am out of it. There is no moral or intellectual justification for choosing part of one context (cell phones, CT scanners, votes for women, champagne on airliners) while rejecting the rest of it in favor of candles, crystals, and cabals. That is mere hypocrisy. Whether Kathleen Lennon is guilty of insincerity, I don't know, but her published statements lay her wide open to the charge with no conceivable defense. She may, of course, be perfectly sincere but not have explored her ideas to their logical limits. That is, she may spend her time wafting around the further reaches of academic silliness and pretension. That would be funny if it were not dangerous.

Because phenomenologists have no agreed discipline and don't appear to worry about consistency, there is no reliability and none of them can be proven wrong. When nobody is wrong, nobody is right, so people must do something else to attract attention. In the absence of reliability, showmanship is trumps. That's why, to a phenomenologist, being boring is worse than being wrong. And that's why, to anybody who believes that there is an objective reality independent of any human bias, phenomenology and its spawn are a total waste of time. Perhaps there are no atheists in a foxhole but there are surely no post-modernists in a speeding ambulance.

I wish to go on record with a prediction: The coming generation will see through post-modernism and phenomenology, and they will discard it. They will turn on it as the rising generation must ever turn on their parents' obsessions, to overthrow them, because that is the nature of human affairs. Enoch Powell said: "All political careers end in failure; that is the nature of politics and of human affairs." All ideologies must end. It is the inescapable duty of all rational youth to shatter their parents' beliefs, as that is the only way they can become their own people. Our children will see that post-modernism is an urban myth, and not just because it will never produce a better iPhone. I have unwavering confidence that our children will soon recognize that what is touted as obscure profundity is profound obscurity, otherwise known as arrant nonsense. Just as the present generation of post-modernist phenomenologists is totally caught up in a race to the bottom of the pits of obscurity, the new generation will learn again the value of clear, incisive thinking. Of course, there will never be as many people in the race for clarity because a race for gibberish allows every monkey to climb down from its tree and join in. The race itself will exclude the inessential.

But oh boy, I wish I could churn out a book a year and have university presses squabbling over the publication rights, disdain the royalty payments, then hire a lawyer to get more from students (as Derrida did), but can I give the 'sexual limit experiences' a miss? Maybe I should practice being thought-disordered....

I've got it, a thought-disordered psychiatrist! What an insight, nobody would ever have thought of that. Let's see...

"My topic tonight is hegemonistic psychiatry's callous attempts to reduce human suffering resulting from persisting neocolonial and modernist repressions of the free expression of the proletarian will to bourgeois matters of bio-, psycho- and social parameters. Starting in Rochester NY (and how bourgeois is that?), Engel's subterfuge was to distract the toiling masses from their true enemy, the capitalist kleptocratic state, fooling them into thinking that their oppressor was a phantom he called 'biomedicine.' His deceit was that he put the biological first, thereby subliminally reinforcing that social factors can safely be left out of the post-industrial equation, fit only for the narcotizing influence of Hollywood and now Silicon Valley. By his emphasis on the arcane biological sphere, he conjured the promise that Big Science would soon deliver a tablet capable of bringing, dare I say it, happiness to oppressed schoolchildren and their struggling mothers in the alienating suburban wildernesses of..."

No? So I can never be a paid up member of the obscuranti?

Mais si je scrive en français....? Non?

Merde!

<table>
<tr><td>

5

</td><td>

Phenomenology and Psychiatry

</td></tr>
</table>

"... at the heart of science is an essential balance between two seemingly contradictory attitudes—an openness to new ideas, no matter how bizarre or counterintuitive, and the most ruthlessly sceptical scrutiny of all ideas, old and new. This is how deep truths are winnowed from deep nonsense."

Carl Sagan

5.1: Introduction

Just in case anybody has been asleep for the past thirty-five years, modern psychiatry has been on course to reinvent itself. By dumping all the flowery bits (Freud, California dreaming, The Meaning of Life) and sticking to a diet of statistics, brain chemicals and scanners, psychiatry hoped to become sufficiently respectable to enter the pavilion of scientific medicine through the front door, rather than slinking around the back lane. So far, this has been outstandingly successful. Funding for mental health research has grown enormously, as have psychiatric publications; there are far more academic psychiatric posts, psychiatrists serve on many more government committees, profits from psychotropic drugs are the equal of any other class of drugs, and court cases may turn on the psychiatric or psychological evidence. The practice of psychiatry itself is becoming easier as the tedious business of listening to agitated people is steadily replaced by self-administered questionnaires. This has all come about because psychiatry has adopted a clear program of finding the biological roots of mental disorder and devising definitive treatments. So who isn't applauding?

At is happens, quite a few people aren't swept off their feet by the reductionist rush. There are plenty of people who believe that the idea of "drugs for the masses" is overdoing it, that we are breeding a drug-dependent culture. Others feel the idea that everything human can be explained by genes is somehow dehumanizing. Within psychiatry itself, people are starting to have second thoughts, and not just querulous provincials:

Since the publication of DSM-III in 1980, there has been a steady decline in the teaching of careful clinical evaluation that is targeted to the individual person's problems and social context and that is enriched by a good general knowledge of psychopathology. Students are taught to memorize DSM rather than to learn complexities from the great psychopathologists of the past... DSM has had a dehumanizing impact on the practice of psychiatry. History taking—the central evaluation tool in psychiatry—has frequently been reduced to the use of DSM checklists. DSM discourages clinicians from getting to know the patient as an individual person because of its dryly empirical approach... validity has been sacrificed to achieve reliability [1].

Another eminent psychiatrist railed against the "... self-justifying and self-sustaining hermeneutic world of today's manuals of mental disorders..." and asks whether the diagnostic manuals have become "... self-sustaining impediments to scientific progress" in psychiatry. However, after taking the manuals to task, he softened the blow: "Those who create these manuals are neither fools nor rogues... They welcome research, debate, and change" [2].

These quotes were taken from a seminar held at the Institute of Psychiatry in London, September, 2005. The participants had come together to consider modern psychiatry's decline into the dehumanized shell of a science of mental disorder. The topic of the conference was phenomenology and psychiatry, and some of the more important papers were published in a special section of the prestigious journal, Schizophrenia Bulletin. It was perhaps an unintended irony that this section, which looks at mental disorder as a psychological phenomenon, was paired with another entitled: The use of endophenotypes to deconstruct and understand the genetic architecture, neurobiology, and guide future treatments of the group of schizophrenias. As an approach, the latter is about as hard-nosed as biological psychiatry gets (endophenotypy is the latest starter in the race to find The Biological Cause of schizophrenia, after the human genome project ran out of wind). However, in view of what I've said in Chapter 4, we need to look at the history of psychiatry to understand why anybody would be interested in phenomenology.

5.2: Psychiatry and Phenomenology

These days, there would be something like 150,000 psychiatrists in the world, but a hundred years ago, there were probably well under a thousand. Thus, it was fairly easy for an energetic young man (I don't know if there were any female psychiatrists then) to push himself up the ladder. All he had to do was turn up to work sober, write a few interesting papers and, in no time, he was the Grand Old Man of something. In addition, many of them had other interests they could pursue, especially psychology, neurology, and philosophy. Indeed, an obsessive interest was a clear advantage. The Austrian neuropsychiatrist Julius Wagner-Jauregg (1857-1940), was awarded the Nobel Prize for medicine in 1927 for his particular obsessive interest. Almost from the day he graduated, he was gripped by the idea that he could treat mental and neurological disorders with artificially-induced fevers ("pyrotherapy"). This led to the fortuitous discovery of the effects of malaria-induced hyperthermia on the progress of dementia paralytica (tertiary syphilis). Purely by chance, *T. pallidum* is highly sensitive to fever. As there was precious little else that could be done for the epidemic of cerebral syphilis, he took the prize.

Another early student of diverse interests started law, swapped to medicine and went straight into psychiatry, but left after four years for a post in psychology. Eight years later, he moved into philosophy where, with a sideline in theology, he remained until his retirement. Karl Jaspers (1883-1969) was one of a small but enormously influential group of German-speaking psychiatrists but, even in that group, he stood out as he made his mark in just four years. He was born in 1883, started law in 1901, changed to medicine in 1902, graduated in 1909, spent four years in the same psychiatric hospital as Emil Kräpelin, then left for academia and never returned to clinical practice. However, in four years, and in addition to several influential papers, he wrote a two-volume work entitled *General Psychopathology*. The current English editions amount to about 1,400 pages and are laden with his extensive knowledge of the burgeoning field of phenomenological philosophy, as well as references to the classics such as Spinoza and Kant. The idea of a newcomer arriving in psychiatry, working in a busy clinic and calmly knocking out a major, almost revolutionary, interdisciplinary work in his spare time, all in four years, is rather breathtaking. Quite clearly, he could spend his nights reading Hegel and Husserl (in German, of course, if that helps) without having to catch up whatever the journals had printed that week on the molecular genetics of schizophrenia.

While Kräpelin was defining the major psychoses from a population basis, and Freud was manufacturing his theories, Jaspers took a pragmatic look at psychiatry, but from the sufferer's point of view, from what it is like to be mentally ill. He wanted to define the phenomena of suffering so that the categories of disorder would declare themselves without being forced into artificial groupings such as Kräpelin's binary model of psychosis. Over the years, his influence on European and British psychiatry was far-reaching but not obvious. Except for the US, which was dominated by Alfred Meyer and then by Freud, Jasper's approach, of letting the patient describe his symptoms in his own language during the course of taking a detailed history, became more or less the normal basis of daily practice.

On the one hand, Jaspers was not influenced by how much a particular patient resembled the next one: the sufferer's symptoms were uniquely his and his life was also one of a kind, which was not Kräpelin's approach. Kräpelin was looking for similarities so he could lump his patients together (and thence determine their prognosis). On the other hand, the anamnesis, or history and mental state examination, formed the basis of practice but it wasn't the practice itself. In this sense, it differed from psychoanalysis, in which the theory was more important than anything the patient may believe, because the analyst could—and routinely did—overturn the patient's self-perception with a single interpretation. In psychoanalysis, the history melded with the corrective practice. Crews described the analytic hour as a matter of "... grinding the patient's conduct and history into the sausage machine of standard complexes, repressed primal scenes and the like" [4, p.xxv].

Nothing could be further removed from Jasper's patient approach to his patients. He took minutely detailed histories to show the patient's world from within, to show how mental disorder evolved in an individual life. His goal was to make a valid assessment of the patient by means of a thorough understanding of his station in life. One of his psychiatric papers, published after barely a year on the job, used this type of information to ask whether paranoia was a result of a degeneration of the brain, the standard view of the time, or of personality factors. This was on the basis of the almost revolutionary idea that the evolution of the patient's history made some sort of sense, that his mental disorder was not inexplicable. However, Jaspers also believed that frank psychotic symptoms in general could not be understood, so he clearly saw the process of psychosis as alienating.

Remarkably, after only four years in psychiatry, Jaspers published his account of how psychiatry should be seen through the phenomenological lens, then left. His approach was to describe in great detail the phenomena of mental disorder (the symptoms) which signal the difference between being glum and being depressed. It was by their specific symptoms that the individual disorders were recognized, so the phenomenology of mental disorder led straight to a valid classification or nosology of the disorders. It was valid in the sense that the patients defined themselves: their symptoms were not seen distantly or through a Freudian filter. Kräpelin looked to the patient's life course to make a diagnosis, the Freudians didn't bother with diagnoses, and Jaspers let the patients declare their own. In time, his stance became increasingly popular and was eventually applied to the Kräpelinian categories of psychosis themselves. It was known that schizophrenia, formerly dementia praecox (i.e. the dementia of adolescence) had a particular course. Naturally, its course could only be determined by watching it for a period of time but this was a concern as it sometimes meant delaying treatment which, for all anybody knew, may have been valuable in preventing the condition becoming chronic.

Before long, practitioners started to look at the patient's individual experience of mental illness to see whether they could identify features which would correlate with the poor prognosis of schizophrenia. Using Jaspers' methods, one diagnostic group was derived by the psychiatrist Kurt Schneider (1887-1967). Schneider's group of First Rank symptoms, which he hoped would be diagnostic of schizophrenia, gave weight to the form of the symptom, not their content. It was the voice itself that counted, not whose voice it was or what it was saying. There were eleven symptoms, including the patient's experience of hearing his thoughts spoken out loud, of hearing voices commenting about his actions in the third person ("Now he's picking up the cup. Do you see the way he picks up his cup? He's putting the tea in it, now he's lifting the cup to drink from it.") or voices arguing in the third person about his personal qualities ("He always wastes things, he's such a wastrel." "That's not true, you're too hard on him." "I tell you, he's no good. You shouldn't defend him", etc). In order to elicit these symptoms, the interviewer had to sit with the patient, sometimes for quite long periods of time before gaining his confidence, as the patients themselves were often acutely aware of how mad it all sounded.

By the post-war period, this approach formed the basis of the nosology or diagnostic categories of mental disorder, especially in Europe, including Scandinavia and the UK, but not in the US, where psychoanalytic concepts prevailed. There, diagnostic groups were defined by psychoanalytic concepts but, by the 1960s, it was clear that American psychiatry was in serious trouble. There was no consistency of diagnosis and even, as the controversial Rosenhan experiment in 1973 indicated, no consistency from beginning to end [5]. After a great deal of internal struggle, American psychiatry was launched in another direction, with Jaspers' phenomenological concepts forming the basis of a new, allegedly atheoretical diagnostic system (DSM-III in 1980). This has since acquired a life of its own but there is no reason to believe Jaspers would be pleased with the chimera that has resulted.

Meanwhile and far away, and whether aware of it or not, anybody starting psychiatry in Australia in the 1970s was a little Jaspersian. In fact, I was aware of it, because one of the few teachers who had any impact on my training had been a student of the British Jaspersian Frank Fish, and was quite convinced that Kurt Schneider was the savior of psychiatry. So talking to patients about their lives, as distinct from assessing them for surveys or for ECT, came naturally to me. Unfortunately, even in those days, the demands of full-time work and full-time study of the orthodox statistical and biological material left no time for leisurely contemplation of the complexities of phenomenology. Then DSM-III arrived and psychiatry entered a Faustian bargain: it swapped validity for reliability. The naïve idea of the patient telling the psychiatrist what he felt was wrong in his life fell victim to the "... self-justifying and self-sustaining hermeneutic world of today's manuals of mental disorders...," those "... self-sustaining impediments to scientific progress."

Now, it seems, the wheel has turned full circle. Jaspers' careful, 'patient-centered' approach has been emasculated by the demands of diagnostic certainty and cost-control. In a brief, impersonal interview, the patient is questioned for a few essential features and is then handed a prescription and an appointment for a "med check" (review of his medication) in a month. Any humanity in psychiatry is out the window, partly because of financial pressures to shove patients through, and partly because it is not scientific. Not scientific? Who cares; it's patients we're talking about, not cattle. Well, therein lies the problem because, these days, good science is equated with good psychiatry; good psychiatry should be cheaper than bad psychiatry (the ghost of Sigmund Freud hovers over this part of the conversation); and good science is distant and dispassionate, impersonal and uninvolved; from which it follows inexorably (and dispassionately) that good psychiatry is also distant and dispassionate, impersonal and uninvolved. *QED.*

By this means (or some equally loopy path), we arrive at the unseemly position where a psychiatry which was once personal, patient-centered, and considerate, is now characterized by some very senior figures as dry and dehumanizing, a self-justifying impediment to scientific progress. For the record, the error of the DSM-III committees was to think that phenomenology, a humanist, mentalist view, could form the basis of a materialist, reductionist science of human behavior. A moment's thought would have revealed that it could never happen but the people trying to jump the lumbering wagon of psychiatry from one wheel rut to another were in a hurry. Bizarrely, some of today's critics have been at the very center of the drive to make psychiatry more scientific, according to an unstated, undefined model of science which tries to reduce humans to brain chemicals. So now their chickens come home to roost.

The first critic mentioned above, Nancy Andreasen, from Iowa Medical College, was the editor in chief of the *American Journal of Psychiatry* from 1992-2005. She was very active in the moves to shift American psychiatry into the biological camp and, under her stewardship, the Journal's publishing program was one of unreconstructed biologism. Her website says: "She has written three widely-praised books for the general public: *The Broken Brain: The Biological Revolution in Psychiatry* (1983), *Brave New Brain: Conquering Mental Illness in the Era of the Genome* (2001), and *The Creating Brain: The Neuroscience of Genius* (2005)." Having heard her speak on her biological research in schizophrenia, I can confirm that, if indeed she is having doubts about the fundamental basis of the biological program in psychiatry, they are of very recent onset. Most unusually, she gained her PhD in English renaissance literature and was a professor of English before she studied medicine. The second, Paul Mullen, is a noted forensic psychiatrist from Melbourne. His own record of welcoming "research, debate and change" can be read in Chapter 8 of *Humanizing Madness* [3].

However, what counts is the question of how people who are allegedly neither fools nor rogues could be so catastrophically wrong as to build a "... self-sustaining impediment to scientific progress", one which has led to the desiccation of psychiatry, and may yet result in its destruction. One would have thought that serious mistakes of this nature could only be affected by people who are either abject fools or unredeemed scoundrels, but there is another group which probably does as much damage as the others put together: the confidently well-meaning. Historically, the well-meaning people who confidently led psychiatry into the Freudian jungle and lost their way were replaced by a similar group of well-meaning and equally confident experts, albeit from the other side of the fence, who bravely led psychiatry out into the stony deserts of biology—and promptly lost their way, too. Both groups lost their way because they ignored Sagan's sagacious advice (see above) on the role of self-criticism in science. They thought they had the psyche on a dog leash and therefore could not go wrong.

A historical example will illustrate the point. In the early 1980s, the world's financial position was very shaky. In Britain, under Mrs. Thatcher, one of the most confidently right wing but very well-meaning governments in that bemused country's history was pressing ahead with the novel program of privatization, reducing services and taxes, and restricting the role of government. Forty-two miles across La Manche, faced by exactly the same financial pressures, the new, well-meaning socialist government of M. Mitterand boldly embarked on a program of increasing state aid, nationalizations, raising taxes, and extending services. One disease, two totally opposed treatments, formulated by well-meaning ideologues. And this, of course, is the crucial term: confident and well-meaning people who lack the capacity for self-criticism are ideologues. They are the most dangerous people on earth (as an aside, thirty years later, the judgment of history so far is that the wily French haven't made such a bad fist of it as their blundering Anglo allies but the jury will be out for a long time on this one).

So back to psychiatry: what evidence did the well-meaning biologists of mind have to prove that they had pinned the problem of mental disorder to their laboratory benches? Well, none. All they knew was that the other mob had made such a hash of it that psychiatry was wandering in circles so, with a bit of support from the new psychotropic drugs, they simply walked in and took over the shop. They threw out the analytically-inspired DSM-II and wrote their own, basing it on the Jaspersian phenomena of mental disorder alone so that it would be atheoretical. In fact, it wasn't atheoretical at all. Jaspers never said that the disorders he identified were categorically different from each other. DSM-III only made sense in the context of a biological model of mental disorder.

Somewhere along the line, they also lost sight of Jaspers' human-oriented psychiatry so that young psychiatrists today wouldn't know a secondary pseudo-hallucination from their *gedankenlautwerden*, just because they aren't in DSM-IV. Thirty years after DSM-III, the judgment of history is that being lost in the Freudian jungle is really no worse than being lost in the reductionist desert. It's still lost. However, all may not yet be lost as, fresh from their Damascene conversions, the phenomenologists arrivées have a plan: go backwards. Psychiatry, they argued, should return to one of its historical roots, phenomenology. My impression is that they are doing a Gorbachev.* All they want to do is improve their reductionist psychiatry by injecting a bit of humanity into its biological rump and all will be well. I have argued that biological psychiatry is a dinosaur; it needs much more than just a needle in the rump.

5.3: Psychiatry as a Failed Science

As Andreasen noted, the DSM exercise has had some unexpected and pernicious effects on psychiatric practice. It has greased the change from a caring profession to one dominated by drugs, stop watches, and cash registers. It has over-simplified the process of making a diagnosis, at the same time promoting it to the most important part of the contact with patients. It has converted psychiatrists into biological demi-technicians, aloof from the hurly-burly of clinical practice (i.e. dealing with people with problems) and more at home in meetings or conferences on epidemiology or brain enzymes. To a large extent, this has resulted in a "deskilling" of the entire psychiatric profession in some critical areas. Instead of actually listening to patients to find out what is wrong, now they hand them a brief questionnaire; then tell them what is wrong. And to fill the gaps, other professions have flooded in.

Today, psychologists claim equal status with psychiatrists, even in the area of using the latest DSM to make diagnoses and to advise on medication, while social workers aren't far behind. Psychiatrists don't even get to see the patients first off; they are well down the queue, only brought in to confirm the provisional diagnosis from the nurse's summary and write the prescriptions and certificates. Psychotherapy has been contracted out, essentially to anybody who wanted it, as has management of mental health services—and management of psychiatrists. The top psychiatrists themselves have become entrepreneurs, skilled at sucking in biological research money for ever-hungry universities (occasionally with some sticking to their hands), or expert consciences of the nation, ever-willing to comment on a wide variety of social questions—all without the benefit of a scientific model on which to base their opinions.

Andreasen gives some superficial reasons why this has been the case but the real reason is this: psychiatry doesn't have a formal model of mental disorder to guide its practice, its teaching, and its research. Biological psychiatry is not a model; it is an ideology. Therefore, anything it does to standardize practice is necessarily and inevitably a "dumbing down" of the profession. Andreasen does not want to acknowledge this. Having been close to the heart of the entire DSM process of turning psychiatry into a sort of half-witted apology of neuroscience, she could have written an editorial at any time, saying, "Hang on, we can't be a science without a scientific model of mental disorder"; but she didn't. Instead, she wrote popular books about genomes and broken brains. Now, unhappy with the direction the psychiatry she helped shape is going, she wants to restart the process, even to the extent of acknowledging that American psychiatry has lost its way and might need to import Europeans to kick start it: "Someday, in the 21st century, after the human genome and the human brain have been mapped, someone may need to organize a reverse Marshall plan so that the Europeans can save American science by helping us figure out who really has schizophrenia or what schizophrenia really is" [1, p. 112].

That is an absolutely devastating admission, essentially an admission that her life's work has failed. What she is saying is that she bet all her money on reductionist neuroscience as the solution to the question of the nature of mental disorder but, after decades and untold billions of dollars, things aren't going forward; they are somehow going backwards. American psychiatry (and Australian, and British, and Canadian, Dutch, Egyptian, and French down to Zulu) is getting worse, not better. To cap it off, medical students are staying away from the profession in droves [6]. After hammering psychiatry into a sterile laboratory, the first few apostates of the DSM project are sheepishly admitting that reductionist bioscience cannot solve the quintessential questions of mental disorder. They are surprised to learn that the subject matter of psychiatry cannot be put under a microscope (or scanner, or gene sequencer, or all the other machines that haven't been invented yet). They are shocked to realize that their reductionist methodology has somehow allowed the essence of mental disorder to slip through the materialist nets they set to trap it. The problem is, the harder they try to turn psychiatry into a branch of the formal neurosciences, the worse it gets for the poor crazies that nobody wants to talk to; but the more sympathetic psychiatry is, the less it fits the reductionist model of science. It's a bit like one of those ghastly little gowns they give you to wear when you're having an operation. If you try to cover your front, your bottom sticks out, and vice versa. So unless and until there is agreement on a formal, articulated model of mental disorder, we can either have a caring and emotionally satisfying but intellectually chaotic psychiatry, or a technically brilliant but soulless biopsychiatry. But, as Professors Andreasen and Mullen found out the hard way, we can't have both. Well, they can't say they weren't warned many years ago.

5.4: To Resurrect Phenomenology

As promised in Chapter 4, it is at this point we come back to phenomenology. Our task is to give an account of human needs (affection, bonding, fear, grief, etc) and mental disorder within a rational model of mind. This sets phenomenology two tasks. I will deal with the first in this section, while the second will occupy the bulk of Part II of this volume.

A rational model will perforce start with the phenomena of mind as its raw material, not with gene sequences. The phenomena of mind (including mental disorder) must give the clue to the form which any solution to the mind-body problem must take because, discarding ideology, there isn't anything else. By using them according to Jaspers' approach, we can define the form of the mental half of the mind-body problem before turning to the larger body of the materialist sciences to see what they can offer for a solution. The clue that emerges, the clue that jumps up and down shouting for attention, is look beyond the phenomena themselves. Granted this is a little radical but phenomena of mind do not spring into being de novo. Nothing comes from nothing. That is the central doctrine of materialism: Everything has a cause. Mental phenomena are not nothing, therefore they have causes too; so, in a materialist theory of mind, those causes have to be material. Phenomenologists overlook that point because theirs is a descriptive account of mind, not a causative or explanatory theory of mind.

In the causative sense, the phenomena of mind that count are not the glaringly obvious ones, like sight, pain, emotions, and so on, because we already know they are causally ineffective. Whatever causes the obvious phenomena of mind cannot be an obvious phenomenon of mind itself. That is, each one of them stands as the surface or overt marker of a causally effective but covert or otherwise invisible (not open to introspection) mental event. The cause of a phenomenon of mind just is a mental event, not a biological event. A causative theory of mind does not end with the statement: 'And so the biological events cause the mental events'—because that's just what a causative theory must explain. However, it is a restricted sort of mental event but we don't know what they are as nobody has ever seen them. Strictly speaking, the unseen events are also 'phenomena of mind' in the broadest sense but we won't call them that because it would break a long-standing tradition. Even though we don't know their form, we know they are there because we experience their results (like we know rats are in the ceiling). Talking of unseen mental events might sound contradictory but we cannot exclude them. Phenomenology just says: 'We will look at the phenomena of mind.' There is nothing in that statement that says: 'And, by definition, there cannot be any hidden mental events which are not open to introspection.'

Every time there is a mental event qua glaringly obvious phenomenon of mind, something else must have happened in the brain's computational space to generate it but it is not a glaringly obvious phenomenon of mind; it is a hidden or covert phenomenon of mind. The hidden mental 'something' just is the effective agency in the causation of both observable human behavior and the experience of being human. It is information.

The phenomena of mind themselves give us the clue as to where we should be looking for their causes. Just as a visible plant constitutes evidence of hidden roots, those overt mental phenomena constitute direct evidence of the existence of something other than themselves, some hidden causative machinery of mind. This directly refutes crude dualism, which states that there are two utterly distinct kinds of substance, mind and matter, each requiring nothing more than itself in order to exist. As materialists, we don't believe that. We believe that the phenomena of mind do not exist in an ontological vacuum; that, in order to occur (as in 'be experienced'), they require a healthy, functioning brain. That is, they are directly the product of certain unseen activities whose basis rests fairly and squarely in the material realm. It is the information we cannot introspect that does the hard work of generating the experiences that we do introspect, namely, all those experiences of being a knowing, seeing, feeling, and hurting person. That is, we cannot introspect our informational state because we are composed of information, and the total experience of being something is generated by that information.

All that remains for psychiatry is to start to think of information as a material commodity. Turing, von Neumann, Shannon and the other great figures of the heroic age of informational theory defined the parameters of a theory of information qua commodity. Information itself is colorless, odorless, and tasteless but, from a theoretical point of view, its particular virtue is that it can be manipulated in a material switching device, such as the brain. It can be treated as a commodity that flows, like water flowing through a pipe, so the brain has no trouble manipulating it. As a commodity, information is malleable: it can be cut up, mixed and sent here and there before being reconstituted in its original or any other order.

At the same time, it also carries meaning which is the raw material of the phenomena that constitute our mental lives. Every perceptible mental event, every perception or experience, is a signal, a marker that something has already happened at the biological level of the manipulation of information in the brain; but the meaning carried by the information is not itself biological. Information as nerve impulses is very biological, but information as meaning is not: meaning is mental, a psychological state, and conscious experiences or mental phenomena signify that the meaning or knowledge state of the mind has just been changed. [A word of warning regarding the expression: "... the meaning carried by the information is not itself biological." Meaning is not an additional substance: I am not trying to sneak crude dualism in through the back door. The meaning of a volley of impulses just is the effect they have on the target organ. Information is a dual function element that bridges the gap between the physical and the mental]

So in order to graduate from protoscience to science, psychiatry has to stop worrying about gene sequences and focus on the reason patients come to us: because their experience of life is painful. It is our job as experts to explain to them why that is the case. Diving into the patient's brain biochemistry will never tell us why he is in pain; at best, it can only ever tell us that he is in pain (and even that would require a science fiction type of neuroscience). That is, brain biochemistry is the agency or mechanism of suffering, not the cause. The cause lies in the totality of the patient's life experiences, his beliefs, memories, hopes, and fears. Specifically, the cause of his mental distress lies in the total informational state which turns him into the unique person he is and not into somebody else. However, and unfortunately, he is blind to the pathogenic factors in that informational state; he can no more introspect them than he can introspect why he likes Italian sausages or how his heart races when he has to speak in public. What he experiences is distress but the causative level of his psychopathology is hidden from his view (OK, unconscious if you have to). How can we be so sure? Because if it were not hidden from view, he would fix it himself before his pain became overwhelming.

Be aware that I am talking about information at different levels. The first level is the level of neurons and neurotransmitters, of gene expression and epigenetic effects. This is the brain level, the level at which dumb data are harvested from the inner and outer worlds and pumped around the brain so they can be processed. This is information as Shannon characterized it. As the data are processed in dedicated brain structures, it generates a higher order informational space or virtual machine which is absolutely unique and private to the individual concerned. Part of that informational space is silent (hidden, not open to introspection) and very fast. This part, Chalmers' 'psychological mind', gives rise to observable behavior while the rest is used to generate another virtual space which constitutes the experience of being something ("There is something it is like to be..."). So information theory gives rise to the phenomenologists' Being; it throws a materialist loop around this most slippery but persistent notion of subjectivity as something real—but eternally private and, of course, mortal.

By this means, we arrive at a materialist theory of mind as real, natural, causally effective, and dualist, both externally (mind vs. body) and internally (causally effective and unreportable vs. causally ineffective and reportable). How can we talk about unreportable mental events? Strictly speaking, we can only guess at them but given the reportable events they trigger, we have a fair idea of the generic processes that must have happened at the meaning level to bring about just those particular mental events.

The job of the psychiatrist then is to interrogate the phenomena exactly as they are experienced by the patient himself, in order to understand the hidden processes (memories, beliefs, rules, fears etc) which, passively or actively kept outside the patient's awareness, are causally effective in his distress. This is the entire rationale for psychotherapy. The job of the therapist is to see the world through the patient's eyes, to get with and stay with the patient's distress in order to understand it from the inside. This is because an agitated person automatically looks outside for causes, the reason being that it is our nature, meaning that is our evolutionary heritage as primates. A frightened baboon does not wander off to sit alone on a rock and start to look for ticks in its fur. As soon as it hears an alarm call, its evolutionary heritage compels it to look outside itself, to scan its environment. Humans are no different. A jolt of fear from whatever cause forces us to look outside our selves, but the human self is a mental phenomenon. Therefore, "looking outside the self" may involve worrying about the heart or the bowel. Distressed people do not attempt to look back into the phenomena of distress; it is the therapist's task to turn them back from whatever feature external to the self they have seized upon, and search for the hidden cause of the fear state.

Once those processes are known and can be accepted by the patient ("brought to consciousness"), real change can take place. There is no prior reason to believe that the hidden processes are always sexual in nature, and convincing reasons to believe most of them are not. Drugs, of course, simply suppress the phenomena (of distress) which constitute the clues pointing to the destructive hidden elements. While the patient remains on medication, his distress is suppressed and so, therefore, is any incentive to examine himself in order to undertake personal change. Unfortunately, drugs are not selective in what they suppress; so, while the patient may be satisfied with his newfound chemical equanimity, it is at a terrible price to his growth and life experiences as a person. While it is possible that more selective drugs with fewer side effects will eventually be found, they can never be any more than stop-gap measures. They suppress distress after the psychological matters have caused it, not before. For obvious reasons, drugs will never be able to act on individual beliefs or other personality factors: drugs cannot selectively eradicate the damaging elements of the total belief system.

Biological psychiatry was ideologically committed to a biological solution to the mind-body problem but that was facile. The concept of information is the only conceivable means of joining the phenomena of mind to their physical substrate, the brain. Reductionist biology cannot solve an informational problem because biology is already one level below the causative level of mental phenomena. Only an informational theory can explain that level.

5.5: Conclusion: The Reality of Mind

Some parts of the rambling, shambling institution of orthodox psychiatry are slowly realizing that their headlong rush into biology is not producing the results they hoped for. In fact, as the former editor of the *American Journal of Psychiatry* has noted, it is starting to have major, unexpected, adverse side effects. Three decades ago, when our leaders opted for a biological psychiatry, they forgot to follow Sagan's version of Popper's injunction: to submit their idea to stringent testing, to try to test it to destruction. It did not occur to them to question the idea that mind is directly reducible to brain because, as doctors, they were raised on a diet of biological reductionism. To them, it was second nature but, to any ordinary citizen, including many of the extra-ordinary citizens who live in philosophy departments, the idea of mind-brain reductionism is deeply counter-intuitive. Of course, that by itself proves nothing; as Dennett has said, the true theory of mind is likely to be counter-intuitive just because we've tried all the obvious ones.

Don't forget that psychiatrists didn't opt for biological reductionism just because it was novel and untried (it had certainly been tried by philosophers—and discarded), they chose it because they couldn't conceive of anything else. Behaviorism had failed; mentalism as psychoanalysis had failed; dualism was anathema as it smacked of the supernatural; that really only left biological reductionism (just quietly, part of the appeal of reductionism was that it left room for the religious soul; if mental illness was a bodily fault, it left the soul untainted, which was very handy for those who believed souls were created perfectly in heaven). In fact, the rationale doesn't matter: regardless of the reason for choosing biological reductionism, psychiatry's first task was to submit it to the most intensive criticism, a task which would normally have fallen to—guess who? The editors of the major journals. Well, that didn't happen. There was no debate. We went to bed one night as good little Freudians (in the US) or good little eclectics (everywhere else) and woke up as shock troops in the war of biology against the rest. If it sounds Orwellian, it was, and still is. Biological psychiatry is dominant only because of a passive conspiracy of the well-meaning to pretend that all the troops are happy, that there is no muttering in the ranks and that it is only a matter of time (and a few squillion dollars, if you don't mind) until the tough nut of mental disorder suddenly cracks open under all the big guns blazing at it.

Talking of nuts, they just stumble along in the rear, totally shell-shocked. Plus ça change, plus c'est la même chose.

The whole biological exercise was fantasy, pure wishful thinking. It would have fallen in a heap at the first sign of the blow-torch of self-criticism but group thinking took over. What should have been self-critical analysis became a conspiracy of the like-minded, a rat race to the top of the academic pile where fast-talkers can pole vault over the sluggards by pulling a huge research grant out of their pockets, and research grants are only given to randomized, double-blind, cross-over, multi-center trials of drugs that are likely to make fortunes, just because the grants committees can understand that particular jargon better than they can talk of using meaningful relationships to rectify emotional deprivation (that sort of talk embarrasses them anyway). The fantastic edifice of biologism stays in place only because nobody questions it. Trouble is, medical students are starting to question it. That's why they are avoiding psychiatry as a profession.

When now we submit the basic ideas of biological psychiatry to a "ruthlessly sceptical scrutiny", as should have been done thirty years ago, all the "deep nonsense" is blown away, leaving just… nothing. It has no deep truths. Realizing this, Andreasen and others proposed we go back to our phenomenological roots but that was just a case of clutching at an old security blanket. Psychiatry needs a model of mind before it can have a model of mental disorder, and phenomenology is only a description of mind, not a model of mind. However, handled properly, it leads to a realization that we can postulate an unseen machinery of mind (because that is what a model is) based on what we know of the experienced mind. What we know is what we get, the glittering realm of phenomena or experiences of mind to which we all have immediate access. Each of these experiences is a marker of something that took place in the very fast and unseen realm of the computational or decision-making mind that runs on the biological substrate of the brain. Just as, in the real world, a sound means 'something just happened' (Schopenhauer's Principle of Sufficient Reason: 'Nothing is without a reason'), so too in the inner, private but still real world of the mind, the perception of a sound means that there has been a lot of activity at the informational level. There has to be: if there were not, if sounds just popped up for no reason, then our experiences would bear no relationship to the external world and we would all die.

The unseen causative level of the mind is a real thing; it's just that it's out of sight. Because there is no mechanism of perceiving this level, we can only intuit it but that's good enough. Similarly, just because we can't pin it on a cutting table doesn't mean it isn't real. I can't pin my computer's programs on a cutting table, either, but they are very real. Information, as Claude Shannon showed nearly seventy-five years ago, is a very real thing. Seventy-five years is long enough for psychiatry to stop chasing dinosaurs and catch up with the real world.

At this point, readers who are doing their duty by submitting these ideas to a "ruthlessly sceptical scrutiny" will have two reasons to object. Firstly, all this talk of mental phenomena might imply an Observer to experience them. That is not the case. Observers lead to infinite regresses, which are lethal to any serious model of mind. The sense of self arises out of the totality of the phenomena: the experienced mind is no more than its sum total of experiences. Take away the experiences and there is nothing, only coma. We are not able to perceive 'mind devoid of phenomena' because if we take away all the perceptions, all that is left in the head is the unseen or silent workings of the hidden machinery of mind, i.e. a clear account of the zombies that are so popular with some philosophers. This means that pure consciousness and all of those other marketing ploys of the mysticism industry are logically impossible.

The second point derives from our understanding of evolution. Evolutionary theory, as we understand it today, argues powerfully against the idea of an organ or behaviour having no functional role in the overall economy of the organism. Thus, if the phenomena of mind have no causal significance, why do they persist? I do not have a definite answer that will convince the hostile critic. I can only suggest that humans are not alone in having minds; that everything we know about mammals and most other animals suggests they too have experiences of the world; that being a bird is not like being a lump of wood. On the other hand, I would say mosquitoes have no inner life; that their very few neurons are totally committed to keeping them in the air and finding food and mates. I doubt they have any more perception than a flower does. There are clever philosophers who like to equate mental life with organization, which leads them to claim that rocks, which have an organized crystalline structure, therefore have some sort of mental life. Unfortunately for them, organization is not enough. Mental life depends on the processing of information; it depends on a doing, and rocks, which are a little bit rocky inside, don't actually do anything. So much for panpsychism, but I should return to the actual question: why an inner life?

I can only suggest the experiential realm plays a critically important part in the functional mechanism of mind. My suggestion, for what it is worth, is that it constitutes the entry point to memory; that the incoming information has to be in a certain form before it can access the memory function and that form just happens to be the form of phenomena. By the physiological process of attending to something, a mental phenomenon is generated which alone is able to activate the memory function. However, just as most sperm don't result in a pregnancy, most phenomena don't result in a memory; otherwise our heads would be so big we would need wheelbarrows to carry them.

* Mr Gorbachev didn't set out to destroy communism, he just wanted to make it work better and thought that injecting a bit of choice would do the job; to his dismay, he found that, given a choice, the people dumped communism.

6	# The DSM-V Project: From Bad Science to Bad Psychiatry

"I do not feel obliged to believe that the same God, who has endowed us with sense, reason, and intellect, has intended us to forego their use."

Galileo

6.1: Introduction

Looking at the different sciences throughout history, it is probably fair to say that systems of classification have tended to generate intense feelings, and psychiatry is no exception. I have previously argued that the categorical system of diagnosis, as seen in DSM-IV, is so seriously flawed that it cannot be improved without abandoning the basic precepts upon which it is constructed [1]. With the projected revisions of the nosology, the psychiatric establishment has a rare opportunity to rectify its errors by enacting a number of major changes to the concept of psychiatric diagnosis.

The project to replace DSM-IV [2] has been underway for more than ten years, involving 600 researchers, as well as unknown numbers of support and other staff. It has cost tens of millions of dollars already and yet the field trials—the largest, most complex, and most expensive part—are still to come. It is undoubtedly the largest single project in the history of psychiatry, dominating the profession's thinking to an extent rarely, if ever, seen in other fields of nosology. Nonetheless, the launch date has been pushed back and back and is currently thought to be some time in 2014. Its progress has been marked by unprecedented controversy, with the chairmen of both the DSM-III and the DSM-IV Task Forces voicing stringent criticism of their successors [3]. There is no reason to believe that the DSM-V committee has any intention of revolutionary changes to its charge: it will be a case of evolution toward the same goal rather than revolution toward another.

In this paper, I will argue that this enormous project is entirely the wrong project for psychiatry at this stage of its development and that the precious resources it consumes should be directed elsewhere. Notwithstanding, even if it were the right project, it would still be wasted effort because its inherent errors mean it is doomed to failure. DSM-V cannot achieve its basic goal of a further "... seminal contribution to patient care and to the scientific study of psychiatric disorders by providing rigorous and reliable diagnostic criteria for (psychiatric) conditions" [4]. Instead, it will continue the process of damaging psychiatry and reducing its importance in the world of mental health, to the point where it becomes a commodity and psychiatrists themselves become irrelevant.

In the first place, I will examine some of the thinking behind the central idea in DSM-V, that separate categories of mental disorder can validly and reliably be distinguished from normality and from each other. I will show that this is wrong in principle, that it cannot be realized in practice, and that it puts the diagnostic cart before the causative horse. Next, using one of the new diagnostic categories, I will show that it is impossible in practice.

6.2: "What is a Mental/Psychiatric Disorder? From DSM-IV to DSM-V"

The heading above is the title of a recent editorial in Psychological Medicine, which outlines some of the DSM-V Task Force's thinking on defining mental disorder [4]. The notion that mental disorder and mental normality are not just of a different nature, but are incompatible (i.e. a person cannot be mentally normal and mentally disordered at the same time), is fundamental to the DSM project. Thus, if mental disorder cannot be defined sui generis, then the project cannot start. The subcommittee suggested the following criteria:

> A: A behavioral or psychological syndrome or pattern that occurs in an individual
> B: The consequences of which are clinically significant distress (e.g. a painful symptom) or disability (i.e. impairment in one or more important areas of functioning)
> C: Must not be merely an expectable response to common stressors and losses (e.g. the loss of a loved one) or a culturally sanctioned response to a particular event (e.g. trance states in religious rituals)
> D: That reflects an underlying psychobiological dysfunction
> E: That is not primarily a result of social deviance or conflicts with society

The first point to note is that, on any measure of human behavior, there are no categories of 'normality' and 'abnormality.' Regardless of the parameter under study, if every human in the world were scored on that parameter, there would be a continuous line from the most normal to the most abnormal. Not at any point would there be a clear, reliable and valid disjunction or discontinuity. Not even death is so clear that we can definitively operationalize its definition. In the field of mental disorder, which is murky and uncertain at best, this is even more true. No mental symptom of any sort can be taken as a certain indicator of mental disorder just because all symptoms grade imperceptibly from absent to florid. Moreover, taking any mental symptom at all, the milder degrees invariably have a wide range of causes which any sensible definition of mental disorder would and does exclude.

Sadness varies from the faintest ennui to a full-blown depressive psychosis in which the patient can do no more than sit mute in a corner, beyond speech, movement, appetite, and tears. Anxiety varies from the slightest frisson of apprehension to a raging panic attack in which the person is unable to move even to save his life. The drive to be tidy and orderly extends from a teenager's bedroom to a person who spends the whole day on his morning ablutions. Even apparently clear-cut psychotic symptoms vary widely, depending on the context (going to sleep or waking, drugs, illness, fear states, loneliness, etc.), the culture and even the subject's wishes (ecstatic religions). Previous editions of the DSM have recognized this by including references to "marked" distress or "clinical significance." That is to say, there are no categories in nature, so any attempt to impose them is artificial.

The DSM-V Working Group recognizes this but seems to think that, because general medicine sometimes has difficulties with categorical diagnoses (e.g. malignant vs. premalignant), it does not reflect badly on psychiatry if it has the same problem:

> Other considerations:
> H: No definition perfectly specifies precise boundaries for the concept of either 'medical disorder' or 'mental/psychiatric disorder.'

There is, however, a vast difference between occasional, transient problems with minutely-defined boundaries in some fields of medicine, compared with the total absence of anything like the most basic concept of a boundary-marker in any of the areas in psychiatry since the beginning of its days. It is the concept of a boundary that is lacking in mental life, as the Committee implicitly acknowledges with its new category of 'Mixed Anxiety Depression'.

We can look at each of the criteria in turn:

6.2 A: A behavioral or psychological syndrome or pattern that occurs in an individual...

This is largely meaningless. In this context, behavioral and psychological are largely interchangeable. The "syndrome or pattern" imposes the requirement that the practitioner find an order in the disturbance, mostly by standing back from the patient and seeing him, not as an individual, but as "yet another example of this condition." It invites the practitioner to elide differences, to overlook the person's individuality, and homogenize his life, so that he matches the simplified model. Yet, this presupposes a utility in this action, specifically a search for common causes in the disorder. That is, from the outset, the psychiatrist must stop seeing his patients as the products of vastly complex and utterly unique psychological careers, the only feasible justification being that the patient's life experiences are not relevant. This automatically implies that mental disorder is not and cannot be psychological in nature. It has to be biological, since this is the only human commonality of sufficient scope to swamp the individuality. So at the outset, DSM-V begs a critically important question of the nature of mental disorder, irremediably biasing all that follows. On this basis alone, I would say that the DSM project is not scientific, but its proponents would plead a second chance.

6.2 B: The consequences of which are clinically significant distress (e.g. a painful symptom) or disability (i.e. impairment in one or more important areas of functioning)

Immediately, we run into the pseudo-objective nature of the DSM project. We cannot define 'clinically significant' in any reliable or objective sense. The criterion is sufficiently elastic to allow for anxious people declaring themselves significantly distressed or clinicians declaring psychotic people 'disabled', even when they disagree. Like beauty, clinical significance is in the eye of the beholder. It is influenced by the patient's wealth and social status, the psychiatrist's interests, the insurer's demands, and other matters such as war, disaster etc.

6.2 C: Must not be merely an expectable response to common stressors and losses (e.g. the loss of a loved one) or a culturally sanctioned response to a particular event (e.g. trance states in religious rituals)...

This is an implicit admission that the notion of the biological basis of categories of mental disorder is spurious. It says that symptoms will be labeled as mental disorder or normality not by their nature or content but according to their social context. This argument has been elaborated at great and, to my mind, entirely convincing length by Horwitz and Wakefield [5] in their elegant monograph on the transmogrification of normal sadness into depressive illness.

6.2 D: That reflects an underlying psychobiological dysfunction...

This is either truism or ideology or, more likely, garbled thinking. It is truism in the sense that, if observable and experienced mental disorder has a cause in the natural realm, then it is going to be somewhere in the psychological and biological spheres, just because there aren't any others. However, I think the authors clearly had something else in mind.

The authors do not define 'psychobiology', but imply that a form or kind of mental-biological reductionism is the correct explanation of mind: "There is a growing awareness of the extent to which all behavior and psychology are dependent upon brain processes..." [4, p. 5]. I am not aware of any serious thinker in the field of human affairs who believes that human psychology is not somehow crucially dependent on the intact, functional brain, the only interesting question being the precise nature of that mind-brain relationship. They continue: "... and the extent to which brain changes have complex behavioral and psychological effects." This preempts the vital question by ignoring the option that psychological changes also have complex effects on the brain: I decide to lift my arm and, behold, it elevates. These days, does any educated person hold that the desire was not somehow causative of the action? Using what Dennett [6] scornfully calls the 'intuition pump', the authors artfully lead the reader away from mind-body causation, down the path of mind-brain reductionism. When one looks at the qualifications of the authors of this particular paper, it is incomprehensible that they should have elected to imply that they know the answer to the nature of mind-body interaction. They do not mention that biological reductionism has been shown to be unworkable in principle [7] and advocating it in this deceptive manner is ideology, not science.

However, the authors further cloud the matter by bringing the psychological back into the equation: "The term 'psychobiological' emphasizes the extent to which these different types and levels (behavioral, psychological, or biological) of dysfunction are intertwined in reality..." [4, p. 5]. With the mental set they have previously established, i.e. mind-body reductionism, this is meaningless. It is not possible to state that "... all behavior and psychology are dependent upon brain processes..." in the implied context of reductionism and then say that psychological matters can also be causative of mental disorder. I suggest that this is just garbled thinking caused by an implicit ideological commitment to biological reductionism.

6.2 E: That is not primarily a result of social deviance or conflicts with society.

In combination with Criteria C (not your usual upsets) and D (psycho-biological dysfunction), this authorizes the DSM committee to name anything they like as a mental disorder and exclude anything else. If a woman becomes distressed to the point of being nonfunctional because she does not want a road bulldozed through her house, she is not thereby mentally ill because she is showing an expectable response to conflict with society. A boy who hates school and wants only to leave and get a job in the bush can be deemed either mentally ill (white middleclass) or socially deviant (poor black). Some behavior was first mental illness, then social deviance, then a harmless eccentricity, and finally, a perfectly legitimate lifestyle choice (homosexual conduct).

6.3: DSM-V is a Bad Answer to the Wrong Question

I conclude that the criteria for mental illness as developed by the DSM-V Committee are incapable of generating a science of mental disorder. They are, in fact, pseudoscience. The reason they failed is just because there is no articulated scientific model of mental disorder which, ab initio, dictates the borders and contents of mental disorder. Trying to derive a classification of mental disorder when we don't even have a model of how it arises is totally back to front.

Some people might object to this gloomy conclusion by pointing to the success of the Linnaean system of classification in biology. Prior to the work of Carl Linnaeus (1707-78), biology was largely an incoherent mess. There were many systems of classification in use but they were often idiosyncratic or based on misperceptions, e.g. dolphins and whales were normally grouped with the fish. It is not, however, the case that Linnaeus boldly imposed Man's civilizing vision on nature's unruly array, bringing order to a "blooming, buzzing confusion". Rather, he chanced upon the supremely elegant innate system of speciation that had evolved throughout a billion years of life. Linnaeus' binomial system firmly established the principle of classification according to relationships. The reason it succeeded was not because it drew lines in the sand and issued fiats, but because it faithfully followed the biological fact of evolution of species. That was Linnaeus' good fortune because, at that stage, he knew nothing of the mechanism of speciation. There had been many equally intelligent and diligent thinkers before him who didn't quite stumble upon the correct model; so biology students today are taught the Linnaean system, not the Baconian or the Stensenian (after Niels Stensen, aka Nicolaus Stenonis). His example is similar to Mendeleev's monumental work on the Periodic Table. He did not draw boxes on a piece of paper and shove elements in them because they looked artistic but, by careful attention to the phenomena of the elements, he found the natural order which the (then unknown) atomic model imposed on them.

In psychiatry, we are still in a pre-Linnaean phase of trying to impose a preconception on the bewildering complexity of human mental disorder, the preconception being that mental disorder must be categorically distributed. In turn, this Procrustean exercise is impelled by the belief that each and every separate mental disorder must have a unique and discoverable, non-mental cause, which is another name for the biological model. That is, the DSM nosology of mental disorder is driven by the need to find a series of specific, internally uniform clinical pictures as the surface manifestation of specific unseen biochemical lesions. I have no argument with the idea that this obsessive drive for etiological neatness results from psychiatry's near-death experience with the Byzantine folly of psychoanalysis, but it is actually the wrong way to approach science. The proper way to conduct science is to find the model and then see what nosology it dictates. Biochemistry is a good example, as is the germ theory of illness. Somewhat further afield, aberrations of planetary motion told astronomers using the Copernican model of the solar system where to look for new planets. That could never have happened with the geocentric model.

Therefore, at this stage of its intellectual development, the correct project for psychiatry is to decide the question of the nature of mental disorder: is it biological or psychological? By answering the question of whether mental disorder is psychological or biological, we will ipso facto answer the question of whether the final nosology of mental disorder will be categorical or dimensional in form. Even though the Committee has not overtly embraced the reductionist, biological model of mental disorder, they have shifted the focus of thinking by implication. Early in the paper, they debate the correct terminology for the subject matter of psychiatry: "'Mental' implies a Cartesian view of the mind–body problem, that mind and brain are separable and entirely distinct realms, an approach that is inconsistent with modern philosophical and neuroscientific views" [4, p. 2]. Without specifying their stance, they clearly imply that mind-body dualism is not scientific. This stance is completely unsupported by the literature, by philosophers, and by psychiatrists. The philosopher David Chalmers [8] has outlined in great detail a convincing case for a rational dualism. My own work has shown that reductionism cannot be a model for psychiatry [9] and that the monist philosophers Daniel Dennett and John Searle have failed to establish their case [7]. The claim that a scientific model of mind must meld or unite mind and body is absolutely without warrant. Given the process Stein and his group have undertaken, of setting the intellectual tone, as it were, of the scientific status of psychiatric theorizing, this is intellectually dishonest. Their duty was to explore the options, not announce ex vacuo that the competition between psychological and biological models was over.

If it emerges that the correct model of mental disorder is psychological in nature, and I have argued at length that it is (2007, 2009), then the categorical system of DSM diagnosis will disappear as quickly as the psychoanalytic model did. Until this question is determined, openly and honestly, we are simply engaged in a vastly expensive exercise of drawing boxes in the sand, then watching impotently as the social winds blow them away. But who would want a categorical system of diagnosis in psychiatry? Only those psychiatrists who have decided that mental disorder is biological in nature, i.e. ideologues who are not prepared to debate the nature of mental disorder just in case they lose. When we consider the industries, both academic and commercial, involved in this debate, as well as the stupefying sums of money, questions over the true nature of mental disorder should not be brushed aside by a committee representing those vested interests who stand to lose most from an unfavorable outcome.

6.4: DSM-V will Lead to Worse Psychiatry, not Better

Anybody who goes to a psychiatric convention will be familiar with the 'keynote' speeches where eminent psychiatrists trumpet the rapid advances psychiatry has made since the dawn of the modern era, more or less since the publication of DSM-III in 1980. Thirty years of rapid scientific progress, they boldly declaim, have brought us to the brink of a complete understanding of mental disorder. However, growing numbers of perfectly sensible psychiatrists are starting to wonder where the progress is, and why we have been hearing the same bravura speeches for three decades. In particular, young psychiatrists and trainees are beginning to question what, to them, sounds suspiciously like propaganda. DSM-V, however, promises to propel psychiatry into a field which is normal for all other fields of medicine but which, for us, has been nothing more than a vague dream: prevention. Specifically, it offers the hope of preventing the most devastating illness of all, schizophrenia. If so, it would be a dramatic transformation of the practice of psychiatry, and of its status in medicine, and a vindication of those who first dreamed of a rational biology of mental disorder.

One of the most important innovations in DSM-V is the concept of the person who is 'at-risk' of developing a psychotic disorder. Initially, the

DSM-V Development Site defined the concept of the Psychosis Risk Syndrome but, on May 17th 2010, this name changed to Attenuated Psychotic Symptoms Syndrome (APSS). The diagnostic criteria did not change. The purpose of the new category of mental disorder is to identify people with a significantly increased risk of a psychotic breakdown, offering early psychiatric intervention to prevent the appearance of the full syndrome. This represents a substantial shift in emphasis from the traditional role of psychiatrists, which was to wait within their hospitals until floridly-disturbed people were brought in by their relatives, their friends, or the police. There are several reasons for paying attention to the prodromal symptoms of psychosis. The first would be to prevent the huge dislocation of life which accompanies a psychotic episode. The second would be the recognition that drugs are not magic; they are expensive, unpleasant, have many side effects, and offer no more than partial remission under long-term supervision with no prospect of cure. Finally, there have been several theoretical developments that indicate the possibility of greater precision in identifying people at risk of psychotic states.

The first of these points is beyond question. A psychotic disorder shatters the lives of not just the patient but even of family and friends. The second point, that the available drugs are nasty, toxic, relatively ineffective, and outrageously expensive, might be disputed in public but not in private. The third is open to debate but one recent development is seen as offering much greater precision in identifying people at risk. The notion of the endophenotype was introduced to psychiatry from insect biology [10]. Researchers screen psychotic people for any sort of abnormality that might be taken as a biological marker of the genetic tendency to the psychotic state, to apply to people who have not developed a mental illness. Thus, if square thumbs were more common in psychotic people and clustered in their families, then screening the population for square thumbs may yield people with a high genetic risk of psychosis. As yet, there are no such reliable indicators but researchers remain hopeful and considerable sums of money are available for this, the most recent development in genetic research of psychosis.

While the concept of the 'At-Risk' individual is still being debated and is far from consensus, there are powerful constituencies arrayed behind it. The suggested criteria are as follows [2]:

> A: Characteristic symptoms: At least one of the following in attenuated form with intact reality testing, but of sufficient severity and/or frequency so as to be beyond normal variation; (i) Delusions (ii) Hallucinations (iii) Disorganized Speech.
> B: Frequency/Currency: Symptoms meeting Criterion A must be present in the past month and occur at an average frequency of at least once per week in the past month.
> C: Progression: Symptoms meeting Criterion A must have begun in or significantly worsened in the past year

D: Distress/Disability/Treatment seeking: Symptoms are sufficiently distressing and/or disabling to the patient and/or others to lead to help-seeking

E: Characteristic attenuated psychotic symptoms are not better explained by another DSM-V diagnosis, and...

F: Clinical criteria for any DSM-V psychotic disorder have never been met.

I believe this is a singularly dangerous idea and should be resisted strenuously by anybody who adopts a humanist stance. It is a case of psychiatry unleashed, and the benefits its planners hope to achieve can never outweigh the potential damage it will do. My case against this rubbery notion is that it is not and never can be scientific. In the rest of this section, I want to look at it in some detail, if not politely.

6.4.1: PRS is not science but is a case of value-judgments masquerading as science

Let's look at the definitions, taken from the official APA DSM-V Development website: (Please note that this site changes rapidly, the following material was available on May 14th 2010 and was changed on May 17th but the significance and purpose remain the same.)

6.4.1 a) "Characteristic symptoms (of PRS): At least one of the following in attenuated form with intact reality testing, but of sufficient severity and/or frequency so as to be beyond normal variation; (i) Delusions (ii) Hallucinations (iii) Disorganized speech."

This is completely self-contradictory. The definition of delusion is: 'A fixed, false belief out of context with the subject's cultural and intellectual background.' There is no room in this definition for 'normal variation', for 'attenuation', or for 'intact reality testing'. The whole point of saying a person has a delusion is that his belief is not just crazy (i.e. his 'reality testing' is not intact), but it cannot be budged (i.e. cannot be attenuated). That is, a delusion is of a nature which is always "beyond normal variation", so there can never be "mild" degrees of delusional belief. I am completely unable to attach any sense to the idea that there could be a "normal variation" of abnormal beliefs. That is like saying there could be a normal variation in the legal definition of theft, or there could be insignificant degrees of pregnancy; either you are, or you aren't.

If the DSM-V Committee wants to break down the boundaries to the idea of psychosis being an alien state, then they are attacking the very basis of the DSM project itself, namely the notion that there are distinct categories of mental disorder, separated from each other and from normality by virtue of their biological causation. Moreover, if we allow degrees of mad beliefs, then the door is wide open for prejudice to blunder through where only objective science should lightly tread.

Everything said so far also applies to hallucinations.

With "disorganized speech", we are treading on dangerous ground indeed. Have the members of the DSM-V Committee never read James Joyce? Did they actually listen to what Governor Palin was saying, as distinct from cheering because it sounded great? Have they never tried to find out from a socially anxious teenager why he doesn't want to go to the class party? Have they not read any of the francophone philosophers who are currently de rigueur in liberal universities throughout the US? What about the various CEOs of Big Banking currently appearing before the Senate inquiries? Christian leaders trying to justify the notion of a "just war"? Politicians trying to argue that we need to borrow our way out of a debt crisis? Fat cat communist leaders justifying their dictatorship of the elite in terms of the dictatorship of the proletariat? Religious fanatics justifying ghastly terrorist murders? Mangled speech, deceitful or self-serving speech, and disorganized speech are universal. Nobody can tell them apart.

For myself, I think anybody who uses expressions such as "sign up to", "wait up", or "made up for by" shows disorganized speech, but I accept my minority status. And that's without even starting on film stars who use the word 'like' sixteen times in a single sentence.

The notion that "disorganized speech" can reliably and validly distinguish between pre-psychosis and all other types of garbled talk is itself evidence of "disorganized thinking". There is no possible way the term can be operationalized objectively. It will simply license repression and dismissal of people who stutter or stumble over their speech. Agitated foreigners, frightened or guilt-ridden teenagers, minorities, hostile or defiant prisoners, the confused elderly, inarticulate country people, the intellectually handicapped, exotic religions, fringe political groups, people locked in mental hospitals against their will... The list is endless.

This is exactly what went on in the Soviet Union. Their diagnosis of "sluggish schizophrenia" was used to imprison dissidents in mental hospitals and pump them full of drugs or stun them with ECT until they simply could not argue. The definition was so loose that it could be used to detain anybody who objected to being detained but in fact, it wasn't used much, only against about three hundred persistent dissidents. In that sense, the proposed DSM changes are much worse, because they won't be used against the state's enemies, but against normal citizens. There will be no end to it.

This is worse than the Soviet Union, worse even than 1984. The idea that we should blur the borders of psychosis, throwing the net over more people, is bad science. As Kingsley Amis said, "More will mean worse."

Let's move to the second criterion:

6.4.1 b) Frequency/Currency: Symptoms meeting Criterion A must be present in the past month and occur at an average frequency of at least once per week in the past month.

In one month, a teenager must show one odd idea ("But how do you know we can't communicate with extra-terrestrials? It says so on the internet"), one odd experience ("I feel out of it"), and one episode of disorganized speech ("Um, it's like, I wouldn't, um, you know, like, can I...? No, forget it. I said forget it"), and bingo! Drugs for life.

I suggest that the people who devised this criterion have very little clinical experience. Five days a week, month after month, year in, year out, I would see a dozen people a day who would satisfy this requirement. They get better, without drugs.

Is it impertinent of me, one of the world's most isolated psychiatrists, to suggest that some of the most eminent psychiatrists in the world today have very little clinical experience? Not in the slightest. They don't. The reason they are researchers is just because they don't actually like clinical experience. They don't want to deal with difficult people; they want to reduce it all to a matter of checklists and prescriptions with monthly med-checks by junior doctors, with teams of nurses, psychologists, and social workers to clear up the messy bits. They want psychiatry standardized and homogenized, the rough edges smoothed down and the individuals bedded into their ready-made boxes. Researchers much prefer orderly conferences and meetings, tidy research seminars, and grant applications; they like civilized committees and university management workgroups, joint government-industry-academic task forces meeting in palatial surroundings, and all that. What they don't like doing is patiently explaining again to a frightened single mother that her 16-yo, 195-cm, 95-kg son (6'5", 210-lb) who works full-time in a metal workshop, is not going the way of his uncle just because he loses his temper and starts to yell that she is ruining his life when she tells him he can't go out with the other apprentices from work, and that the drugs which his uncle was given in a mental hospital twenty years ago, which made him sit peacefully under a tree, are neither necessary nor desirable.

Research psychiatrists don't like dirt under their fingernails. When it comes to dealing with difficult, scary, and/or dangerous patients, their opinions are not reliable.

Next requirement:

6.4.1 c) Progression: Symptoms meeting Criterion A must have begun in or significantly worsened in the past year;

This is meaningless. If you wait long enough, everything you don't like about your relatives gets worse. It does not offer any means of distinguishing between the alleged patient's alleged condition actually getting worse, and my tolerance getting thinner. It licenses the powerful to menace the disempowered.

So much for Criterion C. Shall we move on?

6.4.1 d) Distress/Disability/Treatment seeking: Symptoms are sufficiently distressing and/or disabling to the patient and/or others to lead to help-seeking.

Again, it is just a matter of value-judgment: the lady above, whom I saw yesterday, was becoming very panicky over her son's temper outbursts. She felt he was desperately in need of treatment; her counselor at the women's support center (who had never seen the boy) assured her he was in mortal danger. A quick phone call to his employer showed that they regarded him as their best apprentice. He never lost his temper at work; he could be entrusted with complex jobs and was keen, cheerful, and quick to learn. He only lost his temper at home when his mother, who was a terribly anxious person, tried to make him hurry into the shower or stop talking to his friends on his mobile (cell phone) because it was late and wasted money (with his plan, calls were free after 10.00 pm).

Again, we have the problem that this entire notion legitimizes the idea that somebody can deem a person mentally ill, regardless of what the person himself believes. When a man believes he is Jesus Christ and wants to walk across Niagara Falls to prove it, there may be a case, but stroppy teenagers? Sure, I agree, it would be easier if they were all mentally ill; that way we wouldn't have to reason with them, just say: "Have you had your tablets today, dear?" Oh, that already happens?

Well, not in our home.

Last two:

6.4.1 e) Characteristic attenuated psychotic symptoms are not better explained by another DSM-V diagnosis, and...

6.4.1 f) Clinical criteria for any DSM-V psychotic disorder have never been met.

"Characteristic attenuated psychotic symptoms"—As soon as I saw it, I fell in love with this expression. It sounds so... I don't know, so with it, so punchy. Before long, they'll be known among the in crowd as CAPS: "Oh, his CAPS are up today, we'll have to retitrate his psycholeptics." It conveys that powerful sense of clinical certainty that we all lust for, it seems to lift the user above wishy-washy impressionism ("I don't really know, Mrs. Smith, he could be just a bit anxious, you know, maybe a bit of normal teenage depersonalization or something. Let's just wait and see...") to the exalted status of Somebody With Authority Who Knows About These Things:

> "You don't have to worry, dear, the doctor said he knows what's wrong with you..."
>
> "There's nothin' wrong with me, he's a f....g idiot!"
>
> "Don't be like that, they're only trying to help. They said they've got some tablets that will help you. Same as your uncle."
>
> "I'm not takin' their f...g rat poison! Anyway, what good did it do for him? He strung himself up in the end. Some life, poor bastard snuffed it in the bog in the nuthouse."
>
> "Yes, but they did try. Shh, here comes the doctor, he's got some forms for me to sign..."
>
> "I ain't stayin' in this f....g madhouse, I'm gettin' outa here. Lemme go, you dumb f..ker, stop twisting my arm. Mum, they're holding me down, help me..."

Characteristic symptoms: one thing 35 years of psychiatry has taught me is that there is very little characteristic about psychotic symptoms. Our experts on the DSM-V Committee may beg to differ: "What are you talking about?" they may scoff. "Psychosis is a pushover. It's dead easy to decide when a person is mad. Just give him this questionnaire and it will answer everything you need to know."

Would that it were so easy: what seems crazy to one person makes perfect sense to the next, even on so mundane a matter as politics. What is normal in one culture is lunacy in the next, especially if you bring religion into the equation; what seems cuckoo to one generation is hot fashion to their children. The only way a questionnaire can solve questions of psychiatry is by dumbing down the questions to the point where nobody can get them wrong. Except those who are smart or fluent enough to hide their experiences, while the poor little anxious kid who doesn't want to upset the doctor will answer everything in great detail, steadily digging a hole for himself as he goes.

Attenuated: it means watered-down, weakened, not the real thing. It means maybe, could be, might be, but it also and necessarily means could be wrong, or might not be. So, instead of what used to be called 'masterly inaction' or 'adopting a waiting brief', meaning a matter of knowing when to sit on your hands and wait for nature to declare itself, the psychiatrists rush in firing on all drugs. How many of these symptoms would turn out to be not psychotic in nature? My experience is that the great majority would be of no lasting significance, or might indicate some other disorder, such as anxiety. Some surveys report a misdiagnosis rate of up to 85% with some major questionnaires. That is worse than useless. Useless means 'of no help one way or the other,' meaning 50% error rate. An 85% error rate is far worse than useless.

There's no escape. If you miss out on a diagnosis on the way in (i.e. the so-called 'attenuated psychotic symptoms' aren't better explained by another DSM-V diagnosis), then we'll get you on the way out with a new one called "You look a bit crazy to me." (Purely as a historical note, I prefer the expression "My word, you do look queer." This was the title of a song by the inestimable Stanley Holloway. In the song, a young chap was told by a lot of people that he didn't look well, until he started to feel unwell but, these days, people don't like being called queer). And just remember: if a young person decides to leave a very restrictive religious group, his parents will be able to find a psychiatrist in the group who will earnestly believe that anybody who wants to leave it must be crazy—and will have the diagnostic label to prove it. A young Muslim girl who doesn't want to be clothed head to foot in a burqa, or who resists infundibulation (genital mutilation), would obviously be in an early stage of psychosis; as would be a Hindu man who didn't want to enter an arranged marriage. And what about healthy young Russian men who don't want to be conscripted? (You would need to know how bad the Russian army is to understand this.)

Don't forget that psychosis offers a third path between normality and wickedness. It allows punishment without the same level of hatred. It allows parents to say, "Oh yes, she does those dreadful things but she's not a bad girl, just sick." If she were a bad girl, it would obviously reflect on the parents themselves; biological disorders spare the parental guilt, which is doubly helpful when they are paying the psychiatrist's bills.

The diagnosis of Psychotic Risk Syndrome exponentially enlarges the possibilities for social and political repression.

6.4.2: The idea of an "at-risk" person will spread to all other psychiatric diagnoses

As soon as the diagnosis of PRS is established by fiat of the DSM-V Committee, then its advocates will immediately start trumpeting how beneficial it is, how it is saving so many lives and careers. They have to: they can't possibly say, "Sorry folks, we goofed. The concept can't be operationalized." Schools will pressure parents; prisons will pressure inmates to take drugs for an early release; families will pressure general practitioners; while psychologists will pressure everybody to be given the right to prescribe drugs. The numbers of people on psychotropic drugs will easily treble by 2025, if not much sooner, and drug company sales will go through the roof.

There is, however, a further risk: we will quickly have a revised DSM-V (DSM-V-TR) which will formally establish the notion of a blurred borderland, an anxious antechamber, for all psychiatric diagnoses. The people who brought you Bipolar Affective Disorder will not stand idly by while their target population is eroded by the trendy new diagnosis of PRS, they will want their own. So we will have BADRS, followed in rapid succession by PBDRS (pediatric bipolar disorder risk syndrome, for the children of hopeless parents, so that the diagnosis of PBD can jump by another 8,000% to match the last twenty years), ADD/ADHDRS (if your brother managed to get himself on dexies at school), Substance Abuse RS (if your old man is a drunk), MDRS (in case your dumb mother got depressed over staying married to a drunk), OCDRS (so don't line up your favorite toys before you go to bed so you can see them in the nightlight, little boy), and the crème de la crème of psychiatric diagnoses, the most protean, the most slippery and least provable of all (... drum roll): PDRS.

Personality Disorder Risk Syndrome

Oh boy, can you see the scope of this one? The swarms of psychologists standardizing their questionnaires so they can collect their newly minted PhDs, the probation officers with their check lists, the school teachers moving silently around the hushed and frightened classrooms, chuckling knowingly to themselves as they rustle through the pages of The Teacher's Handbook for Uncovering Personality Disorders in the Under-Fives, the social workers writing reports for courts, the employers smirking as they selectively dismiss the unionists, the insurance companies choosing who they want to insure...

Don't laugh. It's coming to a practice near you, and you might be the first on your block. Your cell block.

6.4.3: There are not enough psychiatrists to administer the newly-widened diagnoses

It is not widely known, but psychiatrists are actually fading out. In Australia, we do not graduate enough doctors for our ordinary needs, so we have to import them (which leaves India and Africa a bit bare, but never mind). Moreover, today's medical students think psychiatry is a bit of a dead loss, so they are not enrolling in the training courses. Those who do are more likely to be older practitioners changing career after having a family, women wanting to work part-time, foreign graduates who see it as an easy path to permanent residency, or clean-cut young men who want administrative or research posts or the well-paying fields of 9-5 office-based insurance psychiatry. Increasingly, psychiatrists are weary people in late middle age who work three sedate sessions a week at a community mental health center and spend the rest of the time in training sessions, committee meetings, clinical meetings, at conferences, or writing research papers showing how more mentally-disturbed patients could be farmed out to general practitioners and psychologists. Private psychiatrists, if you can afford one, have a three- to six-month waiting list.

Your old-fashioned "bin doctors" are a dying breed, the psychiatrists who actually went in on weekends to see people brought in by overworked police or who did ward rounds in the emergency department on Sunday mornings to try to sort out the epidemic of Saturday night overdoses. In a few years, they won't exist. I see 60-80 patients a week, 48 weeks a year. They are bulk-billed patients, meaning people who can't afford private rates, such as manual workers, pensioners, students, young parents, probationers, the chronically mentally ill, and the unemployed. As such, I am a rarity, an anachronism, a figure of mirth, a second rate loser who can't make it in the cut and thrust of academia (just ask my colleagues). When I leave, retire or drop dead, nobody will take my place.

The new diagnostic category of Psychosis Risk Syndrome will mean that psychiatrists will need to screen something like three times more teenagers and young adults than the few who can be seen now. If we add the BADRS and all the others which are certain to follow in DSM-V-TR (due about 2015, I'd say), then psychiatrists will do nothing but screen patients. They will not have time to treat. And all this at a time of impending crisis, as the average age of psychiatrists rises and the numbers of new, young, full-time graduates plummets. So in very short time, the job of screening people for the new disorders will be assigned to people with much less training and experience.

Psychologists, general practitioners, and nurses will be first in line with their clipboards and their questionnaires, closely followed by social workers, school teachers, probation officers, sundry counselors at the many crisis centers and refuges that are springing up, school guidance officers, welfare workers, drug and alcohol counselors, field workers of all kinds, disability support staff, summer camp staff, churches, marriage guidance staff (of course), Uncle Tom Cobley and all. The problem is that if we breach the wall and give the right to one group, the rest will immediately start clamoring and ringing their parliamentarians or congressmen so they can have the right, too. They will say, "It's all or none," but no public official will be able to say: "OK, if that's how you want it, we'll settle for none." They will fudge the matter, as they do with any contentious issue, because the need to be re-elected always trumps science. Soon, we will have armies of well-meaning (read: bossy) people fanning out across the countryside, into every housing estate, school, prison, scout group, church, army base, everything; all of them desperate to prove their worth in finding the elusive At-Risk Child (teenager, prisoner, recruit, you name it). And if the child or prisoner protests, well that proves he is At Risk, because lack of insight is a cardinal psychotic symptom.

In short order, there will be a backlog of patients awaiting review by a psychiatrist for their PRS. Notice how the label sticks. A person who has been referred is no longer somebody who is waiting to find out whether he has a disorder, but he is going to have it confirmed and officially approved. This is not fantasy, it happens regularly. I see a person who has been referred from an agency with the suggestion he "is ADHD" or he "is Bipolar" (we used to be able to say "He is schizophrenic", meaning "He is a person living with schizophrenia", just as "I am Australian" means "I am a person with Australian citizenship." These days, we're not allowed to, as it has become pejorative, but everybody says, "I'm ADHD," or "my brother's Asperger's"). If perchance I decline to confirm the young psychologist's diagnosis (made with the Beck Depression Inventory or the PANSS, or the SCID or whatever questionnaire she found in a book), then I can expect a hostile phone call: "But the BDI said he has extreme clinical depression, you can't..."

"Lady," say I, patient to the last, "there is no such thing as clinical depression. The expression was made up by the Women's Weekly in 1997 and is kept alive by Neighbors. Secondly, he doesn't have extreme anything. The word 'extreme' means 'at the limits of human experience, the point beyond which there is no return.' If he had extreme depression, he would be lying on the floor in a pool of urine and feces, unable to eat, drink, or speak. This man is fairly cheerful. He likes his job and is planning a holiday. He loses his temper at work because of two idiots who don't do any work but they blame him when things go wrong, and then he feels guilty. We can deal with that in psychotherapy. He does not need antidepressants, antipsychotics, or the so-called mood stabilizers, admission to hospital, or ECT. He is safe to have a truck driver's license and a firearms license."

"Well," she says tartly, "we'll see about that."

If PRS is given the seal of approval, there will be a slight pause, then there will be a tidal wave of pressure from psychologists and nurses who will demand to be given the right to diagnose people (with their simplified DSM-IV check lists, they more or less have that now) and then to treat them themselves, without the unnecessary delay of seeing a psychiatrist. Starting in the provinces (such as where I live and work), then in the prisons, then in the Aboriginal communities, they will get it. The reason they will get it was cast in the diagnosis when it was poured in the squabbling foundries of the DSM-V Committee, that the whole idea behind the concept of Psychosis Risk Syndrome is this: Early treatment.

Six months wait for a review does not constitute early treatment. The whole rationale of the PRS project is neatly summarized by the "small puppy" argument. "But daddy," says the tearful little boy, "why can't I keep him? He's such a small puppy." Those who are pushing for the right to diagnose people as At Risk of Psychosis are using the father's case in this argument: "It may indeed be a small and fleeting puppy/delusion, but if we Act Firmly Now, we can Stop It Getting Bigger/Worse." No parent on earth can resist this argument, because of the hidden implication: "And you wouldn't want that on your conscience, would you?"

The psychologists and nurses (and then social workers and all the rest) will correctly say: "The essence of the diagnosis of Psychosis Risk Syndrome is the early identification and rapid treatment of people at risk in order to prevent the full-blown syndrome which, as we all know, is essentially untreatable. What is the purpose of deploying psychologists and nurses to remote or difficult areas where there are no psychiatrists, to detect and identify these unfortunates, if we then have to wait six months or a year for an appointment to have the diagnosis reviewed? And what is the purpose of shipping these patients from their cultural setting, where I am an accepted part of the community, to a city far away which they see as frightening and alien, where nobody understands or cares, to talk to a rushed psychiatrist who has probably never seen an Aboriginal/prisoner/child in his career and who is only doing the job so he can finish his PhD and get the hell out of clinical practice?"

You see the debating ploy, don't you? First state an uncontested fact, then insert a rhetorical question for which ordinary reasonableness allows only one answer, then suggest a very moderate solution that will save everybody a lot of trouble, carefully omitting to mention that the speaker stands to gain a great deal from it. I mean, if they have the huge responsibility of prescribing drugs, then what should happen to their pay? You got it, first time.

There is no politician on earth who can resist that argument. The logic is impeccable, because it is the logic of the DSM-V Committee itself—but turned against them. It is irresistible, especially when it is backed up by a squad of angry parents who have been given all the right websites to look at by the psychologist/nurse/social worker/drug counselor who, of course, doesn't know that drug companies pay for the websites. In short order, there will be PRS Support Groups all over the country using special funds provided by the Federal Government as an adjunct part of the National Mental Health Program. There will be holiday camps for PRS children, insight groups for PRS Prisoners, counselors appointed to the Families of PRS Survivors' Action Committees, PRS-ANON, a separate Veterans' PRS Counseling Service, and so on. The proliferation of bureaucratic meddling is itself a self-sustaining industry. No politician ever dares close a caring agency.

So in no time, psychiatrists will find they are outside the mainstream, just as we are now outside the mainstream of the ADD/ADHD industry. In my area, children are nominated as disturbed by teachers and school guidance officers (who are not psychologists); the parents are brought in for a meeting so they can be scared witless by the well-meaning teachers; the child is then referred by the family doctor to a pediatrician who will prescribe the drugs after a ten minute interview. At eighteen, when the former child patient wants to join the Army, he will, for the first time in his career as a mental patient, see a psychiatrist about his alleged psychiatric disorder. That is, there is a huge psychiatric underworld where DSM diagnoses are made, drugs prescribed, therapies administered and whatever, but which is closed to psychiatrists. The alienists have become aliens themselves. Just as an example, in 1987, when I moved from Perth, Western Australia, where I had trained in medicine and then psychiatry, to the far north of the state, the diagnosis of ADD/ADHD was quite rare. Within fifteen years, the number of children receiving stimulant medication rose from next to nothing to 18,000. Almost all of these had been prescribed the drugs by a small number of pediatricians. Following a publicity program and tighter prescription procedures, by 2009, the number of children taking the drugs had dropped, even though the state population continued to rise quite rapidly. It is now about 6,000. It's amazing how a disease of the brain can be eradicated just by making it more difficult to prescribe drugs.

How will parents be able to resist this pressure? They won't, especially if a recent precedent is followed where a couple nearly lost custody of their child because they refused to allow the school to send their offspring to a pediatrician who invariably put every child on stimulant medication.

By their lack of intellectual rigor, psychiatrists are losing control of psychiatry. With the notion of the Mental Disorder Risk Syndrome, they will actually shove the whole field into the hands of people with less training and less experience. I'm not suggesting that psychiatrists are blameless, but bad psychiatry will not be improved by recruiting and deputizing swarms of poorly trained apprentices (i.e. poorly trained in psychiatry) who freely use psychiatric concepts and treatments but who bitterly resent and actively sabotage psychiatric oversight and discipline.

More Will Mean Worse, on the indubitable basis that More Cannot Mean Better.

6.4.4: A psychiatrist who does not diagnose Psychosis Risk Syndrome will be culpable

The momentum to classify people as At Risk will become irresistible when lawyers start suing doctors for not diagnosing PRS in somebody who later shows some sort of disorder. That is, the entire balance of proof will shift, from assuming that a person is mentally sound until proven otherwise, to assuming, on the slightest suspicion, that he must have treatment. Even if a person refuses treatment, he will later have grounds to sue the doctor who went along with his wishes at the time, on the basis that psychotic people and therefore prepsychotic people are insightless. So general practitioners (GPs) will find they are assailed by psychologists, social workers, teachers etc. who want people put on drugs but, if the person refuses, the GP will have to sign an order transferring the case to the Mental Health Tribunal which has the authority to order community treatment orders, to be administered by the GP who requested it.

If the GP says he doesn't see any reason for the drugs or doesn't want to prescribe them (including the clearly ridiculous reason that he doesn't believe the case for the At Risk Syndrome has been made, who is he to argue with all those experts from Yale and Harvard?), he will not be able to refuse the psychologists etc. because they will then have grounds to urge the family to lodge a complaint with the Medical Board. If the Medical Board doesn't act, then there's always the Health Complaints Commission, the Ombudsman and, quel horreur, Sixty Minutes, capped off with an action for negligence which will take a minimum of three years, if not closer to seven.

GPs will not be able to resist this pressure. I resist it, but I am an obstreperous OWM (Old White Male, if you don't know), one of a dying breed. Good, you may say, but I spend a lot of time reversing false positive (wrong) psychiatric diagnoses made by non-psychiatrists. The patients are invariably and pathetically grateful.

A medical practitioner who does not make the diagnosis will be sued ten, twenty years in the future if and when something goes wrong, even if it was totally unrelated to the earlier episode. If the person commits suicide (as people are wont to do), somebody will be able to find one odd idea, one funny experience and one bit of garbled speech in his last month and say it was the psychosis rearing its ugly head again but, if the doctor had done his job all those years ago, it would have been prevented by the wonderful drugs that everybody reads about in the daily press.

How can they be so sure? Well, if the APA says PRS has to be identified and treated, and all those clever telegenic psychiatrists who are so adept at getting their faces on TV are talking about it as a matter of national urgency, it has to be true. So the doctor will be sued, just as obstetricians are now routinely sued decades after the delivery. The dice are, however, loaded both ways. If a patient is forced to take the drugs against his will, he will not be able to sue for damages because the doctor's clever lawyers will say: "Ah yes, but if you hadn't had them, you would now be severely disabled by psychosis so you cannot show an injury from having the drugs. Thus, your case fails."

A diagnosis of PRS is a triple whammy: "You're sick but you don't know it, only we specialists can know it; you must take this treatment to stop getting worse; if you don't develop the disorder, that proves how effective our treatment was but, if you do, then you obviously had a bad dose of it so we can't be blamed."

The diagnosis of PRS will become a self-reinforcing industry.

6.4.5: The diagnosis of PRS will carry huge and unpredictable social consequences

In my work, I regularly assess young men who have applied to enlist in the Defense Forces. During their intake interviews in the Recruiting Center, they have revealed that they were prescribed stimulant drugs while at school. My job is to determine if they have a mental disorder which is likely to interfere with a military career. I interview the applicant, talk to his parents, check school and medical records, and then write a report. Without exception, I find no documented evidence that they have ever suffered a primary disorder of attention which required stimulant medication. Quite often, I find an anxious or insecure boy from a dysfunctional family background but that would describe half the recruits in your modern army, so my report usually says something bland like 'He will not fall below the general standard of recruits' (my colleagues in the medical section of the recruiting office know perfectly well what this means). My job in this process is to reopen the gate that sprang shut as soon as they mentioned ADD. The default setting is closed: 'The likes of you may not pass this way.'

A person with a major psychiatric diagnosis is ipso facto handicapped, even if the diagnosis is wrong. Numerous careers are restricted to such people, including the military, police and other emergency services, commercial pilots, pharmacists, nurses, teachers, and others. Professional people such as lawyers, medical practitioners, school and kindergarten teachers etc. with a diagnosis of a psychotic disorder are automatically under restriction, so the same will apply a fortiori to PRS. Why a fortiori? Because PRS is subtle; that's its essence; the patient isn't obviously mad so we have to take extra precautions to make sure that none of them slips through. In psychiatric terms, that means increasing the rate of false positive diagnoses. There will be major social consequences of being given this diagnosis, including restrictions on commercial passengers' licenses on sea, road, and in air; firearms and explosives licenses; permits to handle or transport toxic or explosive chemicals; life and health insurance, maybe even entry to medical and law schools; and imagine what it would do to a political career? It is perfectly feasible that passports will require mental health endorsements in the near future, so we can expect Muslims with a diagnosis of PRS to be under close scrutiny, and so on.

6.4.6: Folly Multiplied

In my view, the suggestion of a diagnostic category called Psychosis Risk Syndrome is manifestly a case of psychiatry running riot. It has no scientific validity whatsoever; it cannot be operationalized, meaning it can never be reliable; it cannot be put into practice and it will have huge unforeseen consequences.

As I have said so often, the reason this is happening is because modern orthodox psychiatry does not have an articulated, scientific model of mental disorder to guide its daily practice, its teaching, and its research. The whole concept of the PRS is testimony to the failure of the DSM project. In the absence of science, pseudoscience must flourish.

This is the clearest example I know of pseudoscience in the modern world. Not since Walter Freeman drove around the USA in his "Lobotomobile," shoving ice picks in the brains of the mentally ill, has psychiatry stumbled so far from the principle of *Primum, non nocere*.

First, do no harm.

Note: The expression "Psychosis Risk Syndrome" was the term offered by the DSM-V committee when I first came across this notion in early May 2010. I thought it was not just pseudo-scientific rubbish but actually dangerous, and wrote the first version of this lecture. However, on May 19th, when I wanted to check something, I found they had changed the name of the new category of "illness" to "Attenuated Psychotic Symptoms Syndrome".

This is Orwellian. The term "risk syndrome" clearly implies that the person is in danger of developing a major mental illness, and that in itself further implies that treatment is urgently required. However, simply calling it "attenuated psychotic symptoms syndrome" changes that perception to some extent. The diagnostic criteria haven't changed. All they are trying to do is head off some of the (well-deserved) criticism they are receiving. They will now try to say, "Oh yes, but we don't mean they have to be treated." This is rubbish. There is no such thing as a mental disorder which doesn't get "treated." Simply being given the label will cause intense anxiety in the patient and relatives; then somebody will find a wonder-drug (extract of sun-dried sea urchin) that they say cured their nephew, and the stampede will be on.

One does not have to be a psychiatrist to show that the concept of the 'psychosis risk syndrome' is unsound. The reasons it is unsound are not in themselves of a scientific nature. The arguments in its favor are delivered with a welter of high-sounding technobabble but, stripped of the verbiage, the arguments are nonetheless false. The only reason it could ever get through the wall of skepticism which is supposed to surround all science is that it plays upon the fears of the general public. People, especially parents, are inclined to give credibility to people who claim to be knowledgeable in frightening fields—and what field is more frightening than insanity?

I can think of something that is more frightening than insanity. It is declaring a sane person potentially insane.

6.5: Conclusion: More Will Mean Worse

In 1962, the British author, Kingsley Amis, objected to plans to open universities to half the adult population on the basis that it would necessitate an irremediable and pointless lowering of academic standards. "More will mean worse," he bellowed, and he was absolutely correct: more has indeed meant worse. The DSM-V project is a case of "more of the same", but more of the same old, failed DSM ideas will inevitably mean worse psychiatry. It doesn't matter if the language is updated, it is of no account if categories are reshuffled, broadened, blurred, or loosened; the faults are conceptual, not operational—a case of old wine in new bottles. The DSM-V Task Force has spent some three million hours so far (600 people at ten hours per week for ten years), and the biggest jobs are still to come (Frances, 2010). It has been three million wasted hours, just as all those psychoanalytic textbooks and conferences, plus the therapeutic hours on the analyst's couch, were wasted. It's the wrong model.

The faults of the DSM project stem from the fact that it is not a scientific project just because the profession of psychiatry does not have a declared, articulated scientific model of mental disorder to guide its daily practice, its teaching and its research. It has nothing on which to hang its observations. We have libraries full of observations, of male and female, young and old, from hundreds of cultures, and yet we have no catalogue to tell us where everything should go. This is why the DSM project will eventually be declared bankrupt. We should be working on the model of mental disorder; once we have that, the system of classification will fall in our laps, just as, in 1846, the planet Neptune gave the clues of its presence to Alexis Bouvard, who had the model to understand them. Without a formal model of mental disorder, psychiatry cannot "read" the symptoms and understand what is happening beneath the surface manifestations. Absent understanding, there can be no cure.

<table>
<tr>
<td>

7
</td>
<td>

A Life of its own:
The Strange Case of the
Biopsychosocial Model
</td>
</tr>
</table>

"Genuine progress means the continuous destruction of myths."
George Orwell, *Collected Essays 1945-50*

7.1: Introduction

Nobody has ever claimed that modern technological medicine is anything other than spectacularly successful at what it does. With its base rooted very firmly in biological reductionism, Western medicine attempts to explain the full complexity of human existence as matters of molecules, or less. Most people would never think of questioning this goal [1, 2]. The amazing success of reductionist medicine is seen as its own justification for the program to continue indefinitely, until all questions of human behavior have been fully explained in terms of molecules. In turn, the molecules which make us are based in the genome so, the optimists believe, a full account of the genome will explain everything there is to know about humans [2, 3]. However, not everybody is satisfied with this view, especially when its partisans argue that it will apply outside the material world of matter and energy interactions. While many influential authors are happy to speak of the reduction of mind to brain molecules, there are others who feel this is too glib. One of the earlier critics of reductionist biomedicine, the American psychiatrist George Engel (1913-1999) believed that questions of psychology and sociology should be given equal status in the causation of illness. In a series of papers spread over twenty years from about 1960, [4-8] Engel outlined the place for what he called a biopsychosocial model to replace the blunt instrument of the dominant biomedical model.

His main paper was published in the prestigious journal *Science*, in 1977. Subsequently, he expanded on his ideas and, over the years, his model became increasingly influential, especially in English-speaking countries outside the US. The reason for this unexpected following was probably a national preference to be seen as moderate rather than "too biological" [9]. Engel's broad conceptual approach to mental disorder satisfied this need very well. Increasingly, over the past twenty years,

British, Canadian, and Australasian psychiatrists have identified themselves as upholders of the biopsychosocial model of psychiatry. The website of the Canadian Psychiatric Association (CPA) shows that the Association's first objective is "... to uphold and develop the biopsychosocial approach to the practice of psychiatry..." [10] Similarly, "The *Canadian Journal of Psychiatry* includes peer-reviewed scientific articles analyzing ongoing developments in Canadian and international psychiatry. Regular features include... psychiatric research on a broad range of biopsychosocial topics." [11]

In Britain today, it would be fair to say that the idea of psychiatry as a self-contained specialty hangs on this model to the extent that, without it, psychiatrists might start to lose their reason for existing [12]. The argument is given that, since general practitioners (family physicians) are trained in biological medicine to manage chronic biological disorders, such as diabetes, arthritis, asthma etc., and given that mental disorder is biologically-determined and mostly chronic, it follows that GPs are fully qualified to manage mental disorders. Effectively, if psychiatry embraces a wholly biological model of mental disorder, we will be without a job, so we need to retain a firm grip on the psychological and sociological aspects of medicine. The biopsychosocial model offers that, because nobody else has it.

Similarly, for many years in Australia and New Zealand, the biopsychosocial model was taken to define psychiatry as the point of demarcation between our field and all others. Thus, a president of the Royal Australian and New Zealand College of Psychiatrists (RANZCP) stated: "The biopsychosocial model is fundamental to our profession... (It) underpins every aspect of our training (... and) day to day thinking and action within our own practice." [13] This was later placed in an official RANZCP Position Statement [14] and then on the College website, where it remained for five years until October 2003. In 2002, three years after Engel's death, the *Australian and New Zealand Journal of Psychiatry* (ANZJP) published a series of commissioned articles on his contribution to medicine and psychiatry. The first paper, by his son and daughter-in-law [15], was a personal account of his life's work and how this could be related to the disaster in New York on September 11th 2001. The second [16] was a historical outline of the influence of psychoanalysis in the development of Engel's ideas while the fourth [17] was described as "personal reminiscence."

The authors of the third paper, Smith and Strain [18] had no doubt: "Medicine in Australia became biopsychosocial without knowing it... A generation of Australian medical students and psychiatry trainees have been taught (the biopsychosocial method)" (p. 458). This followed naturally from their view that: "Engel's biopsychosocial model... stands as one of the most influential ideas in Medicine in the 20th Century" (p. 459). His model, they believed, was wholly scientific, in contrast with "counter dogmas" such as holistic or humanistic medicine. The latter "...qualify as dogmas to the extent that they eschew the scientific method and lean instead on faith and belief systems handed down from remote and obscure or charismatic authority figures." They also saw deficiencies in static, descriptive models, such as the DSM-IV system, in which the different axes are essentially separate domains: "The integration of biology, psychology, social issues and behavior, and the interaction among them, is the hallmark of the biopsychosocial model of disease..." Singh, who knew Engel well enough to visit him at home, stated: "What no one can deny is that he did leave a towering edifice...." [17, p. 471].

Readers of these papers would feel that psychiatry is moving into a more humane phase. It is reassuring and apparently reasonable. It should be a source of pride for psychiatry, except for one point: there is not a word of truth in it.

7.2: The Myth of the Biopsychosocial Model

Early in 1998, I established that George Engel never actually wrote his model [19]. All he ever did was issue a call for such a model. He showed where it might fit in general medicine, and how it would be nicer to patients than treating them as biological preparations, but that is the limit of what he did. My case was that at no point in his writing did he set out a series of propositions that could, in any sense, amount to a model to integrate the biological, the psychological, and the sociological aspects of human life. In the years since then, I have repeated and expanded this argument but no person, not even Engel's son or daughter-in-law, has shown that my basic case is wrong. It is now an unassailable fact that the 'biopsychosocial model' attributed to George L. Engel does not exist. Nor, for that matter, does a biopsychosocial theory, or biopsychosocial approach, or a biopsychosocial medicine or psychiatry, or anything. The whole thing is nothing more than a three-word mnemonic which persists only because everybody agrees not to question it. It has the force of a moral injunction only because, as a matter of scientific fact, it doesn't exist.

Was it just the case that his many avid supporters made an honest mistake? I don't believe so. Most of the references I have given to show the spread of this "model" were published after my critique of April 1998, not before it. The comments by the President of the RANZCP were printed late in 1998, six months after my paper. She may have been encouraged by the fact that the editor of the *ANZJP* commissioned two critical commentaries of the original paper and published them in the same issue, without offering me the right of reply [20, 21]. When I tried to rebut what were highly derogatory and misleading commentaries, my paper was rejected without explanation. In 2002, years after Engel's death, the same editor commissioned the embarrassingly effusive papers on Engel's "contribution" to psychiatry and rejected another criticism of the many misquotes and misattributions of my original paper. This was getting a bit peculiar. Why was everybody so determined to make holy writ out of something that didn't even exist?

In 2004, at the Christchurch Congress of the RANZCP, I presented a paper with the explicit title 'The biopsychosocial model and scientific fraud' [22]. This detailed what was starting to look like a deliberate attempt by a small group of people to inflate and maintain a fiction:

> A Medline search of the word 'biopsychosocial' over the past three years yielded nearly four hundred references, not one of them critical. Indeed, the *Journal of Psychosomatics* now uses the terms 'psychosomatic' and 'biopsychosocial' interchangeably....

Psychiatrists have long attempted to convince the general public, the funding bodies and, most significantly, the younger generations of students and psychiatrists that the profession has articulated a rational model which grants it special and unique knowledge of the etiology and phenomena of mental disorder. Yet all along, we have known, or ought to have known, that there is no such model, thereby exposing ourselves to charges of intellectual turpitude. It is my view that a reasonable person could claim that we are guilty either of the grossest intellectual neglect or of outright scientific fraud. For myself, I can see no defense against either accusation.

That seemed to be fairly blunt, not a lot of room for misinterpretation there. It must have hit a tender spot because nobody spoke to me again at the conference. My intention was to draw a line in the intellectual sand, so that the ordinarily cautious psychiatrist (and psychiatrists are mostly very cautious) might think twice about making the claim without providing some sort of justification, but it seemed I was too late. The program to make Engel the patron saint of moderate psychiatry throughout the world appeared to have acquired a momentum of its own. The ANZJP has continued to publish papers referring to the biopsychosocial model as though it were a reality, although it has long since stopped requiring authors to provide references to it. In a letter to the editor in 2005, entitled "The myth of the biopsychosocial model," I pointed to the folly of this intellectually sloppy approach:

Science is conducted according to rules, one of which states that people cannot believe just what they like. We are compelled to adjust our ideas according to the evidence, yet the frequent defenses of Engel's mythical model indicate little general awareness of the discipline required to advance the science of psychiatry. Instead of an objective neutrality, we see an inexplicable partiality which serves only to retard model development in psychiatry. [23]

Nothing has changed much. On May 2nd 2010, a Medline search for "biopsychosocial model" yielded 1114 citations. Not one of the first sixty could be considered critical, and references to my 1998 paper, which showed that the concept doesn't actually exist, are themselves non-existent. Interestingly, practically none of these papers actually cited Engel's original work, as though it has now moved beyond questioning. I will admit that this causes me no little worry: have I misunderstood Engel's work? Am I the only person on earth who can't see how valuable his model is? Every year or two, I have to go to my filing cabinet and pull out my dog-eared copy of his 1977 paper to search it laboriously. No, I haven't misunderstood it at all. You can see perfectly clearly where he changes from talking about how such a model will do this and that to talking about it in the past tense:

> "The development of a biopsychosocial medical model is posed as a challenge for both medicine and psychiatry... The proposed biopsychosocial model provides a blueprint for research, a framework for teaching, and a design for action in the real world of health care."

It's all there in black and white. He jumps from talking about how, if somebody ever developed one, an integrative biopsychosocial model might help medicine, to acting as though he had just done that. But he hadn't.

In another paper, he talked about the clinical application of his new idea:

> "(The) biopsychosocial model enables the physician to extend application of the scientific method to aspects of everyday practice and patient care heretofore not deemed accessible to a scientific approach... The biomedical model can make provision neither for the person as a whole nor for data of a psychological or social nature..."

But where is the model? It isn't in his reference list. Nobody has ever referred to it, not even his son and daughter in law. It is a phantom, a "towering edifice" of self-delusion.

7.3: How Myths Survive

In November 2009, the ANZJP marked the sesquicentennial of Darwin's Origin of Species by publishing a section of six commissioned papers on evolution and psychiatry. These were introduced by an editorial penned by the editor-in-chief of the journal and a colleague. The editorial noted that, because evolutionary concepts play practically no part in psychiatric theorizing, psychiatry remains apart from the mainstream of biological sciences: "Psychiatry still manifests a reticence... that would have done Bishop Wilberforce proud" [24]. While this may overstate the case somewhat (His Grace was not exactly reticent in his views on evolutionary theory), the authors suggested that an evolutionary approach to psychiatry might allow the long-anticipated but much-delayed integration of mind and body: "While biopsychosocial psychiatry is widely espoused, the reality is that the three domains of the biological, the psychological, and the social are too often conceived of (sic) as unrelated." (p. 992) They offered an example of how a defeated chimp shows similar behavior to a depressed person, asking: "Where is the separateness of biology, psychology, and sociology?" Finally, they issued a challenge for "... psychiatry to take up the task of integrating our clinical practice into an evolutionary framework... Much may be gained by exploring neglected domains, for many new ideas and lines may be revealed."

Leaving aside their fanciful wish that an empirical theory of evolution might settle a metaphysical question (mind-body integration), my interest was sparked by their naked claim that "biopsychosocial psychiatry is widely espoused." I say it was naked because, following in the tradition they had helped establish, they didn't bother to give references to prove that this new specialty called 'biopsychosocial psychiatry' is now the model of choice of thinking psychiatrists. In a letter to the editor, dated April 12th 2010, I stated:

In the history of psychiatry, there never was a biopsychosocial theory, model, approach, or whatever. The whole thing is smoke and mirrors. Perhaps this is why Cantor and Joyce did not bother to provide references for their claim that '... biopsychosocial psychiatry is widely espoused...' They knew there aren't any. It is a matter of the gravest concern that, in their misdirected attempts to provide an intellectual framework for their singular view of psychiatry, they resorted to a device which had previously been characterized as '... the grossest intellectual neglect (if not) outright scientific fraud...' Granted (ANZJP) does not have a scientific publishing policy (see Instructions for Authors), but that does not excuse printing such a wildly misleading claim...

The cosmologist, Carl Sagan, said:

> "... at the heart of science is an essential balance between two seemingly contradictory attitudes—an openness to new ideas, no matter how bizarre or counterintuitive, and the most ruthlessly skeptical scrutiny of all ideas, old, and new. This is how deep truths are winnowed from deep nonsense."

Twelve years ago, I showed that the biopsychosocial model is 'deep nonsense.' Six years ago, I said: '... scientific truth is not established by dint of repetition of a falsehood.' To my knowledge, that ethical rule still applies—without exception.

To clarify that point, the publishing policy of ANZJP states: "The acceptance criteria for all papers are the quality and originality of the research and its significance for our readership" [25]. This could, of course, be the publications policy of any extremist religious or political group in the world. It is not and never can be a scientific publishing policy. My numerous attempts to help the editorial board by pointing this out haven't borne fruit yet, but doubtless, I will one day get a letter of thanks for being the only person ever to have read the publishing policy and found that it contains this awful error.

In a non-standard email received two days later, the editor-in-chief (i.e. the author who had been criticized) stated: "Thank you for your letter. Unfortunately, we do not consider it suitable for publication in this Journal." That appeared to be somewhat less than fair. Of course, having a rubbery publishing policy, with no requirement that authors actually address a model of mental disorder, allows the editors to publish what they want for any reason they want, but ignoring a serious error like that seems to stretch the rubber to perishing point. Are there rules, or aren't there? It seemed very simple to me, so I snapped off an email:

The publications policy of the college journal is based on 'quality and originality of the research and its significance for our readership.'

My work is original: I exposed the biopsychosocial model as spurious in 1998 and have added to my case since then. Nobody in the world has shown errors in my argument, and it stands as the final word on the topic.

The quality of my research on the topic of the scientific status of psychiatric theories is considered impeccable.

There is no doubt that a considerable portion of the readership would regard a false claim in an editorial as highly significant. You cannot deny this, just because you have never polled the readership. Moreover, as the (unelected) editor-in-chief, your job is to guard against false claims, not shield them from criticism, especially when the claim is your own.

You do not have the authority to decline a letter on the basis that it is 'not suitable' for publication, just because that term cannot be defined scientifically. However you attempt to define it, you will leave yourself open to accusations of a partisan publishing policy.

I reiterate my statement: "The claim 'A biopsychosocial psychiatry is widely espoused' is wholly without scientific justification and can only mislead the profession..."

That didn't attract a response, so I wrote the paper that forms the bulk of this chapter, and submitted it for editorial review. Two weeks later, the paper was rejected over the signature of the editor in chief on the basis that it too was "unsuitable for publication."

It should be noted that the Instructions for Authors continue: "The Editorial Board reserves the right to refuse any material for publication... Final acceptance or rejection rests with the Editorial Board." That's pompous talk for "Nick off, junior, it's our party and we'll decide who we'll let in." For the record, the Editorial Board of the *ANZJP* is not elected by the general membership of the college. On the rare occasions when there is a vacancy, the board itself advises the college executive who it feels should be appointed to fill the vacancy. The executive then asks the general council of the college to ratify this appointment, which duly happens. Board members, who are selected from the reviewers, are appointed for unlimited terms. The board decides itself whom it will appoint as reviewers and also chooses an international advisory board. The editor in chief is also nominated by the board members from their own number and is confirmed by the executive. The whole thing is totally incestuous but, more to the point, there is nothing an outsider can do to break this cozy monopoly. Nobody will ever get a seat on the board if the existing board doesn't like him, and not one of the reviewers or the so-called international advisory board could be considered a critic of the status quo. And it's all perfectly legitimate. (See end note)

This self-reinforcing approach to science is shared by the editorial policy of *The Canadian Journal of Psychiatry*, the stated goal of which is to advance a non-existent model of psychiatry. The CJP publishes letters only if they address papers published in the journal. However, it rejects papers criticizing its editorial policy as based on a fantasy as "outside their brief"; whatever that means (Parris, J. editor-in-chief, pers. comm. 2009).

Chomsky has summarized this in a similar context:

> "Still, in the universities or in any other institution, you can often find some dissidents hanging around in the woodwork—and they can survive in one fashion or another, particularly if they get community support. But if they become too disruptive or too obstreperous—or, you know, too effective—they're likely to be kicked out. The standard thing, though, is that they won't make it within the institutions in the first place, particularly if they were that way when they were young—they'll simply be weeded out somewhere along the line. So in most cases, the people who make it through the institutions and are able to remain in them have already internalized the right kinds of beliefs: it's not a problem for them to be obedient, they already are obedient; that's how they got there. And that's pretty much how the ideological control system perpetuates itself in the schools" [29].

Myths survive because a small group of people make it their business to keep the myth in currency because of its particular utility to their purposes, mostly relating to maintaining their hold on the power base. Without their energetic efforts, myths will simply fade away just because they are of no explanatory value. Left to their own devices, the rising generation will always see through their teachers' myths unless they have been submitted to a process of indoctrination. So I would say that it is not an honest mistake, but the sort of mistake that desperate people make. However, I admit that is just my opinion.

7.4: Scientific Myths and the Progress of Science

The historian and philosopher of science, Thomas Kuhn, established that science is rather less rational than its practitioners would like to think [30]. A scientific model or paradigm, in his particular sense, is a 'best effort' to explain and understand the world as the scientists of the day experience it. Quite clearly, the model explains some things quite well; otherwise it wouldn't be accepted, but, to a large extent, it also determines what will be seen as matters to be explained, and ignores the rest. Gradually, however, anomalies build up until somebody looks at the whole picture of the prevailing model plus the observations it can't explain, and makes a leap of intuition to a totally new approach which gives a better account of the anomalies than the old. Initially, the new model may struggle to answer certain questions as well as the old one seemed to, but its strength and its appeal lies in its ability to explain the observations that the old model dismissed as irrelevant, just because it could not explain them. New science is bigger than old science, reaching further with a simpler model.

Scientists, however, are only human, and people who have devoted their lives to working on a particular theory or model may strenuously oppose the new view: "In science," Kuhn said, "... novelty emerges only with difficulty, manifested by resistance..." (p. 64). Kuhn and other philosophers of science have detailed the irrational opposition of scientific communities to new ideas. It means that, for a time, there will be two or more competing models in a particular field. It is a hallmark of the pre-scientific stage of any field of research that it will have incompatible models vying for attention, but only one can survive. Classic examples from the history of science include the Ptolemaic (geocentric) and the Copernican (heliocentric) models of the universe, the Newtonian and the relativistic models in physics, and the creationist vs. Darwinian models of species development. Gradually, the new model is developed and expanded until it sweeps the old approach away, and a new generation of scientists simply accepts the new view as 'this is how it is.'

Psychiatry does not have an agreed model of mental disorder. Instead, we have at least three competing paradigms, the psychodynamic, the behavioral, and the biological. Each of them seems to explain a bit of mental disorder, but not one of them can give an over-arching view. Given the failings of the psychoanalytic and behavioral models, psychiatry has, by default, rushed to the biological camp but without explicating its consequences. I have examined these three approaches in much greater detail elsewhere [26, 27, 28] and there is no question that not one of them, including the biological model, approaches the minimal standards of a scientific model of mental disorder. Psychiatry is therefore in a pre-scientific or naïve stage of development and our scientific duty is to criticize these models in order to move beyond them. Quite clearly, the unthinking attachment of modern psychiatry to the inchoate biological model of mental disorder means that, when a new model arrives, many brilliant academic careers will come to a sudden halt. Such is the nature of progress: science has no favorites.

However, in the classic Kuhnian analysis, psychiatry represents an anomaly because we have a wild card, as it were. Not only do we have the three formal models listed above, but we also have an informal one, the biopsychosocial model, which isn't even a model. As shown above, a number of professional psychiatric bodies in the world, bodies which ought to be of the very highest academic and intellectual integrity, actively foment the notion that they have an agreed, articulated scientific theory of the integration of body and mind, but it is one which the scientific literature explicitly states does not exist, and never has. The biopsychosocial model is an unredeemed myth. If it were not slipped regularly into papers and editorials, it would simply fade from view. Its persistence needs to be explained but, manifestly, it cannot be explained on rational grounds. There are several possible explanations.

The first possibility is the crudest, meaning the conspiracy mode. In this view, editors of psychiatric journals are actively engaged in a coordinated program of deceit specifically designed to entrap psychiatric trainees into supporting their view, all the while establishing a monopoly on research funds and public attention for themselves. I don't believe this, because psychiatrists are incapable of coordinating anything.

The second possible explanation stems from their own biological model: Editors of psychiatric journals are all suffering a chemical imbalance of the brain which compels them to hold a fixed, false belief out of context with their cultural and intellectual backgrounds, i.e., a delusion. They have a shared delusion that the biopsychosocial model is a reality. I think we can reject that on epidemiological grounds although the self-selecting nature of the editorial system in psychiatry means that it isn't impossible: a case of assortative mating, as it were. The simpler explanation would be that they share a cultural delusion, but a shared, culturally-determined delusion which is conventionally protected from criticism is another name for religion. This is not incompatible with my assertion that psychiatry is pre-scientific, but I don't think it is the answer. There is a vast difference between insightlessness, as in 'incapable of seeing', and the third possibility, the 'neurotic scotoma', as in 'doesn't want to look as it may prove to be embarrassing.'

My preferred suggestion is summarized by the following quotes:

> I know that most men, including those at ease with problems of the greatest complexity, can seldom accept the simplest and most obvious truth if it would oblige them to admit the falsity of conclusions which they have proudly taught to others, and which they have woven, thread by thread, into the fabrics of their lives (Leo Tolstoy).

One of the saddest lessons of history is this:

> "If we've been bamboozled long enough, we tend to reject any evidence of the bamboozle. We're no longer interested in finding out the truth. The bamboozle has captured us. It is simply too painful to acknowledge—even to ourselves—that we've been so credulous" (Carl Sagan).

Reasonable psychiatrists (and most psychiatrists are very reasonable) have been led astray by their need for a moderate face. Unhappy with the crude scientism of biological psychiatry, repelled by the excesses of psychoanalysis, and disappointed by the sterility of behaviorism, psychiatrists have yearned for a model that retained their humanity, kept the psychologists at bay and stopped the real doctors laughing. Engel's plan for a scientific but humanitarian psychiatry seemed to fill the order, and such was their desperation that psychiatrists "wove it, thread by thread, into the fabrics of their lives," but without checking on the details. Had they looked, they would have seen, of course, that there were no details. Now, having nailed the biopsychosocial model to their mastheads, none of them has the courage to break ranks and admit it is a sham. By this means, it has become a convention or shibboleth, an incantation to act as a moral brake on the frantic activities of the extremists but it is not and never will be a valid scientific concept.

This might explain their behavior, but it will never excuse it. The road to scientific damnation is paved with good editorial intentions.

7.5: Exposing bias and Prejudice Masquerading as Science

A few weeks ago, my daughter asked why doctors are called 'quacks'. The answer, according to Wikipedia, comes from the US of the late nineteenth century. Orthodox medicine of that time was brutal, venal, and a definite health hazard; so the scene was wide open for non-medical people to sell their own remedies to the frightened and desperate population. A person who had a salve 'quacked' his wares; so he became known as a 'quacksalver'. Later, this was shortened to 'quack', meaning an unreliable or untrustworthy doctor, especially one pushing a false remedy or explanation. This was the era of the 'snake oil' salesman, which became a byword for political dishonesty (it is of interest but no relevance to psychiatry that there is still a goanna salve on sale in Australia which claims to be 'Of great benefit to man and beast', although perhaps not for the goannas).

Psychiatry claims to have a special model that justifies its existence, a model that nobody else has or understands. This claim has been adopted, supported, and protected by a powerful constituency at the very core of the profession. It is unmitigated quackery. Anybody who claims, for example, that "biopsychosocial psychiatry is widely espoused" is a quack, i.e. an unreliable or untrustworthy doctor, especially one pushing a false remedy or explanation.

One thing is quite clear: the psychiatric establishment, which is very largely self-appointed and self-perpetuating, cannot be trusted to act self-critically. In the US, highly influential figures at the very heart of the profession have been found taking fees to produce results favorable to the drug industry. Down here in little-known Australia, we don't have a separate psychiatric drug industry but there is still plenty of money available for anybody who wants to do any sort of research on possible biochemical causes of mental disorder. One of the most powerful ways the myth of biological psychiatry is perpetuated is through the psychiatric publishing industry, which is firmly in the grip of the establishment. Journals selectively publish papers supportive of their unstated positions and actively suppress criticism of those papers. Let's have a look at just one recent example.

In the volume of the ANZJP devoted to evolution, the introductory paper was contributed by an American psychiatrist, C. Robert Cloninger. Cloninger is professor of psychiatry, genetics and psychology at the Washington School of Medicine, in St Louis, Missouri, his highly-rated alma mater, where he was greatly influenced by Samuel Guze [1]. Earlier in his career, he followed the well-trodden path of statistical analysis of personality factors, inheritance of alcoholism, and other conventional fields but lately has branched out into spirituality. He is closely involved with a group called the Anthropedia Foundation which concerns itself with health and well-being and is now the director of its research institute. His paper was entitled: "Evolution of human brain functions: the functional structure of human consciousness" [31]. In briefest terms, he tries to relate (note that word) five stages of neocortical development in mammals to five elements of human self-aware consciousness, namely: sexuality, materiality, emotionality, intellectuality, and spirituality. Each of these is then related to the five special senses and thence to five basic motives or emotions: fear, anger, disgust, surprise, and happiness/sadness. From this, he claims to have derived a matrix which gives "a general and testable model of the functional structure of human consciousness that includes personality, physicality, emotionality, cognition, and spirituality in a unified developmental framework."

It is not possible to summarize the special quality that permeates this paper. It has the form of a scientific paper (he has written enough of them to get that right), replete with Methods and Results, lists of the evolutionary ages, "geologic timeline of coincident events in human evolution", then it moves across to emergent structures and functions (not forgetting amphibia and cladogenesis), finally losing itself in the five planes of being and other esoteric stuff. But it is all completely, joyously mad. If Prof. Cloninger ever had any critical faculties, he has let them fly away as though releasing a handful of colored balloons and watching them twist and turn gaily into the summer sky. Then, unfettered by the boring ballast of any form of intellectual discipline, he has turned his prodigious but piecemeal knowledge to creating a gallimaufry of giddiness, a wild celebration of pulling the wool over his own eyes in the hope that the public will whoop with delight and pull it over theirs so they can all run around in the pre-scientific darkness, bumping into each other, and crying out that they have found inner harmony; or something. It is pure, unleavened pseudoscience, exactly the sort of hollow intellectual pretension that Sokal pilloried in his magnificent hoax (see Chapter 4).

Unmoved by this abuse of the scientific process, I dashed off yet another letter of complaint to the editorial board:

> (Cloninger's paper) is a breathtaking example of the very worst kind of pseudoscience, one that has no place whatsoever in the scientific canon. It is devoid of even the most elementary features which distinguish science from whimsy. Anybody who reads that paper and decides that it yields some new understanding of the problem of the nature of mind is a victim of self-delusion. It insults the intelligence of the readership.
>
> It is a monumental indictment of the current editorial board of the journal that this paper, apparently solicited, was received and accepted on the same day without any attempt to correct its profound intellectual errors. It is truly remarkable that people entrusted with advancing psychiatry could ever allow this essentially incoherent piece a place of honor in an edition devoted to Charles Darwin. I am convinced that it was published just because of the author's name and his connections with the editorial board. If I had submitted it, there is not the slightest doubt that it would have been rejected on the same day.... Science, as I pointed out many years ago, is not a matter of "anything goes" and this applies to editors too. The burden of proof of how and why this paper constitutes science rests with the board: those who approved it must show why it meets the criteria for scientific thought—but they will inevitably fail, not the least because none of them are aware of the criteria.

I believe that any member of the editorial board who cannot see the overwhelming flaws in this paper is not fit to hold office. I call for the resignation of the current editorial board so that we, the members of the RANZCP, can reconstitute our journal as a legitimate journal of scientific record.

Rather predictably, the rejection slip was back in a few hours: "You may wish to send this letter directly to the College President," intoned Prof. Peter R Joyce, editor in chief of the journal, "and request my dismissal as Editor. However, it is not suitable for publication in this Journal, while I am Editor."

Since I share the editor's rock-solid conviction that college presidents can be trusted not to act definitively, the matter rested there until the March 2010 edition of the journal arrived. Among the usual riveting offerings was one entitled "Self-mutilation and suicide attempts: relationships to bipolar disorder, borderline personality disorder, temperament and character". The authors were Peter R Joyce, Dr X, Dr. Y, C. Robert Cloninger, and Dr. Z. Although separated by the Pacific Ocean, Joyce and Cloninger have a sufficiently close relationship to collaborate on long-term epidemiological studies.

Let us look at the facts. As editor in chief, Joyce chose or authorized the topic for the special edition. He chose or authorized the contributors and their topics. He approved Cloninger's contribution in a few hours. He then rejected a valid criticism of that paper in a few hours (which suggests he probably didn't have time to get a second opinion on the letter). That, in my opinion, gives the perception that the editor acted in a position of conflict of interest, which is inexcusable. His motives in rejecting my letter are unknown, not the least because the editor is unaccountable.

Readers may complain that, in finding fault with a third tier or minor national journal of psychiatry, I am trying to tar the whole psychiatric publishing industry with a small brush, but I disagree. Bearing in mind how difficult it is to get anything out of this particular journal (essentially, impossible), I admit I have not approached any of the more prestigious journals, but first impressions indicate they are just as guilty. Somebody else will have to establish the case.

The problem with the psychiatric publishing industry lies in its history. Psychiatric journals were started in the mid to late nineteenth century as the 'in house' publications of the various national associations. I do not know how many psychiatrists there were in the US, Germany, or in the UK in, say, 1880, but it would not have been many. They had little or no formal training, as Jaspers' record shows, and essentially learned on the job. The tiny associations were concerned to raise standards and the journals were an essential part of that. In each case, a few people at the center of the group offered to review papers contributed by members and, slowly, this was formalized into regular editions supervised by an editor with a board to assist him. The central idea behind each journal as it exists today is that a small group of experts decides what the larger membership needs to read. However, times have changed. Just as a modern medical student knows far more physiology and biochemistry than the most eminent professor of medicine from a century ago, so the readership of a psychiatric journal no longer consists of a bunch of provincial hicks and drunks who need to be told what to read—if they read at all. Times have changed, but the idea behind the journals hasn't changed one iota. It is still a case of a group of (largely self-appointed) experts telling the readers what they need to know and, implicitly, what they should ignore.

There is, however, a very powerful statistical case to say that the experts are more likely to be wrong in their judgment than the readership [32]. Multiple judgment averaging (to give it one of its names) relies on the difference between systematic bias and random error to reduce or minimize errors. While the mathematical application of this technique was devised for quantitative data, it also can be applied to qualitative. Consider a case where four experts collectively arrive at a decision about a particular matter, then a thousand people who are familiar with the matter but don't necessarily claim to be experts are individually asked their opinions. The median opinion of the thousand non-experts is much more likely to be closer to the truth than the consensus of the four experts, and the reason is very simple. The experts are more likely to give an opinion which is systematically biased just because there is no inherent self-detecting or self-correcting mechanism. On the other hand, the large group comes with a self-correcting mechanism, called random error. If (and only if) the choices of the non-experts straddle or bracket the true measure, then their errors will cancel each other. The larger the sample, the more likely it is that the errors will self-correct just because their errors are not subject to a single systematic bias. The very fact that they are random means that they distribute around the true measure in a highly predictable manner. As the sample group increases in size, so the median opinion tends inevitably to the truth.

Even if there are groups with systematic biases within the large group, they will tend to balance each other or, if they don't, they will be readily detectable. If the group is large enough to include a cabal of feverish radicals, it will most likely also include a gaggle of nay-saying conservatives who negate them. Systematic bias in small groups can arise from many sources. In specialist areas, two of the most important include biases induced by training and from self-selection. Training errors can be seen in the different diagnoses reached by, say, psychiatrists trained in Britain compared with those trained in the US. Another example was the difference between psychiatrists trained in psychoanalysis compared with those from a biological or even behaviorist background. Each group "saw" the cases from a different, incompatible viewpoint.

The problem is that we humans see what we are trained to see. It is given to few to peer through the distorting lenses of our schooling yet still find the unbiased truth. That, however, is an honest error: there is a difference between getting it wrong and doing it wrong. Self-selection bias is a matter of doing it wrong, which arises just because the experts reject the idea that they may in fact be biased, as Chomsky described in the quotation above. Their view is that, because they agree, they are more likely to be right than a group of people split by disagreement, so they make sure there is no disagreement by the stunningly simple expedient of allowing only their friends to join their group. By this means, they fail their fundamental scientific duty of self-criticism: they "do it wrong", which is inexcusable. In practice, their "expertise" is just a form of tribalism.

7.6: Two Heads are Better than One…

Just to check the validity of this conclusion, we can go back in history to a notable case where the powers-that-were were utterly wrong. In 1633, the Renaissance scientist, Galileo Galilei (1564-1642), was charged by the Holy Office (Inquisition) with disobeying a papal order by 'teaching' the Copernican concept of a heliocentric universe. His judges were ten cardinals, princes of the Church, whose concern, as history shows, was not so much the physical structure of the universe but papal authority and the social stability which they believed that particular authority guaranteed. Under threat of ghastly punishment, they demanded and received from the frail sixty-nine-year-old philosopher his assurance that he abjured the heliocentric model. We now know Galileo's judges were completely and irredeemably wrong.

The cardinals represented the 'peak body' of the church: the pope was chosen from their number while he and his favorites chose new cardinals to fill vacancies in the college. In order to be eligible for appointment as a cardinal, a young man had to enter the church and undergo years of training and indoctrination. If he proved his reliability and had the right connections, he rose through the ranks but, at all times, in all places, and in every conceivable form, he was subject to the most intense supervision and restriction. Nobody who was not absolutely loyal and subservient to the whole of the intellectual, moral and social structure of the church's authority made it up the ladder. This is what Chomsky meant when he said: "… the people who make it through the institutions and are able to remain in them have already internalized the right kinds of beliefs: it's not a problem for them to be obedient, they already are obedient; that's how they got there."

And it is precisely because the cardinals had been through the mill, as it were, that they were so catastrophically wrong. Their system could not correct itself. There were so many reputations built on the Ptolemaic model, so much authority vested in the idea that the earth could not move and that the sun and other heavenly bodies were created perfect, that news of empirical facts (spots on the sun, Jupiter's moons) had to be suppressed (their authorities are Psalm 93:1; Psalm 96:10; Psalm 104:5; Chronicles 16:30; Ecclesiastes 1:5). Whatever his motivation, each of the ten cardinals on the judicial bench knew he was right and Galileo was wrong. Why was he so certain? Because cardinals had the education, they had the ancient authorities, they had divine authority, and they had the executioners playing dice in the dungeons beneath the palace. Once the trial started, once the charges were read, the judges could not reach a verdict other than guilty. That could not happen as it would negate the first principle of any power structure: self-preservation. They were incapable of detecting and correcting their own errors because they did not entertain the possibility of being in error.

To paraphrase William Hearst, nobody will ever go wrong by over-estimating the vicious self-righteousness of closed groups of men—and their capacity to obstruct progress. We humans do not know how to guarantee intellectual progress; we only know how to obstruct it. We know that humans are intensely curious and creative creatures and that, left to their own devices, they will usually find a way around most problems but the operative expression is 'left to their own devices'. Left to his devices, Galileo first invented a telescope then turned it to the skies where, lo and behold, he found that things weren't quite as the people without telescopes had supposed. However, there are always people around who don't like others being left to their own devices. They want to interfere and control and obstruct, to tell people what to do and what to believe. Sometimes their motives are venal, sometimes just old-fashioned power, sometimes fear of change bringing something worse, it doesn't matter. Obstruction is obstruction; progress will happen despite the authorities.

The psychiatric publishing industry is little different from the Inquisition that decreed Galileo was wrong. The industry is controlled by a small group of people who have undergone a long apprenticeship (six years medical of school, five years of psychiatric training, many years sitting at the foot of an eminent professor doing his bidding without demur), who enter the academic/ publishing stream of the psychiatric profession (as distinct from the hard work stream, the social gadfly stream, or the making-money stream, etc) and then serve another grinding stint patiently pushing their way up the slow-moving escalators of the profession. Eventually, if they know the right people and go to the right conferences and introduce themselves to the right speakers and ask the right authorities to review their papers, they might be asked to act as a reviewer for a journal. This goes on and, if they approve the right papers and reject all those the editor wouldn't like, write the appropriate editorials, and cultivate suitable international authors, they might somehow (nobody actually knows how) be invited to fill one of the rare vacancies in the college of cardinals, sorry, the editorial board. The final jump, from the board to the post of editor in chief, will go to the individual who best exemplifies the qualities the board considers desirable. The post of editor in chief will not go to Chomsky's dissidents who are "... too disruptive or too obstreperous—or you know, too effective... they'll simply be weeded out somewhere along the line."

And in the process of weeding out dissidents, the Establishment will weed out those "... intensely curious and creative creatures (who), left to their own devices, will usually find a way around most problems." That is, the entire process by which a psychiatrist gains the stamp of approval of the Establishment is also the process which eliminates the creative spark that offers the only chance of dragging the profession from the nineteenth century to the twenty-first. Two heads are better than one, because one head will probably not know it is wrong (and will never admit it is wrong), and the dialectic of thesis-antithesis-synthesis can only take place when one person places himself in opposition to the party line. A chorus of yes-men (and, sorry to say, yes-women), which is what an editorial board is, will never find fault in its own views: "... it's not a problem for them to be obedient, they already are obedient, that's how they got there..." The central problem is that, by virtue of their three-decade apprenticeships, the editorial board members have lost sight of the possibility that they may be wrong. They do not lie in bed at night, worrying over some arcane point of theory; they sleep easily, as Galileo's tormentors did. The current system filters out the thoughtful and replaces them with the faithful. When everybody is thinking the same thing, nobody is thinking at all. Unless there is some institutional process of self-criticism (a contrarian on the board with right of veto, alternating boards in opposition, open elections to the board, etc), then all the board can do is dish up the same dreary pap, year after year, and call it progress.

In science, progress is the goal but competition is the mechanism. Without the free, open, competitive interplay of opposing ideas, of people shouting at each other rather than middle-aged clones purring their anodyne, recycled monologues at gently dozing conference audiences, then we will never have the slightest idea of where the truth lies. Just ask Galileo's cardinals—by the way, does anybody remember their names?

7.7:... And a Hundred Thousand are Better Than Six Clones

In the endless search for truth, two heads are better than one, but only if they disagree. The psychiatric publishing industry has long outlived its value. It has become an obstruction to progress; it has become part of the problem, not the chance of a solution. It is time to bring it to heel and make it serve the profession and the patients rather than serve itself. The only way this will happen is if we destroy it. Its essential structure, that of a board of censors (because that is what they are) reading submissions and deciding in camera what the readership will see, is the source of obstruction to progress.

At present, papers are submitted; they are reviewed by anonymous people chosen by the editors; and are accepted or rejected according to standards the editors do not publish. Allegedly, reviewers are blind to the authors of the papers but one would have to be particularly obtuse not to recognize, say, one of my papers. The process is very slow—it can take up to two years for a paper to appear in print—extremely expensive and, coincidently, is extremely profitable to the publishing companies (a letter I submitted to Australasian Psychiatry was recently accepted for publication. The acceptance letter advised that it would be available online to all subscribers but, if I wanted to make it freely available online to the general public, then I would have to pay the publishers $3250; for 250 words. I would dearly like to be able to claim that my words are worth $13.00 each but, sadly, they probably aren't). It also uses a lot of paper

We can correct all of these deficiencies by the very simple matter of reversing the whole process. I propose an electronic system of publication similar to the on-line auctions which are transforming business. That gets rid of the paper and the long delays. Second, anybody can publish anything, as long as it isn't obscene. Even nonsense can be published (much as Cloninger's paper was published), but it will be given a grade. Third, the readers review it and grade it, not the editor's friends. The fact that something has been published doesn't prove that it is worthwhile. Only the readers' opinions count, because they will be random and, if there are enough of them, they will necessarily approximate the truth. Finally, the authors will be anonymous during the review process but the reviewers won't.

The process starts with a website. Authors load their papers with all identifying marks removed. If a reader recognizes a paper, it will be removed for editing. Readers then give the paper a score but, to ensure objectivity, readers and their comments must be identified. Only accredited people can register to give grades although it would help to have a secondary board where the general public could have their say as well (some people are not keen on this idea but it is salutary to recall that, until he had published several papers, Albert Einstein was a member of the general public). For six months, authors remains anonymous, during which time they can amend the paper as the critical comments come in, but the probation period starts again (perhaps just three months). At the end of the sixth month, if the comments are too bad, the authors can remove their papers but if they leave them on the board, their names will be published. From that time, the score is the paper's claim to authority in the literature. Instead of citing a paper as Smith and Brown (2010), publishing in The Journal of Big Psychiatric Egos, the paper will be cited as Smith and Brown (2010) [0.82 at 09/10], where 1.00 is the top mark and anybody scoring below 0.50 would withdraw if he had any sense. There would need to be strict operational definitions for readers to use but that would be an improvement over the present system where editors decide on the basis of their perception of "... its significance to our readership" (ANZJP, where else?)

It would, of course, take a little time for psychiatrists to learn how to be honest. A psychiatrist I knew many years ago, who had grown as close to the establishment in this country as I have grown apart from it, once said to me: "I don't know why you take the ANZJP so seriously. Getting your work published in it is just a game." He thought the journal was a joke, but it was good for getting his statistical stuff in print so he said nothing. Under the proposed scheme, it will not be possible to say nothing. Can you imagine the tears and recriminations if Prof. Smith's golden-headed boy panned his mentor's latest effort? Or what if McLaren's malicious criticism of Cloninger's evolutionary musings attracted support from the unknown unknowns (i.e. the psychiatrists who are presently told what to read and whose opinions are totally ignored by editorial boards)? Psychiatry would move in directions its present controllers couldn't predict. The young Turks might even move it in directions they didn't understand. Horror of horrors, like the Inquisition, it might even come to pass that they would lose their authority.

Well, good. That's what science is all about. It's about attacking the status quo and demolishing it; it's about stopping colleges of cardinals telling the philosophers that the sun moves around the world. It's about clearing the site to build something new when the clones fail to deliver.

Science is about progress, not stasis. Some more about an online publication system:

1. Authors would have to choose to list their work according to a system of classification, such as PubMed, and nominate half a dozen key words so readers could be notified by email that a topic of interest had been listed.

2. Readers would have to agree to grade a certain number of papers, say ten papers in six months, or their access reduced or denied.

3. Authors would have to grade a number of papers before their papers were listed.

4. Authors who took offence at reviews or grades and tried to exact vengeance would be barred for five years.

5. Authors who attempted to cheat or manipulate the system would be barred for life. Clear rules would need to be established for what constitutes manipulation, in order to prevent the Biederman-Nemeroff type scandals.

6. This type of system requires a lot of storage and quite a powerful server; pay-per-click advertising would almost certainly be necessary, with advertising slots auctioned to users and a certain number of public interest slots free.

7. It might require special sections for papers by students and psychiatric trainees, non-psychiatrists, etc, even the general public. There would be a particular benefit in having a section for individuals to contribute their life experiences.

8. A system of this type would make it very easy to keep track of citations etc. Every paper would remain linked to the site and its grade could be amended daily. It would also be possible to drop a paper from the literature, something which is now impossible.

9. Users (readers and authors) would have to agree to serve on a supervising committee from time to time. This would have to be on an alphabetical or similar basis to prevent people having themselves appointed.

A major advantage of this type of system is that it would immediately make the entire psychiatric literature available to any person in the world who wanted to access it (me, for example: I have had practically no access to the scientific literature for nearly a quarter of a century. Only recently have I gained online access to the full literature through the good offices of an American university). The whole purpose of the literature is to foster openness, accessibility, and accountability. Currently, the structure of the psychiatric publishing industry is such as to achieve exactly the opposite ends: secrecy, restricted access, and evasion of responsibility.

7.8: **Conclusion: To Destroy a Myth**

I have no idea how to destroy a myth. In religion, politics, and mythology, the theory is more important than the facts. In science, facts must finally trump the theory but it has been said often enough that traditions are not killed by facts. Experience shows that, when it comes to justifying their prejudices, editors set up their publication policies so that they simply cannot be shamed. Max Planck's memorable quote, about waiting for one's intellectual enemies to die, doesn't seem adequate when the rising generation of psychiatrists is relentlessly indoctrinated with the idea that they are practicing a psychiatry based in an agreed scientific model—which not one of them has ever seen.

I remain of the view that "the general public (including the mentally-ill), the funding bodies and, most significantly, the younger generations of students and psychiatrists" deserve better than an empty rhetorical flourish masquerading as "one of the most influential ideas in Medicine in the 20th Century." Sooner or later, we psychiatrists will be charged with scientific fraud, but will the editors and their friends then stand up to take responsibility? I doubt it. By editorial fiat, the editor's decision is beyond criticism.

Note: In order to prevent needless conflict, I submitted a copy of this chapter to the RANZCP so that they could verify the accuracy of the facts. My letter specified that they should confine themselves to the facts alone as I took responsibility for the opinions. About two weeks later, a letter signed by a junior employee of the college advised me of the college's functions and noting that checking academic papers was not one of them. I replied immediately, asking them to read my referring letter properly as I did not wish to publish any errors of fact. Two days later, a circular arrived from the college informing that the editor in chief of the *ANZJP* had resigned. In typical style, no reasons were given. I would like to think my complaints had something to do with it but, sadly, they probably didn't.

"Everything faded into mist. The past was erased, the erasure was forgotten, the lie became truth."

George Orwell, *1984.*

PART II:
The Many Voices
of Mental Disorder

Part II of this book will focus on the experience of being mentally-disturbed, or the phenomenology, if you want to make it sound as though you actually have a theory. There are different ways this can be done. The easiest would be to pull together some writings by people who have suffered mental breakdowns of various sorts but that isn't easy for several reasons. Firstly, ordinary people mostly don't want to talk about their experiences, they just want to put it behind them and get on. Second, all too often, "confessions" are written with the purpose of putting up a smoke screen. A reviewer of the autobiography of former Australian Prime Minister, Bob Hawke, said: "Autobiographies are rarely written from the standpoint of taking a critical look at their subject, and this one is no exception to that rule." They may have something to hide; they may have an ideological ax to grind, or relatives to get even with; but the end result doesn't give a balanced look at the question. Finally, most writing is by professional writers and misses the point of the very ordinariness of a troubled life. A simple phobia becomes poetry or operatic drama when the experience of fear is universal.

In the remaining chapters, I want to show how to approach mental disorder so that the person speaks subjectively for himself yet the outsider can retain an objective stance. There has to be a meeting across the subjective-objective gulf; otherwise there can be no change. If psychiatrists restrict themselves to a purely objective viewpoint, as Kräpelin did, then they will not see their patients as humans, only as rather noisy and unruly cattle. On the other hand, if we try to submerge ourselves totally in the experience of being mentally-ill, we will end up quite as lost as the patient. As we reach one hand to a drowning person, the other must have a firm grip on something solid, otherwise we both go under.

Because there are so many sides to the experience of being mentally-disordered, these chapters will look mostly at the role of anxiety. I do this for several reasons. Anxiety is very common; it is a very serious disorder which ruins lives and causes a multitude of other problems and, with very few exceptions, it is profoundly misunderstood by orthodox psychiatry. For mainstream modern, institutional psychiatry, anxiety is a nuisance, a contaminant which is dismissed with the label 'comorbidity'. These cases will show that it is more than a contaminant. Because it is the only truly recursive human emotion; it amplifies and reverberates throughout mental life, so that understanding it gives the clue to what is going on.

Part II will show how the phenomena of mental disorder can be used to understand the mechanisms of mental disorder. This approach is based in the theoretical stance I have outlined in the first two books and in Part I of this one:

1. In the first place, my case is that the experience of being mentally disturbed is very real and has to be taken seriously. It amounts to something to be gripped by a terrible sadness or to be frozen by a nameless fear. Nobody chooses the path of mental disturbance. Telling the sufferer "Pull yourself together" or "Get over it", or something equally dismissive, like "Take these tablets and come back in a month", is not taking it seriously (I don't mean to imply that every little flutter of anxiety needs to be treated as a national calamity. There are times to say to somebody: "You'll survive; don't worry about it.")

2. Everything has a cause. The experience of being mentally disordered has a cause, and that cause lies in or is itself part of the mental realm. It is not the case that the sufferer's distress can be ignored while we wait for the blood tests to arrive, and not just because there aren't any blood tests for mental disorder (and never will be). The nature of the suffering tells us how it arose in the first place. Mental events have mental causes; there is no way that physical (brain) events can cause rational mental events. That includes the mental event known as suffering, which is the rational outcome of certain mental imperatives. Mental matters can only be approached on the mental level. This is because the neurophysiological substrate of mental disorder is the agency of the disorder, not the cause. So in order to understand what is causing his distress, we have to talk to the sufferer as a mentally capable being.

3. With very few exceptions, the causes of mental disorder lie in the psychological or informational realm of the mind. Some cases are just normal reactions to abnormal events and will get better with the passage of time, but most of these don't need to see a psychiatrist. The great bulk of mental disorder, however, defies logical explanation, and these cases are rightly the province of a biocognitive psychiatry. The complex interaction of mind and body points to the unseen causes of the breakdown. The causes consist of information coded into the brain at the subneuronal level which acts rapidly and silently to induce the powerful emotional and cognitive changes we call mental disorder.

4. A diagnosis gives little or no information about the precise causes of each case of mental disorder. It tells us what state the person has reached, but does not say why he got there. Psychiatry's standard approach, which is to suppress the symptoms, does not address the causes. Therefore, they remain in place, ready to cause trouble as soon as the suppression is lifted. This is because drugs work in the experiential realm of mental phenomena, while the causes reside in the informational realm. Antidepressants, for example, may relieve the experience of misery but, as soon as the drugs are stopped, the causes will begin to exert their effects again and the symptoms will return. This is why psychiatrists now are saying that depression is a chronic illness. Any problem is a chronic problem if the causes are not tackled directly.

5. Most people do not understand why they are suffering. The causes are essentially hidden from them just as the causes of their beliefs and their dislikes are hidden. Even when they do know what the trouble is, it may seem overwhelming or shameful, so they try to reject it. The historical causes of any particular state of distress are potentially infinite but the causes qua current mental mechanisms are in the present. The mechanism of a particular mental state is a very different thing from the historical antecedents of that mechanism. It is not possible to say to somebody: "You're depressed, that means you were sexually abused as a child." He is depressed because of what he believes about himself and the world now, and how he sees himself fitting in with and managing his bit of the world. His self-perception arose in a historical context, but the relationship between particular life events and the mental outcome is not close; it depends on so many variables that there is only a correlation on a population basis, not individual.

6. The role of the psychiatrist is to identify the precise mental causes of the patient's suffering and to correct them. This is where the real difficulties start because the causes may be buried under layer upon layer of fear, suspicion, distortion, shame and guilt, hostility, genuine amnesia, and ordinary lack of insight (some people just don't think in psychological terms). The therapist's job is to understand the patient from the inside, from the phenomenal or experiential realm, in order to be able to detect the tiny clues that reveal what is hidden in the psychological or informational realm. An insight-directed psychotherapy, therefore, starts with the patient giving a full and true account of his distress, but this depends on a high level of trust from the patient, when trust may be one of his most deep-seated problems. So anybody who wants to get to know the patient, at levels he himself may not even realize to exist, will have to find a path through the minefields.

7. The therapist has to use his own experience as a human being to understand what could be going on in the disordered mind to produce just that effect, and to deal with it. He has to see the patient's experiences of the world, see the world itself, and work out how this mental experience could have arisen from that event. Only another human being can do this. Effective psychotherapy will never be computerized. Only another human can understand the subtle clues the patient gives which allow entry to his innermost, inchoate beliefs and attitudes. For example, the experience of being depressed leads to the concealed, coded information which is causing the depression. The therapist has to get with the patient and stay with him, even though this type of close contact with another person may be profoundly disturbing to the patient. However, since a lot of psychiatrists aren't exactly paragons of mental stability themselves, their own fears have to be resolved in advance, i.e. during their training. In this model, a psychiatrist who hasn't undergone psychotherapy will be about as effective as a surgeon wearing dark glasses and thick gloves.

8. Formal psychotherapy consists of a total assessment of the patient's mind-body state which demands the very broadest training and experience in the therapist. The therapist must have a very broad and intuitive knowledge of normal mind and body functioning in as many cultures and subcultures as he sees. He must be able to put himself in the other person's shoes and show his understanding at every point of the contact. It is impossible to learn psychotherapy out of a book. Similarly, it is impossible to practice psychotherapy without a detailed knowledge of how mind and body interact. In this schema, the idea of a therapist with no medical knowledge is self-contradictory.

8	*Madness from the Inside Looking Out*

8.1: Introduction: The Semi-Structured Interview

In my training, half a lifetime ago, we were allocated one hour for each new case. During this time, we had to take a history covering the patient's presenting complaints, his recent history, then his family background and personal history—including education, work, and social history—a personality assessment, and then the mental state examination. As part of the mental state, we were required to conduct a brief cognitive assessment and then a quick physical examination. It was a directed interview, what is now called a "semi-structured assessment". There are three kinds of assessments: structured, semi-structured, and unstructured. A structured interview asks exactly the same questions of each patient and is tightly controlled by the interviewer. The outcome is restricted to a limited range of options and there is no room for the interviewer to vary the questions to suit the individual. Most structured interviews are given by questionnaire for research purposes. I do not know anybody who would use a genuine structured interview for treatment purposes.

In an unstructured interview, the patient talks as he sees fit, and may even not talk if so inclined. It is often thought that the psychoanalytic hour was unstructured but that was not the case. The patient certainly talked but was questioned by the analyst and brought back to important areas. The non-directive counseling of Carl Rogers probably came closer to a true unstructured interview. There is no reason to believe that a person with a genuine mental disorder will approach painful topics unless given some impetus to do so. If it were that easy, I am sure all mental disorders would be cured before they reached the mental hospital—or the suicide's grave. Nobody puts up with mental pain if there is an easy cure available.

A semi-structured interview follows a standard format but is varied to take account of the details of the patient's life. The purpose is to gain as much information as possible in addition to letting the patient speak fairly freely about his problems. A full semi-structured interview covers all aspects of his life and present functioning in as much detail as time permits, noting which points the patient considers important for further attention. A partial semi-structured interview focuses attention on certain aspects that the interviewer regards as important. I use a full interview, so I always refer to partial interviews as incomplete. I have seen world-renowned psychiatrists arrive at a diagnosis after as little as twelve minutes of what seemed like vaguely directed chat , but I couldn't do that so I would never try. My initial interview takes an hour but over the years, I have had to drop the cognitive assessment and the physical examination as the questions have become more detailed. I never go over an hour because the patients have had enough and so have I. The questions I use are absolutely standard. There is a reason for this, which will become clear.

My office is in a small, ground level complex in a quiet part of the town. The nearest parking space is about eight meters from the door, the furthest would be about twenty. I have a large picture window looking over the parking lot, across a wide lawn and a road to a nature reserve. I sit at a desk looking out the window; so I soon learn what cars people drive. I see them getting out of their cars before they even know which is my office, which is helpful when they are claiming disabilities. I work alone with only a receptionist in the waiting room. The office is small and quiet and there is no security of any sort. For a new case, the receptionist takes his details over about three minutes, and the patient will normally walk into the office within one or two minutes of his appointed time. Nobody is ever kept waiting more than a couple of minutes. I regard that as terribly important, especially for people who have come from work.

Because of Darwin's tropical climate, my office is somewhat sparsely furnished. The floors are tiled with a rug under the furniture to reduce noise. There are some pictures of dolphins on the walls, three rather upright cane chairs, a potted palm, and a small table against the end wall. It is meant to look like an ordinary, tidy suburban home. The patient sits on the right side of the desk, his back to the window and facing the wall behind me. This way, he can look at me or look away, as he sees fit. For the first fifteen minutes of the interview, I glance at him only every few minutes or so, until he seems comfortable, then watch him more closely but never in a direct manner. Physically, he sits about 1.5 m (5 ft) from me so if I want to touch him, say to look at scars, I have to stand up and take a couple of steps to do so. The desk declares a formality which is lost when patients sit in armchairs. Under the billing agreement, my fees as a private practitioner are reimbursed by the government at a lower rate than the normal private fee system. Apart from some medicolegal reports, patients do not pay me, so money is not an issue.

With few exceptions, I do not refer to patients by their first names and introduce myself as "Dr McLaren". This is done to preserve the air of formality, that they are seeing a specialist for their benefit but not for their entertainment. It is important not to lose sight of the fact that seeing a psychiatrist is a professional matter and decorum will be preserved on both sides. At the first interview, people can be very apprehensive and a moderately formal approach settles them more than a feigned friendliness, which can provoke intense agitation in a patient with bonding anxiety. It is easier to relax later than it is to try to regain formality with a panicky or manipulative patient. From time to time, somebody will demand to know my religion or politics. My answer is always the same: "I have no religious or political views at work."

This prosaic approach developed from experience very early in my training. My first psychotherapy supervisor belonged to what even his friends would have called the 'charismatic inarticulate' school. If he had a theory of mental disorder, he never explained it because he never explained anything. His approach was to encourage patients to sink into their psyches and emote. He had an adoring clientele although most of the other psychiatrists thought he was barmy. When I tried to follow his example, it quickly became clear that something was going seriously wrong: quite often, the patients seemed to slip into a trance-like state. Several times, there seemed little doubt that, in states of altered suggestibility, they were simply feeding back what they thought I wanted to hear so that it was not possible to tell fact from fantasy. It was from experiences like this that my interest in a scientific psychotherapy grew. Years later, when I first saw reports of ritual satanic abuse, alien abduction, and multiple personalities, it seemed there was a perfectly good explanation waiting.

Occasionally, somebody doesn't like my approach. In the past fifteen years, I can recall three patients who left during the initial interview. One was a most manipulative 58-yo schoolteacher who left within a few minutes because all the psychiatrists he had seen in Sydney wore Armani suits whereas, by not wearing a tie, I showed that I didn't respect him (nobody in Darwin wears ties). The other two were women who were patently psychotic and could not have been managed in the private setting. My approach to work is much the same as my approach to everything. Patients can see through a façade in a few moments, and they do not like it. Honesty is critical. If patients don't detect honesty in the interviewer, they will not be forthcoming themselves.

8.2: The History: My Life as a Nut Case

This is a transcript of an actual interview with Mark Jones, a 24-y/o man who had recently returned to Darwin after trying to study at a university in a southern city. He arrived a few minutes late on an extremely hot and humid afternoon in February, 2010. He was flustered and sweaty when he entered the waiting room, then found he had left his Medicare card in his car and had to go back to get it.

I have included the mental state examination at the end, even though it isn't part of the transcript. The headings I use during the history are Presenting Complaints, which covers vegetative functions, cognitive function and mood; History of Presenting Complaints; Family Background, covering parents, siblings, family history, education, work record, social history including relationships, children, reasons for separation, alcohol and drugs, gambling, police record, and general health; then Personal Assessment and finally Mental State. As it may not be clear from the transcript when I move from one section of the interview to the next, I have marked the changes. The primary questions are absolutely standard and do not vary from one interview to the next but the secondary questions follow the patient's leads.

My questions are printed in italics while the patient's answers are in normal print. Square brackets indicate my additions to the transcript. All supporting details have been changed except for the time and place of the interview: Darwin, Australia (February 2010).

Introductory questions

Sorry I'm late, I went to the private hospital, wasn't thinking. I used to see Dr. M there.

Don't worry, two minutes we can manage. Come in, please, have a seat there.

Thanks. It's nice and cool in here, damned hot outside. Sorry if I stink.

It's warm. I'm Dr McLaren, I'm a psychiatrist. Who's referred you? I don't know... Oh, he's in Sydney.

It's actually my dad. He's a GP in [names a fashionable suburb on the far north coast of Sydney]. That's OK, isn't it?

Yeah, it's a valid referral. How much information do you want me to send him? You know I have to send a letter back.

Whatever you reckon. He's heard it all before and doesn't believe it, so what the hell.

You can see the letter before I send it if you like. Anyway, you tell me what's the trouble, why you're here today, and I'll have to write while I'm talking to you.

Yeah, no worries. Why am I here? I'm here to sort out whether I'm bipolar or just a borderline but my mum found an old report on me and checked it on the internet and now she reckons I'm Asperger's. Alex K [names a renowned professor in Sydney who runs a prestigious academic clinic] says I'm...

Don't worry about what anybody else says, you tell me yourself why you're here.

[Pause] Dunno. I've got to get my tablets sorted out. I stopped the lithium when I found out how dangerous it is in a hot climate.

OK, what sort of work are you doing?

I'm helping in my mum's business, ordering, deliveries, that sort of thing, until uni starts here next month. That's if they accept my application.

So where are you living?

I'm living at my mum's place, in a granny flat downstairs.

It's self-contained? You get your own meals?

Sure I do, that way I don't have to talk to her boyfriend. It's easier than putting up with his shit... Sorry, shouldn't talk like that.

I didn't come down in the last shower. So what tablets are you taking now?

I'm on Seroquel 400 mg a day [quetiapine] and Zyprexa 15 mg at night [olanzapine] so I can sleep. They had me on Valpro about 2000 mg a day [sodium valproate] as well but I couldn't stay awake so they gave me lithium.

How much?

One tablet, 450 mg a day. I stopped taking it.

That's subtherapeutic. It wasn't doing anything but I won't prescribe it in this climate. Too dangerous.

Good, I won't take it anyway; messes with my head.

OK, so... Oh, when did you get back to Darwin?

About August.

Oh, you've been here what, eight months? Who's been prescribing your drugs?

The clinic, they've been posting my prescriptions.

They shouldn't do that. They should have referred you as soon as you left the state.

Vegetative questions

So over the past few weeks or so, how have you been feeling in yourself?

Shit. Like shit. I reckon I'm losing it.

What's your sleep been...? It's OK, don't worry about it.

[Fighting back tears] Sorry, you must think I'm such a bloody girl...

Men cry. It's OK, there's some tissues there.

Thanks [grabs a handful of tissues and sits forward, elbows on his knees, jamming the tissues hard against his eyes] Sorry, I hate this; most of the time I can control it but... You reckon I could have a drink of water?

I'll get some.... [leaves room]

... Thanks [gulps half a glass of iced water]. That's better. So what was the question? I've forgotten already.

How have you been feeling lately? He feels terrible [writing]

Terrible's not the word. I don't understand it. They said I've got a chemical imbalance of the brain; take their bloody tablets and I'd get better but I'm getting worse, mate, you gotta believe me [starts to sob again]. Oh, shit, I knew I shouldn't have come, it's easier just to take the tablets and shut the fuck up... sorry.

Don't worry, I was working in prisons before you were born. I've heard everything. There's more tissues. So what's your sleep like?

Shit. I'm such a fool, why can't I keep it together? You must think I'm a real loser [jerks back in his chair and presses his fists against his temples, groaning in distress].

Take it easy, we'll sort it out. So what time do you go to bed?

Two, three, any time.

And what time do you get to sleep?

An hour or two later. I stay up until I'm nearly fucked but I still can't get to sleep.

What time do you wake?

I gotta get up for work, so seven.

How do you feel when you get up?

Shit.

Is it solid sleep or restless?

Restless isn't the word. More like world war three; bed's wrecked when I get up.

Broken sleep. Do you have dreams?

Not really, the tablets stop them mostly.

Do you have naps in the day time?

Sometimes I have to; just can't keep my head alive. I worry if I'm driving.

Sure. Do you sleep in on the weekends?

Not really; bloody Jim's up there crashing and bashing; that's my mother's boyfriend, or he starts the mower next to my window. He's like that. I just give in.

So what's your appetite like?

It's terrible. I just eat because I have to.

And what's your weight doing?

I've put on a shitload of weight since they put me on these fucking tablets. Zyprexa, I read about it. I was real fit; now look at me. 98 kg; I used to be about 80.

It does that. I don't like people taking it long term.

Yeah, but I can't sleep at all without it.

We'll sort that out. So what's your level of energy like?

Terrible. I just feel washed out all the time, like drugged. And weak. If I have to pick up something to deliver, I think I'm going to pass out.

And your level of activity? Do you exercise?

In this climate? I try; I go to gym a bit but it doesn't help.

You can't lose weight at a gym but it's mostly the tablets. We'll sort it out. Now, what about your level of interest in things, firstly in your private life?

Bugger all. Or maybe I play some computer games with some guys I know from Sydney; that's about it.

And your interest in your work?

None, I just do it. Keeps the old lady quiet; keeps her not-so-tame gorilla off my back.

And your study? What do you want to do?

I started in maths but I failed; so now I'm looking at accounting. Bloody boring.

And your motivation to do things, what's that like?

You gotta be joking. None. I can hardly put one foot after another. All I want to do is lie down; these bloody tablets [starts to cry again]. I'm sorry, this isn't normal. I used to see Alex K and I didn't cry. I'd make him laugh.

You saw him yourself?

My old man and him were in medical school together, so I got to see the top dog himself. But you hardly get to see him; he's so busy; rushes in, asks how you're going, but he's writing a new prescription before you've even answered. I didn't say anything; just tell a few jokes to make him think I'm OK. He's never there, anyway. Doesn't stop him sending his bills, though. How much is this going to cost me?

Nothing, it's bulk-billed.

You're joking. I thought that died out years ago.

I'm the last hold-out. So you're motivation's terrible. What about your social life? Do you mix with people?

Oh, I'm good at it, just ask the old lady. I can talk to anybody; just wind me up and let me rip.

But do you have a social life?

No, I don't. I get on the chat rooms at night and talk to a couple of blokes in America but they're as mad as I am. Maybe worse. They can't get any treatment; they're poor. I'll tell them I get to see a specialist here for nothing.

Could be worse. And your sexual interest? What's that like?

None. Zip. Dead.

The drugs don't help.

Cognitive section

What about your memory?

Old lady's always at me for forgetting her fucking deliveries. God knows how I'm supposed to study; I can't even stay awake to read; then I can't get to sleep at night. What a mess! They said I'd be better.

The hospital? That clinic? Well, obviously you're not.

Yeah, but that's why they said I'm borderline. You know, an arsehole. I know it sounds weak but when I was 19 or 20, I took some overdoses; I felt so bad. And they won't let you forget it. How long have I got?

You've got 46 minutes left. And your concentration? What's that like?

Terrible. Can't concentrate on anything but dumb computer games.

Does your mind drift and wander, or are you distracted by everything?

Oh, that's right, I'm ADD as well. I'm a dreamer; always been. My mind wanders around; I never know what I'm thinking. So what was the question?

You just answered it. Are you able to make decisions?

No, I put them off; then I get into more trouble.

Do you put them off because it's too much hard work or because you're scared of making mistakes?

Both, but mostly scared of fucking up and getting the shit blown out of me. You must think I'm a real wanker.

I've seen worse. Are you able to think clearly, with one thought leading on to the next?

Not really.

What does that mean? Can you think clearly or do you get confused and flustered?

Flustered, that's the word. If people leave me alone, I'm OK but as soon as there's any pressure, my mind turns into a spin dryer. Zoom zoom!

You mean too many thoughts tumbling in your head, or...?

Too many. Everything crowds in on me and I start to feel like nothing's real. I try to keep thinking of what I have to do and what I'm likely to get wrong and then I panic.

OK, we'll come back to that. And what do you tend to think about, what's on your mind?

When? At work, all I can think about is stuffing up something else again, losing this package or misfiling that order; then the old lady gets on my case and before long, we're in a screaming match and then Jim sticks his bib in and threatens to send me back to Sydney to the nuthouse, so I have to get out, like go home. Maybe I have a few cans or a couple of cones to get me head back together and that gives them something else to go on when they get home. You're an addict; you're an alcoholic; you have to go to counseling; go into rehab; whatever. Listen, you're not going to stick me in the crazy ward are you? If that's why you're writing that down, I'm leaving.

No, I don't admit people to hospital. And when you're not at work, what do you think about?

Good. What? Think about? At night? After they've all gone to bed and it's quiet? I put on some music and just think what a fucking mess I've made of my life; how'm I going to get out of it?

You mean out of the mess or out of your life?

Both. Don't worry, I'm not suicidal.

And have you had any peculiar experiences, like hearing or seeing things that didn't make sense?

You mean hallucinations? No, not lately. I did once; I'd failed my exams and was doing a shitload of dope and somebody gave me some eckers (ecstasy), and I was out of it for a couple of days; couldn't sleep. Really hearing things, like voices telling me I'm a loser. They told me it was a drug psychosis but I know they told my old man it was schizoaffective something. Then they changed it back to bipolar.

But that's not happening now?

No.

What about that sense of things seeming unreal?

Yeah, that. It's like I'm sitting in a tunnel looking down at the world; it all seems too far away and so, like, I'm not part of it or anything. Other people are part of it; they're real, but I'm a freak.

Alien?

Yeah that's, that's good. Alien. I feel like the alien. I should get one of those shirts. Oh hullo Gloria, come in, have you met our little alien? He lives here. Mark, be a darling and say something in alien for our dinner guests, but don't do your usual trick like scaring them or we'll have to put you away again [his eyes fill with tears]. What's wrong with me? I've seen the top professors in the country and all they can say is chemical imbalance of the brain. I take their fucking drugs but why aren't I better? Can you help me? [Leans his head on his hand and wipes his face] What a dumb question! This is fucking Darwin; we're not in Sydney now. End of the line. End of the world [tries to laugh] Sorry, I don't mean to be rude but this is a long way from things, isn't it? Come to Darwin, get your head sorted out. You've probably got as many problems as I have, ay, that's why you're here. That's what they said in Sydney. That's why they posted my prescriptions, because there's nobody here.

I'm here. So you feel the world is real but you're changed. Do you have it the other way around, you're normal but the world has changed?

No, I'm the weirdo. And that's another disorder, Dissociative Disorder. How many of these fucking disorders can you have?

Anything else? What about time? Do you have the feeling of time speeding up or slowing down?

Sometimes. When I'm up against the wall, time seems to slow down; a minute lasts about ten minutes. Seems like that; anyway, I know it can't be true.

Your body? Does that ever seem strange?

Yeah, well look at me. I used to be real fit but now I'm just flab. No, just seems normal.

Section on Mood: depressive

OK, so most of the time, most days, how would you say you feel in yourself?

Shit. Worse than shit. Dead shit.

I'll put that down as terrible. You actually feel low and miserable?

Most of the time.

How bad is it?

Bad.

You get to the stage of saying I'm sick of the way things are?

All the time.

Sick of life itself?

[Pauses uncertainly] Yeah.

Get to the stage of saying if I dropped dead, it would be a relief?

Yeah, relief for everybody else. But I'm not suicidal.

You get to the stage of saying I could finish my life, it's that easy? Maybe look at a branch on a tree and think it would be strong enough, or just say I could jerk the wheel and it would be all over?

Yeah, I do…

A lot?

Um, yeah, most days.

Do you have any urge to act on those ideas or do they just drift in and out?

Just drifting. I don't really want to die. I been through that. I just want to get a life.

Sure. And what's the cause of your unhappiness?

What? I'm bipolar. Chemicals in the brain or something.

No, the actual cause. Why are you unhappy?

Oh you mean…? Like, no job and no career and no girlfriend?

Yes. So why do you not have a job and a career?

I failed. Couldn't study. Borderline or something.

So you don't know?

No. Dunno. Does that mean I'm crazy?

No. Crazy is voices. So you don't know the actual cause?

No. I've had voices. Not now though, but I still talk to myself. Is that crazy?

No, you have to get some sensible answers sometimes. Do you ever feel the opposite of…?

Hey, that's good. Talk to myself to get some sense. Do you know that Prof. K?

I've met him once or twice but he probably wouldn't remember me. They're very busy people.

Section on Mood: Elevate]

Do you ever feel the opposite of depressed; you feel fantastic, full of energy, and on top of the world for no good reason?

Sometimes I feel good... but it never lasts. Maybe I get the idea I could get a job on a mine and save lots of money and suddenly everything seems clear, then reality bites. Like I'd have to eat in the mess with the other blokes, fly in and out in small planes. Then I crash for a while, almost like I gotta pay double for feeling good.

So it never lasts. Do you ever overspend or do silly things when you're...?

No. I don't go manic.

It's actually hypomanic.

Section on Mood: Anxiety

Now, in your ordinary daily life, is there anything you are frankly scared of, like heights, confined spaces, wide open spaces?

Not real good on heights; I always have the idea I'm going to jump over so I have to keep away from the edge.

See that roof there, could you walk on that?

Maybe, but that would be the limit. What else? Confined spaces, not good. That's why I don't like small planes, you can't get off. I was locked in a cupboard once, my brother...

Everybody was, children are like that. You probably locked some other kid in a cupboard.

I did. I remember him screaming and I was glad because he had it like I did. Wide open spaces, no, I love the bush and empty beaches. No people.

Thunder and lightning, electricity...

No.

Water, darkness, dirt, disorder, contamination, do they scare you?

Not keen on dirt but you should see my room.

Weapons like firearms and knives?

No, I'm a good shot and I've got fishing knives.

Any animals scare you? Rats, bats, frogs, toads, snakes, spiders, cockroaches...

Nah, I had a pet python. Animals are fine.

What about dealing with people? Do you become nervous in crowds...?

No way. Can't do that. That was the problem at uni; I couldn't go in the big lecture theaters.

Standing in a queue with people straight behind you?

No, never. I put my things down and walk out. I do my shopping early; Darwin's great; the shops open at six on Sunday mornings.

Public speaking?

You gotta be joking. No way. Couldn't do it.

Appointments and interviews, tests and exams...?

No, none of them. I shit myself with interviews; I can't sleep before exams.

Public transport?

Not good at it. Not here; can't stand those gangs of black kids; shouldn't say it but they look you up and down and you know they mean trouble.

Threats or criticism?

I lose it, totally. Criticism I never know whether I'll burst into tears or go apeshit and want to punch the bloke's lights out.

Arguments and disputes, confrontation and saying no to people?

No no no. If there's an argument at work, like my old lady and Jim have a few words, I have to get away. And saying no to people? Never. Can not do that. It gets me into terrible trouble but I can't do it.

OK, what about the thought of letting people down or causing trouble, does that scare you?

Yeah, the whole lot. I just...

The thought of loneliness, humiliation, disapproval?

Loneliness, I'm used to it. I don't like it but it doesn't scare me. Humiliation? Far canal, you'd think I'd be used to it now, but no. And disapproval, I hate it, although it's all I seem to get.

What about the thought of making a mistake or failing at something?

Ah, mate, that's the worst. Failure. I can't stand being a failure. I'll take crucifixion any day.

So it's bad enough to stop you doing something?

Absolutely. I used to walk off the sports field at school or not turn up to exams because I couldn't stand the thought of failing. My brother was brilliant at everything but I was so fucking useless, you got no idea.

And illness or death or mental illness? They scare you?

Again, they do. I don't want to die; it keeps me awake at night. And mental illness terrifies me; that's the pits. You know why? Because nobody can help you. They say they can, they say they got all these fancy drugs and shit but it's crap. I've seen people come in and out, in and out, they never get any better. Sorry, it's your job...

That's OK, truth isn't always pleasant. Hospitals or dentists, blood or needles, they scare you?

Nah, don't like hospitals but I'm not scared of them.

What about groups of people, like police, military, bikies...?

Cops I'm not keen on; they've dragged me off to the nuthouse a couple of times. Army? Nah, they're cool.

Bikies, blackfellas, drunks, gangs, aggressive people...?

All of 'em. Have to get right away. Those gangs of half-caste kids are a nightmare; sounds bad but it's true.

And people in authority?

If they're nice and take an interest in me, I'm fine; but if they look at me like I'm the grub that dropped the plate, I can't take it. My knees shake; they really shake.

Section Paranoid ideas

OK, so when you're out and about, do you have the feeling people are looking at you or talking behind your back...?

Always. I have to leave.

Strangers, or people who know you?

Both. It depends on where I am. I can't go to parties unless I've got a skinful of piss. Then I carry on and make a complete idiot of myself.

Do you have the feeling people are judging you?

They are. Everybody, all the time. Oh, look at him, that's Ivan Jones' son; he's mental; such a pity for his parents, lovely people. And his brother and sister, so brilliant, but that Mark, he's a loser. Must be masturbatory insanity; it couldn't be hereditary.

Do you have the feeling people are a danger to you; they're likely to have a go in some way?

Always, especially if I'm nervous, then everybody who looks my way is going to come over and call me a dickhead. I can't stand near the edge of the railway platform in case somebody pushes me over. They'd do it for fun, just to laugh.

Do you ever have the feeling you're being watched or spied on, you're under surveillance or bugged?

Sometimes, when I'm really at my worst, I think the neighbors are collecting evidence to give to the Mental Health Tribunal to have me locked up. I checked once with a couple; they said they weren't. Made me look pretty stupid.

Do you have the feeling people are plotting or conspiring against you, they're telling lies or spreading stories, or holding information back from you?

Sometimes. Holding things back. I feel people know something I don't; or they've got some sort of message about self-control and they're all laughing because I'm such a dickhead and I don't know it. It comes and goes.

Section on Obsessive-Compulsive behavior

Sure. Now are you a person who checks things all the time, doors, locks, keys, switches, gas taps, that sort of thing?

Oh, yeah, I got OCD real bad. Depends on how I feel. Sometimes I'm just too tired to bother.

Why do you check?

I feel if I've made a mistake and the place gets robbed or it burns down, I'll be blamed. I'm terrified of being blamed.

And if you don't check, what then?

That's it, trouble. If I'm feeling good, I can tell myself nothing will go wrong and it doesn't; but if I've got one of my panics, then I have to go and check ten thousand times because I can't stand the thought of somebody else getting on my back.

Are you very fussy about cleanliness, tidiness, order, punctuality, and efficiency?

I am, but if you saw my room now, you wouldn't think so. If I live with anybody else, I drive them mad, fussing around, cleaning things.

Do you have special ways of arranging and ordering or cleaning things, it's got to be done just so, by a ritual?

My things. Anybody touches my things, I go mad.

Do you count things or color code them or touch them in certain ways?

I color code clothes when I hang them on the line. Touch things? Yeah, I touch them as I walk past and it annoys me if I miss them.

Do you have thoughts popping into your head all the time that you know are silly but you can't resist them?

I got a head full of shit, drives me mad.

Like what?

Like suicide, or getting even with people who made fun of me years ago.

But you don't think it's silly at the time, do you?

No way, I'm serious. I don't mean that, I'm not a danger; but I often dream of all the kids that made fun of me at school and how I'd like to cut their balls off. Then I could laugh at them like they... [starts to cry]. All my life... I just dunno.

Section on Recent History

That's OK. So how long has all this trouble been going on?

First time I was put in hospital...

No, all the trouble. All the fears, feeling strange, everything.

Oh, all my life. Long as I can remember. I've always been fucked in the head. Born like it, I reckon.

So there was no particular incident that started it?

No.

Section on Personal Background: Family

OK, you tell me about your background. Where were you born and raised?

I was born in Sydney and raised in the eastern suburbs. I moved here when I was twelve after my folks split and...

OK, so how old's your father now?

He's 56.

And he's a GP in Sydney. How old were when they separated?

Eleven.

Who raised you after that?

Some with my mother, some at boarding school, some with the old man, here and there. A mess.

So what's he like as a person?

Oh, he's popular.

But as a person?

He was always working, and soon as he got home, he'd want to see our school books and check how we were going at sport. He's mad about sport, if you weren't on the school team for everything, you weren't trying.

So he's demanding...

Very.

Controlling?

A control freak? Not to look at, he's always bouncing around, laughs a lot but you know he's watching you. He doesn't miss a thing. If you don't laugh with him, he gets snaky and wants to know what's wrong with you.

And how did you get on with him?

Sort of OK if we weren't in the same state. He thinks I'm a loser. Like, lazy, never trying. I mean, he's a doctor but he doesn't believe in all this psychiatry shit; you're either lazy or crazy in his book. I think he was kind of glad when Alex said I was schizoaffective, it meant he hadn't raised a lazy son.

And your mother? How old is she?

She's the same age. She moved here after they separated, came straight up here to join her boyfriend. He was in the Army then and they stayed here after he retired.

So what's she like as a person?

She's OK, but she's always trying to please Jim. So if I'm annoying Jim, like say I'm breathing, she'll be on my case [affects an upper class accent]. Mark, do you have to breathe so loud? Look at the way your nose moves when you breathe. And do you have to scratch yourself when I talk to you? I've got this habit, see, if I'm standing up and somebody is telling me off, I have to scratch my nuts. Drives her mad.

Do either of them drink?

The old man, no, not now. It would interfere with his half-marathons. Oh, and he's a fitness fanatic, always running around in his little dinky shorts and runners, no shirt. If he sees me with my Zyprexa flab, he just shakes his head and turns away. He's into every sport known to man; he's the club doctor for half a dozen clubs. I think he's a sports groupie.

Was there a stepmother?

Yeah, she's not too bad but she's the same; she's got these high-energy sons. They just make money. Like harvest it. It's obscene. I think they invite me to Christmas just so they can all look down on me.

The stepfather we know about.

Oh, he's just never got over leaving the Army. I don't think they should be allowed to retire. They should just give them a medal and shoot them in the head, one after the other. He's got two daughters; you think I'm a mess, you haven't seen them. One's a complete headfuck; the other's a drug-addled whooer in Perth.

Were you raised with them?

No, thank Christ. One of them tried to seduce me when I was eighteen. I nearly pissed myself with fright. By the way, I've never been sexually molested and I'm not a fag.

Why do you say that?

Because at that fancy fucking clinic in Sydney, the doctors pump you full of drugs; then they send you off to see the psychologists who are convinced that everybody with anything has been screwed by the priest. I wasn't. Nothing like that. They can't understand that you can go mad just by being left alone.

So how many brothers and sisters were there altogether?

There's three of us. I'm the second.

So your brother's first? How old is he, where is he, and what's he do?

He's a genius, just ask him. He's two years older than me, he's a doctor, of course, and he's in the Air Force. Dunno where he is now, over firebombing the Afghans, I suppose. He's a pilot, too. He's married and he's everything I'm not. He'd be 15 kg underweight from doing marathons; he got all the prizes at school; he was in every sport; he loves everybody and everybody loves him. He'll be the chief medical officer for the defense forces; that's his goal and he'll do it. And on the way, he'll make sure he's in every combat zone there is, pass every test, beat everybody in the interservices marathon, lecture at ADFA, you name it. [ADFA: Australian Defence Forces Academy, the military university in Canberra].

You're pretty good at this, aren't you?

You noticed? Hey, that's cool. I've been wanting to say these things for half my life but nobody ever asked.

What do you mean they didn't ask?

Nobody asked me.

You've been to the most prestigious center in the country. That's actually a World Health Reference Center, did you know that?

Course I know that; I can read. When you go in the main doors, there's this huge banner about a mission statement or some shit; then all the things they belong to and all the big dicks who visit them. Alex K is a consultant to the DSM-5 committee, you know what that is?

I do know. Anyway, you've got a sister.

Yeah, she's 21. She's in Sydney, blitzing the law school. She's a musical genius, artistic, brilliant, beautiful, goes out with Cameron V, you know about them? They're worth more than this whole shitheap town put together. I hate his guts. He pretends to be nice to me, asks me how I'm going when any fucker with half a brain can see I'm getting ready to jump.

He may be genuine. Quite often, the truly wealthy have no idea what it's like to be down and out.

He hasn't. None at all. He's so dumb, it's written across his stupid forehead. Drives a supercharged Jag sports. And he calls it a syooper-charged Jag-wah, the fucking cocksucker. I dream of gouging his eyes out.

Is there any family history of mental illness?

No way, I'm the first to tarnish the escutcheon.

Anybody drinking too much or using illegal drugs?

I do drugs sometimes, just dope. The old man hit the bottle a bit after they separated but not for long, and I was up here by then, anyway.

Anybody got a criminal record?

No.

Section on Personal Background: Schooling

So where did you go to school?

St. Patrick's by the sea [names a suburb]. You know about it? It's the most exclusive boys' school on the north shore. Cost a fucking fortune and I didn't even get groped by the sports master.

How old were you when you left?

Eighteen, finished Year 12.

That's normal in NSW, isn't it? What sort of marks did you get?

You're pretty thorough, aren't you? My marks weren't actually bad; they just weren't top. My brother's were, and my sister's were but mine were mostly Bs, a few As, and they got worse as I got older, not better.

Why?

I was depressed. First of all, they said I was ADD because I didn't pay attention, so they took me to see this pediatrician who put me on drugs, but I hated them, so I stopped them. I got caught swapping them in the playground and they were going to expel me so my mum said I didn't have to take them. She would've drowned me in the pool if I'd been expelled.

How did you get on with the teachers?

Mostly I didn't. I didn't take much notice of them at all. If they yelled at me, I just fell in a heap but if they were nice to me, I'd do well, except all the kids would tell me I was just sucking up to him which proves he's a fag.

How would they know?

Don't be so dumb. Rich kids know everything. So do poor kids; they have to. A couple of the brothers were fags and I got on fine with them; they didn't threaten me and I didn't play up. I remember... no, another day.

And how did you get on with the other kids?

Mostly no good. I had a couple of friends but they were even sillier than I was. I used to boss them around; made me feel better. I went through a stage where I was bullying a couple of them but I nearly got caught so I stopped that one.

Were you shy or nervous?

Both. I couldn't speak in front of the class and I'd blush and stammer if anybody yelled at me.

Did you get into fights?

Almost never, I was too scared. Once or twice I went berserk because kids were needling me in the classes so I was taken back to see that pediatrician. Second time I refused to go, I jumped out of the car at a traffic light and got a bus back home. Boy, was I in the shit when I got home; they were just about to call the prime minister to borrow the army to look for me.

Did you play sport?

Not much, I was too uncoordinated. They said I had hand-eye dyspraxia, whatever that is.

Dyspraxia. It's nothing. It means you hadn't found the sport you liked.

Well, that's true. I took up scuba diving at uni [university] and loved it but I was smoking too much dope by then.

What were your main interests at school?

Nothing much, I liked music until I worked out that all the other kids reckoned it meant I was a fag. I liked history, and maths, of course, but the teachers were hopeless. They were only interested in pushing the kids through the matric [the matriculation or university entrance examination].

What was your home life like?

Not good. Before they separated, they were always bickering. Not really bad arguments and no fighting, just snaky comments; we could hear all the angry whispering every night, and always trying to get us to take sides. My brother was on my mother's side and my sister was daddy's pet, so I was nowhere.

That's actually quite common. So what did you do then?

After they separated? Mum came straight up here; I reckon she was seeing Jim before but he was still in the army, so I don't know how they managed that. My grandmother moved in for a while; the old man was drinking a bit and I wasn't having a good time at school.

What was she like?

Nana? She was old. My father was the youngest of about six kids, so she's nearly ninety now. She's OK, I don't dislike her. So I had to come here. I wasn't doing any good at school in Sydney but this was a disaster. They put me in [a Catholic school for rural Aboriginal youth]. I shat myself. I have never been so scared in all my life. I'd never seen a blackfella and these kids were fullbloods from the bush. They hardly spoke English; they couldn't use a knife and fork. Some of them wouldn't even shit in the dunnies; they'd wait until lights out and sneak out into the garden for a shit. The gardener just buried it next day. And fight, god help us, I wasn't very big; I was a late starter, and they were all a couple of years older. I put up with it for six months, then I told my mother I'd run away to the mangroves if she tried to send me back. So she took me to see Dr M. Where's he now?

He had a mixed career, as they say. He died in disgrace.

Suicide? They say psychiatrists are sillier than their patients—no offence.

Well, look at you, how silly would that make me?

Ha ha, I deserved that. Anyway, I went back to Sydney, stayed with the old man and the stepmother, but that didn't work out, so I boarded at St Patrick's for a couple of years. That was sort of bearable. Boarders were higher in status than day boys and the brothers were a bit more friendly; they seemed to think some of us might join their order. I just kept on drifting. I spent most of my time at school doodling in my school books and looking out the window at the yachts on the harbor. Somehow I managed to get through the matric and was accepted to do maths but not at the old man's uni, the other one. The cheap one.

You went straight to university?

No, I thought I'd have a break so I came back up here to get some work. Worst thing I ever did.

You didn't get a job?

I did. But they were all dopeheads and I started in no time. Grog and dope, it calmed me. Things went downhill. I was living with my old lady and they were forever threatening to chuck me out. It's not that I was doing much wrong, I just couldn't do anything right. I fell over the barbecue once. I wasn't even pissed. Way they carried on, you'd think I did it deliberately. Nobody bothered that I had a huge scald on my thigh but I wouldn't have shown them anyway. So they went out to the yacht club for dinner leaving me the steak with the sand on it. So I gave it to the dog and got pissed instead. I can't do anything right. But it was so lonely. That's the problem with being a problem child; it's so lonely [eyes fill again]. Anyway, I went back to Sydney and started studying. The old man wanted me to live with him but that was crazy, too far to travel; so I shared a flat near the uni but that was no good. I was just getting worse and worse, too scared to go to my classes; every now and then, I'd hit the grog. I met this girl but she was half out of her tree and that went nowhere. I failed first year, repeated, failed again, took an overdose, went to hospital yahdi yahdi yah. How we going for time?

I'm watching it. So why did you come back?

Grass is greener, I suppose. When you're in Sydney, you long for the laid back tropical lifestyle and when you're here, the sandflies and heat drive you mad and you need to see an art film or go to a concert. There's nothing here. I go mad.

Section on Personal Background: Social

So you've always been single?

Yep.

How much do you drink?

Not much now; couple of beers a couple of times a week but if I'm feeling too bad, I'll get hammered for a few weeks.

And any other drugs?

Just a bit of dope every now and then. The old folks upstairs go bananas if they smell it. Jim threatened to have me arrested once.

Do you gamble?

No.

Do you have a police record?

Resisting arrest, I think. Nothing much.

And your general health is OK? No hepatitis?

Nah, I'm fine.

So what sort of sexual experience do you have?

You have to ask. I'm a virgin. At twenty four. You can laugh if you like.

I'm not laughing. This should be the best time of your life. You don't get a rerun.

[Sits up abruptly, looks to interviewer, starts to cry openly and angrily] You think I don't know that? You think I don't pace up and down all night, trying to work out what's wrong with me and fix it up? Going mad is just so lonely. I'm sorry, I shouldn't yell at you; you're just doing your job.

It's not just a job, it's...

Well I'm fucking glad to hear that because that's all it was to those shits down in Sydney. Just a fucking job so they could get up the ladder. They didn't give a shit about us crazies. Shit I hate crying, makes me look such a wuss.

Section on Self-Assessment

Crying is OK, it's a safety valve. Now how would you see yourself as a person?

As a person? You mean, not a mad person?

I mean the person you see yourself to be. Not who you would like to be, or who others would like you to be.

Well, I... I don't really know. I like to help people. I think I'm fairly bright; sometimes I can make people laugh...

Would you see yourself as a nervous person?

Nervous? Not really.

But you've said you get anxiety attacks.

Oh, yeah, I suppose I am. Don't like to say it, though.

Would you say you're able to stand up for yourself or do you get pushed around?

Anybody can push me around. I'm broke but if you ask me for my last dollar, I'll hand it over.

Does that cause you trouble?

Oh yeah. I give in and give in; then I go mad and get them all back. That's why they said I'm bipolar. Mood swings.

We'll talk about that. Would you say you are easily bothered by guilt inside?

Guilt? Oh man, yes, I do guilt. I do guilt with nobs on.

The brothers won after all. And shame?

Real bad shame. Biggest shame, that's what the black kids say.

And self-consciousness?

It's funny you should say that, I'm not ugly but if anybody turns around and looks at me, I nearly die. Hate it.

Would you say you trust people readily or you're wary of people?

I trust too much, I get into trouble.

Overtrusting is a fault, especially in this part of the country. And would you see yourself as a tidy, organized sort of person? You sure do. Patient or impatient?

It depends. If I'm out to lunch, like in a dreamy mood, I don't take any notice of anything but if I'm nervous, don't keep me waiting. I fly off the handle over nothing.

Do you tend to follow rules?

Rules? Yeah, I do. Safety rules, money, that sort of thing. Not dope, of course; I break that one.

You're no orphan there. Would you say you're a social sort of person or you can get by without people?

That's hard. I actually like people and I'm good at talking one on one but groups terrify me. Especially rich people. People I was brought up with. Poor people I'm not so bad. I can actually talk to the blackfellas.

You be careful of them, they'll start asking for money.

I know. I keep away now.

Are you inclined to be jealous?

Yeah, I'm jealous of people who are calm and sensible; is that what you mean?

No, that's envy. Jealousy is possessive of people.

I used to be. If I had a friend, I didn't want him to talk to anybody in case he liked them better. But girls? No, I've never really had a girlfriend. And this is where you write a note but I'm telling you I'm not gay.

It's not really my business if you are or aren't. It's not psychiatry.

What? But isn't it a disease? A chemical imbalance of the brain?

No, that's just a theory and not a very good theory in my view. So how come you're still virgo intacta?

I just can't. I'm too scared of making a fool of myself. Truth is, I watch porn sometimes and I can, you know, get it off but when it comes to actually talking to a girl, I just sweat and blush and dribble and while I'm making up my mind, some other bloke moves in and I miss out. Again. Either that or I get pissed legless and fall over and spew my guts up.

A great romantic. And you still don't think you're an anxious person?

Shy, is that the same thing?

Same thing. Social anxiety.

Oh, Social Phobia, yeah, I've got that too.

Do you hold grudges.

Oh yes. Grudges I do, big time. Hmm, I think about getting even but when it comes to doing something about it, I feel sorry for them and say, Oh don't worry, you didn't mean it, let's be friends. And they do it again and I hate them and plot their death.

How do you rate your temper?

No good. People don't see it much but it's there.

How do you rate your intellect?

I'm not dumb. I can read maths easily and work it out but dealing with people? No, I'm people dumb.

How do you rate your self-esteem?

Shit.

Why? What do you see as your major failing?

My major failing is failing. I never finish anything. I give in and walk away.

Why is that?

I suppose that's what bipolar Asperger's borderlines do.

Section on Personal Assessment: Insight

And what would you say is the nature of your trouble?

I dunno. I'm a head fuck. Chemical imbalance of the brain, I suppose.

And what's the cause of it?

Oh, that's easy. Genes. But it doesn't make sense. I'm the first one in the family, the rest of them have got it together.

What do you think?

I dunno. I've always been off the planet, a space cadet. I was born screwed and if I don't look out, I'll die... oh shit [starts to cry].

So what do you think should be done? What's a suitable remedy?

Besides shoot me? I dunno. I've tried their fucking drugs and it just gets worse. I've been to their counseling and that was just... just talk. I've had their CBT from Prof. W, he's supposed to be the leading expert in the country; he goes overseas to lecture. I dunno. I don't know what to do. It's not real good, is it?

Mental State Examination showed a healthy, somewhat overweight young man of about his stated years dressed in clean casual clothing including buttoned shirt, board shorts, and sandals. He had short hair and was clean shaven but had a day's growth. He had a single visible tribal style tattoo on the left upper arm, a small gold ear stud, and a quality gold neck chain but no visible scars. He spoke clearly and openly with an odd mixture of a private school accent and Darwin street slang. In general, he was good-looking and neatly-presented. At the beginning of the interview, he was hot and sweaty and smelled of sweat and tobacco. He was flustered, flushed, and agitated, and quickly became distressed and weepy but tried unsuccessfully to laugh it off. At times, he could hardly talk for crying. He was not anxious about the interview and was clearly experienced in medical appointments. He was very unhappy with high guilt, self-abnegation and some despair, and vague suicidal ideas, but with no urge to act on them. He was not hostile or suspicious. There were no signs of a psychotic disorder and nothing to indicate an organic impairment of brain function. He was clearly of superior intellectual ability but educated below his potential.

8.3: *Qui Bono?*

It should be noted that this is an absolutely normal case history. The only difference was that the patient was clever, talkative, and experienced in the ways of psychiatrists.

This man had been treated for a number of years at one of the country's most renowned psychiatric centers. Over the years, he had undergone half a dozen EEGs, at least three CT scans, two MRI scans, and an unknown number of blood tests. At different times, he had been given the following diagnoses: Attention Deficit Disorder, Pediatric Bipolar Disorder, Character Disorder NOS, Complex Partial Epilepsy, Dysthymia, Major Depression, Bipolar Disorder, Social Phobia, Generalized Anxiety Disorder, Panic Disorder, Obsessive-Compulsive Disorder, Schizoaffective Disorder, Post-Traumatic Stress Disorder, Substance Abuse, Drug-Induced Psychosis, Sleep Disorder, Borderline Personality Disorder, Schizotypal Personality Disorder, Narcissistic Personality Disorder, and Autism Spectrum Disorder/Asperger's Syndrome.

Between the ages of twelve and twenty-four, he had been prescribed methylphenidate, dexamphetamine, lamotrigine, fluoxetine, fluvoxamine, imipramine, clomipramine, venlafaxine, promethazine, pericyazine, olanzapine, quetiapine, haloperidol, droperidol, diazepam, clonazepam, lithium carbonate, carbamazepine, sodium valproate, gabapentin, and at least two other drugs that could not be determined. At the time he left Sydney, he had been told that he would be considered for ECT. It was a factor in his abrupt return to Darwin.

From the psychologists, he had received cognitive-behavioral therapy, relaxation training, eye movement desensitization and reprocessing (for the PTSD from the sexual abuse he was adamant he did not experience), drug education and counseling, self-esteem building, psychoeducation, sexual identity counseling, some form of meditation training, stress management, and anger management.

His case records from the internationally-regarded psychiatric center showed that at no stage had anybody taken a detailed history covering his life experiences or a personality assessment. He had never been assessed cognitively. A proportion of the diagnoses appear to have been made on the basis of his responses of various questionnaires, although the originals were not available as they were used in research programs. He had signed consent for this purpose and wasn't concerned about it.

It is my view that there are features of this case which go to the very heart of the modern psychiatric industry. It raises critically important questions about the nature, the goals, and the methods of a medical specialty which is accorded unusual status and powers by the larger society.

The first question we need to answer is this: What is the nature of the intellectual process in psychiatry which can confidently claim that a person is suffering twenty-one separate diagnostic conditions? What does it say of the concept of diagnosis as it is used today; what does it say about the deeper concept of mental disorder itself? My answer is that anything it says about the patient is accidental: what it says about psychiatry is that the notion of separate diagnostic categories is incoherent. To spell out twenty-one separate diagnoses in one young human being is to stretch far beyond breaking point the utility which justifies making diagnoses. It is self-contradictory in the sense that, by aiming to improve our knowledge of the patient, it offers only an ersatz understanding, a make-believe or sham science of mental disorder. The psychiatrists are more interested in making arcane diagnoses than they are in helping the person. It has become a process of one-upmanship, where psychiatrists compete with each other to find the most abstruse diagnosis that the clinical facts can support. Because DSM is so badly conceived, it lends itself to misuse so that the process has become an absurdity, an embarrassment and an impediment.

What justifies the idea of endlessly proliferating diagnostic categories? What makes it worthwhile; what is its point and value? To ask Prof. K on one of his stops between his international conferences would simply invite an incredulous smile. As it happens, I spoke to him years ago on just this point and he brushed the question aside. For him, the idea of minutely teasing out any and every strand of diagnostic significance is its own justification. His attitude would be similar to the botanists who argue over how many species of eucalyptus trees there are in Australia. Most of us don't care whether there are 682 or 712 eucalypts but, among the plant sniffers, it is a matter of great import. Finding a new species is a source of kudos—and hubris—but there is a difference between their self-involved hobby and psychiatry's headlong rush to microscopic pseudo-precision:

the process of finding species in biology has an end. The definition of a species is that individuals can reproduce by means of fertile offspring. One day, the count stops. There is a finite number of species in the world. It can't go any further than the point at which the individuals stop reproducing.

Psychiatry, however, is different. We just keep on going. The silliest example of all is the modern approach to personality disorder (see Chap. 7 in Humanizing Madness). Here, there is no limit. We just keep dicing and slicing the human pie until we have one personality type for each living person. Reductio ad absurdum. Depression is the same. We can cut and recut the depressive spectrum and keep pulling out valid clusters based on the notion that each individual in the cluster is more like the other members of that cluster than like a member of any other cluster. All you have to do to keep splitting the clusters is include more and more factors in your cluster analysis. The race is to the most creative, not to the most sensible. In the psychotic disorders, we started with Kräpelin's dyadic split between Dementia Praecox (schizophrenia) and the manic-depressive psychoses. That was very comforting and intellectually undemanding until it was realized that it didn't actually fit the cases terribly well. Leonhard found his cycloid psychoses, Färgermann uncovered the psychogenic psychoses (also known as reactive psychoses) and Christiansen described the schizophreniform psychoses (all of these are plural); then there were the hundreds of symptomatic psychoses and the puerperal psychoses, and so on. Finally, the whole structure sagged and buckled as schizoaffective psychoses were added to the list. The split had failed. (For interest, see Karl Leonhard's remarkable nosology listed under his entry in Wikipedia. Experienced psychiatrists will recognize most or all of the types he described.)

There is an infinite number of ways of dividing the set of all mental disorders in the world, not the least because there is no firm border (no demarcation criterion) between mental order and mental disorder. As DSM-V will surely show, the number of mental disorders keeps breeding because the keepers of the psychiatric laboratory keep splitting their categories like amoeba.

Finding twenty-one separate diagnoses in one unhappy human proves nothing. It does not prove he has the disorders, or that they are real things. By listing them, all the psychiatrists had done was show that they could reliably follow a flow chart. The validity of the diagnoses—that is, whether they were in fact real things—wasn't even considered. I say it wasn't valid. Their purpose was to look at the "mere surface" of the disorders and then class them that way, roughly akin to classing animals by color and size. The alternative is to classify mental disorders according to their causes but, since orthodox psychiatry doesn't have causes, only gaps in the chain which biochemistry is supposed to fill in one fine day, it can't do that. However, the biocognitive model of mental disorder is a causative model. It looks at inner causes of the surface manifestations. My view is that, for example, Social Phobia, Generalized Anxiety Disorder, Panic Disorder, and Obsessive-Compulsive Disorder are simply manifestations of the same underlying problem. As his history showed, he was and always had been a most anxious person. The single underlying problem of anxiety accounts for the many and diverse clinical pictures which were mistakenly thought to be entities in their own right.

Similarly, anxiety is a powerful cause of day-dreaming in schoolboys. Anxiety produces erratic, inconsistent behavior in the absence of a formal mental illness, meaning it can account for personality disorder; it has a devastating effect on the individual's achievements, meaning it is likely to cause depression, and anxiety itself can produce over-excited, irrational behavior, which mimics the hypomanic states. Anxiety is intolerable, so people will use drugs and alcohol to calm it; it can be manifest as irritability and aggression (more personality disorders), and it can eventually lead to psychotic states, as the stress-induced psychoses attest.

The question is whether we keep splitting his symptoms into minute categories, trying to find just one drug that will "cure" each of them (by acting on the supposed specific biochemical deficit for each of the disorders) or whether we stop the whole, ridiculous process and look at the psychological causes of the different behaviors the diagnoses label.

So, back to the question I posed above: "What is the nature of the intellectual process in psychiatry which can confidently claim that a person is suffering twenty-one separate diagnostic conditions?" The nature of the process is to force the vast complexity of mental disorder into a model found useful for physical disorders, without first establishing whether the same process in psychiatry is homology or analogy. I contend that it is mere analogy, that the current diagnostic process in psychiatry is not and never can be scientific as it was devised for an entirely different class of phenomena. What suits, say, the pneumonias does not suit psychiatry because there is a finite number of pneumonias, and pneumonia is sufficiently delineated from hepatitis, for us to say that the categories and subtypes exist as real entities. Nobody has ever done that in psychiatry. DSM-V, for example, can't even convince itself that categories of mental disorder exist.

The next question is: What is the utility of making all these diagnoses? The question has to be approached from a number of points of view, the patient, the psychiatrist, the drug companies and insurers, the family, the hospital, government, society, and perhaps some others. I will look at these issues in the subsequent chapters.

8.4: Conclusion

In Mark Jones' case, the psychotropic drugs were soon withdrawn and he was commenced on specific treatment for the personality-based anxiety state which was crippling his life. Over the next four months, he showed a good response and was able to start studying. He lost the weight which the drugs had caused and resumed gym training. He has stopped using marihuana and is drinking moderately. There are no suicidal ideas. At present, he is seen weekly for half an hour but this will reduce to fortnightly appointments in July, when he changes to full-time study by taking two extra maths units. He has a long way to go, with at least eighteen months formal treatment remaining, but he is gratified by his response so far and expresses considerable determination to continue treatment. In order to be sure the new treatment has been effective, a case like this should be followed for a minimum of three years. Ideally, the period of follow-up should equal the period of disability, so that he becomes his own control in a naturalistic experiment.

In my view, anybody who reads a history like this and concludes that it says something very bad about psychiatry is at no risk of contradiction. This also applies to anybody who recognizes his or her own life in this case. Mark Jones' previous treatment failed just because orthodox psychiatry (and that center is very orthodox) has not articulated a model of mental disorder to guide its daily practice, its teaching and its research. The notion that we can label mental disorders without knowing how they arise is pseudoscience. It is dangerous and destructive and I believe medical students are absolutely correct to reject psychiatry as a specialty. What we need is a genuine model of mental disorder to build a better psychiatry.

One thing is certain: it won't come from the Prof. Alex Ks of this world.

9 | *Accepting the Unacceptable*

9.1: Introduction

The experienced mental contents do not bring themselves into being. Just as smoke says there's probably a fire somewhere, so the overt phenomena of mental disorder give the clues as to what is happening in the silent, causative realm of mind that has generated the distress and disturbance. Every mental event has a cause but, just as in the real world of matter and energy, what you see is not what did it. For any observation, the causal or explanatory events are not part of the observation itself; they are shifted back one step from the observable events that need an explanation. The cause of any event is always an event of a different nature. In the mental world, the observable mental events of mental disorder are generated by mental events of a different nature, namely, unobservable mental events. Just to nip an infinite regress in the bud, the cause of unobservable mental events will be... non-mental events. Ultimately, events of a physical nature (i.e. neuronal events) underlie the unseen mental events because the perceived events of the real external world have to be transduced into the (real but different) internal world, and back again. So, just as in so many other fields of science, we can track back along the causative chain, from what we can see to what we can't see, using various techniques to ensure that what we imagine to be the cause of an event is most likely right (in the first of these books, I said we may never know the actual codes by which the mind-brain complex works).

For biological psychiatry, the unseen events causing the observable events of mental distress are biochemical events. That is, the line of causation jumps straight from molecules to mental events, with no intervening processes. Intervening processes are actually forbidden by biological psychiatry, because if there were any, they would have to be mental, and that would allow points of error to creep in, becoming themselves the mental causes of mental disorder, which biological psychiatry forbids. Quite clearly, their claim makes no kind of sense.

On the other hand, the biocognitive model says that observable or experienced mental events are caused by unseen mental events. Thus, if I am swimming in a waterhole and I see a crocodile slide into the water, I will feel a jolt of fear because my mind has calculated for me that I am in mortal danger. Note how I said "my mind has calculated for me..." In this context, it means the same as "I have realized..." If I say "I have realized I am in mortal danger", it is not a mental event of the same kind as saying "I have decided to raise my right arm". They are very different and one of the tasks of the biocognitive model is to tease out the minor differences in usage which indicate huge differences in psychophysical causation.

The following case history will demonstrate several points. Firstly, it will show the folly of trying to understand a person's life simply by taking a distant look at the outside of his life. This approach will miss the vastly important point of what is going on inside to cause what we see on the outside. For biological psychiatry, that is a silly point to make because the inner causation just is biochemical; there is nothing to understand about it and it will be rectified at a biochemical level with no psychological intervention.

I believe this is completely wrong and hope the different proofs I have offered in this and the preceding books are convincing. Observable mental events are caused by hidden mental events; this single statement determines the nature of the basis for an effective psychological treatment of mental disorder. If we don't like the experienced mental events, we have to change the hidden events. There is a crushing simplicity in this but the devil lies in the details. Before we can change them, we have to know what they are, which isn't quite as easy as it sounds and not just because they are hidden.

Once again, my questions are printed in italics while his answers are in normal print. Square brackets indicate my additions to the transcript. All supporting details have been changed except for the time and place of the interview: Darwin, Australia, March, 2010. Sean Collins arrived about fifteen minutes before his interview. From my picture window, I watched him park his motorbike and walk to the office. He was limping slightly on his left leg. I could hear his voice from the waiting room where he was speaking loudly to the receptionist but I couldn't understand what he was saying. He laughed once. A few minutes later, he went back to his bike and collected a manila folder from the saddlebag. Shortly, I went into the waiting room to see a healthy man who was standing upright while looking closely at a large military photograph on the wall. He told the receptionist in a loud, firm voice how highly he thought of the picture. While I was getting his file, he stood at the door and talked about the very pleasant weather; then I showed him into my office.

9.2: **The History: Damaging a Knee Damages The Head**

Yeah, good morning, I'm Dr. McLaren, I'm a psychiatrist. You're Mr. Collins, I see you've... Oh, yes, nice to meet you [with a broad smile, he firmly thrust out his hand to shake hands, which I don't normally do at the beginning of the interview]. Have a chair. So, ah, Dr. Vincent referred you; is he your normal doctor?

Yeah, mate.

And you're 33 now. I see you've got a compensation claim. We've got the claim number; who's your case manager there?

Michael Cousens.

I don't know him; they seem to change them very fast.

He's about the twelfth I had in three years.

Great. So anyway, you tell me what's the trouble; why you're here today; and I'll have to write while I'm talking to you. When was the injury, for a start?

Three years ago next month.

What sort of work do you do normally?

Yeah, I'm a plant operator, mate. I drive anything. I was on a big Cat front end loader when I fucked up my knee. Jumped out of the cab, landed on a rock, and rolled [brittle laugh]. Now my dancing days are over.

And who's at home with you?

My wife and our baby; she's ten months.

Oh, that's good, it's a great age. And what tablets are you taking?

I think it's called ibrofen, couple a day.

Ibuprofen. Is that all?

Maybe some Panadeine, I don't like drugs.

And what income are you on now?

[Long pause. His eyes fill with tears] I'm on nothin' mate, fuck all. They bloody cut me off. I'm working 38 hrs a week on my feet, running in and out, up and down fucking ladders. I'm fucked mate; I can't go on. How'm I supposed to support my wife and baby on $540 a week? She works but the child care takes most of that, we pay $360 a week rent. I'm sorry mate, you must think I'm a real soft cock but I… I've had it. Doc Vincent says I've got major depression but I don't want to kill myself; I've got too much to live for.

There's tissues here, man. It's OK, don't be embarrassed. There's nobody in the waiting room.

Thanks mate, I hate my wife to see me like this so what do I do instead? I scream my fucking tits off at her until she says she's had enough. So've I. I've had enough of myself.

So how you feeling generally in yourself?

Shithouse. I'm tired and run down; I'm unwell, and I'm angry.

What's your sleep like?

Terrible.

What time do you go to bed?

Different times. Sometimes nine if I'm feeling OK, but on a bad night, one or two.

What time do you get to sleep?

I lie there for hours, but I'm always awake after three. Leg hurts; I can't get comfortable.

Do you get back to sleep?

Mostly no, or maybe for half an hour; I have to get up at six to get to work.

When you're asleep, is it solid sleep?

No, mate, restless. I toss and turn. Sometimes I go to the spare room because my wife has to feed the baby and I'll keep them awake.

Do you have naps in the daytime?

No.

Do you sleep in on the weekends?

I try not to; my wife needs the sleep, so I get up and feed the baby and get her ready.

And what stops you sleeping earlier?

Worries. Soon's the light goes out, bang, my head fills with shit. Money, the future, these bastards in the insurance company, work, what's going to happen to me and my family. [Leans back in chair and starts to cry again].

So what's your appetite like?

No good. Mostly can't be bothered. I only eat because my wife cooks.

And what's your weight doing?

I've lost 10 kg in a month.

That's a lot of weight to lose. Were you trying?

I got overweight because I couldn't exercise; I've never been that fat in my life. The orthopedic doctor said I had to lose it because it was no good for my knee, so I did. No effort at all.

And your level of energy? What's that like?

Oh, drained. None.

And your level of activity?

I'm on my feet all day at work. This job is supposed to be for rehabilitation but it's making me worse. Soon's I get home, I fall in a heap. My knee's killing me and I'm sick of it. But my wife's had the baby most of the time and I haven't got any energy left for them [cries again, unable to talk]. And I... I just lose it. The place isn't clean so I start yelling and chucking things around. Even the baby, she threw her drink bottle on the floor after I'd picked it up, and I yelled at her. Couldn't stop. My wife told me to get out of the place for a couple of hours until I could be a man. That was like a knife in my guts... I'm sorry mate, I just can't help it.

It's OK, bro, men cry. So you don't do any extra exercise?

I do what the physio says but I can't do anything else. On the weekends, I used to be so active but now I'm dead. On Saturday, I hardly get off the couch. My wife has to do the shopping herself. She used to leave the baby home for me to look after but since my temper's been so bad, she takes her. I sit there by myself and wonder what the fuck's come over me.

And what about your level of interest in things? Firstly, in your private life?

Only my family. Nothing else. It's all gone.

And your interest in your work? What's that like?

I like work, the job's OK, but I just can't keep going.

And your motivation to do things, what's that like in your private life?

I want to do things, so I push myself but I'm useless. Even mowing the lawn knocks me out for about half a day.

And at work? Sounds like you're keen enough.

Yeah, I want to work. I've always loved my work. And I gotta work, that's all there is to it.

Now what about your social life, your private social life? Are you able to mix with people or are you avoiding people?

I see my mates, they come around but I can't go out with them, like fishing and four wheel driving. If I bog my vehicle, I'm done. No way I could dig it out.

And at work? How do you get along with the other staff and the customers?

Yeah, good. I'm good with people but it's draining when my knee hurts.

And your sexual interest? What's that like?

No good.

So what about your memory?

It's not so good. I forget things at work, put things down, and lose them.

Does anybody comment?

Boss has once or twice but I'm my worst enemy there.

And your concentration?

Ah, that's not good, my mind wanders in conversations.

So are you able to make decisions or do you put them off?

I put them off or just give them to my wife. She's good with money.

Are you able to think clearly, with one thought leading on to the next, or do you get confused or flustered?

I can't think straight [crying again]. Soon's there's any pressure on me, I'm ratshit. Head full of mush.

And what do you think about? What's on your mind most of the time?

Just... all these problems. Money. The insurance company. That first doctor who didn't see my knee was actually broken. Just goes on and on.

Have you had any peculiar experiences lately, like hearing or seeing things that didn't make sense?

[Pause]. No, not really. Few dreams, that's all.

No, don't count them. So most of the time, most days, how would you say you feel in yourself?

I'm overwhelmed and drained; I'm always tired.

Do you have bouts of feeling actually low and miserable?

Yeah.

How much of the time altogether? Half the time, quarter, three quarters?

About 70% of the time.

How bad is it?

It can be really bad.

Do you get to the stage of saying I'm sick of things as they are?

All the time.

Sick of life itself?

No, I just want all this shit to be fixed and go back to what I was.

So you haven't got to the stage of thinking you'd be better...?

I'm not suicidal. I told you.

That's OK. So what's the cause of the unhappiness?

All this shit. Never ends. Never ending story.

I think that had a happy ending. [he scoffs] Is there any other problem in your life likely to cause unhappiness now?

No, just all this shit going on and on. I'm not in debt but I had to borrow $2500 from my father the other week to pay our bills. Can you imagine how that made me feel? I'll pay it back but we have to watch every penny. I work long hours but the pay's shit and the insurance company stopped topping up my salary. I was earning big money with Consolidated Goldmines.

Aren't they supposed to pay the difference?

Hah! They sent me some letter but I couldn't understand it, something about section 54 of the work health act. [crying again, barely able to talk]

I think I know that, you'll need to see a lawyer. Now do you ever feel the opposite of miserable, you feel fantastic, full of energy, and on top of the world for no good reason?

Sometimes I feel good, it's a nice day and we've paid the bills and got a few dollars, then I think it will all come good, so we go out for a while. But the moment something goes wrong, whammo. Like last week, we come out of a shop and some drunk blackfella said he wanted five bucks off me. I lost it. Good thing my wife was there, she dragged me away. I was screaming at him to go and get a fucking job and all, I would've smashed him. Fucking useless drunks; they're all on the dole; never done a day's work in their lives. And I want to work but I can't. She was so embarrassed and upset, the baby was crying. I felt such a fucking dick for ruining their night. [convulsive crying].

In an ordinary day, do you have bouts where you get very tense and jittery?

Sure do, all the time. I feel like I'm ready to get into a fight.

Do you get shaky anywhere?

In my hands. Hopeless at work trying to put tools together.

And sweaty? Sticky palms?

I sweat all the time at work, there's no air con, but my hands were sweaty before I came in here.

Good. I've managed to scare somebody today. Does your heart race when you're very agitated?

It goes mad.

And does your stomach churn?

... churn?

Like hollow, hungry, empty, knotted, or butterflies feeling?

Butterflies. Terrible.

Do you get short of breath, you feel you want to go outside for fresh air?

It's as hot outside as in but I feel tight in the chest.

Do you feel light-headed and unsteady on your feet, dizzy, or clumsy?

Clumsy. If I have to go up the high ladder, my head swims, and I have to hang on tight.

You shouldn't be going up any ladders. Wasn't that in the rehab program?

Probably was, but they cut them off too, not that they were any help. I got this job myself.

And when you're agitated like this, how do you feel inside? Do you feel frightened or angry, how do you feel?

I'm so angry, I lose it. I try not to but it just gets me.

How often does this happen?

About three times a week.

And how long does each bout last?

Oh, hours, all day. I'm a wreck; I have to get away.

And what causes them?

Things going wrong at work; people don't do what they're supposed to and they leave it all for me.

What about delays or being held up, minor upsets in your routine?

Hopeless. I see something that nobody else would notice and I pick it up and chuck it to the shithouse. Like I threw the baby's bottle... Oh, what's wrong with me? I was never like this. The doc said I've got a chemical imbalance of the brain. I'll kill my fucking self if that's true. You're not gonna put me in the nuthouse, are you? I'm not going, I'll tell you now.

None of my patients go to hospital. We'll get you better here, don't worry. We've just got to sort out what's wrong, first.

Yeah, I'm sorry; I shouldn't tell you your job, should I? So what was the question?

You answered it. So money gets you upset?

Course it does. I feel like I'm being punished. Listen, they order me to go to all these fucking doctors appointments; I've had to go interstate; I'm away three days, and they won't pay me. I don't get paid at work if I'm not there; and if I don't go to Sydney, they cut off my benefits. Well, they've cut them off anyway. I can't get over this, where's the justice? I broke my knee at work and now they're punishing me, like I'm the bad one. I did nothing wrong, I was their top worker; all my life, I've worked hard. [rubs his hands over his knee] It's finished now, though. But mostly, I go apeshit over thinking of all this. The injustice, that's what gets me. The injustice for my baby... I get so fucking angry. I know why that bloke blew up TIO [a recent incident where a discontented claimant wheeled a barrowload of petrol into the insurance office and lit a match]. Don't write that down, that's enough for the cops to come after me.

I didn't hear anything. So in your ordinary daily life, is there anything you're frankly scared of, like heights, confined spaces, wide-open spaces?

Nah, that's OK.

Thunder and lightning, water, darkness, dirt, disorder, contamination? Any weapons scare you, like firearms or knives?

Nah, nothing like that.

What about animals? Rats, bats, frogs, toads, snakes, spiders, cockroaches, creepy crawlies?

Nup.

Centipedes, scorpions, worms, leeches, maggots? Birds, cats, dogs?

No, I'm fine with animals.

What about dealing with people, do you become frightened in crowds, standing in a queue with people straight behind you, or with public speaking?

No, I'm fine with people. Nobody scares me.

Appointments and interviews, tests and exams, public transport, they're OK?

Yeah.

What about threats and criticism, do they jangle you badly?

Criticism, I'm not good with that.

So you get edgy? Arguments or disputes, confrontation, or saying no to people?

Nah, that's fine. I don't like arguments but I don't run away.

Letting people down, causing trouble, or giving offence, does that bother you badly?

Don't like letting people down; hate that, never do it. Can't do it. And I'm letting my family down [cries again].

Loneliness, humiliation, and disapproval, do they scare you?

Disapproval. That's bad.

What about making mistakes or failing at anything, how does that affect you.

No way. That's no... no, can't do that. I'll never admit failure.

So you'd walk away from something rather than be seen to fail?

Probably. I'd hate myself. Normally, I just won't give in. I just keep going and going till I drop.

Any other fears, like illness, death or mental illness?

No, not scared of death.

Hospitals or dentists, blood or needles?

No.

What about groups of people, such as police, military, bikies...?

No.

Drunks, blacks, teenage gangs, or aggressive people generally? Do they scare you?

No, I can handle myself.

Can you now?

Well... maybe...

And people in authority, do they scare you?

Nup.

Alright, when you're out and about, do you have the feeling that people *are looking at you or talking behind your back?*

Yeah, sometimes. I get real paranoid.

Do you feel they are judging you?

Maybe. Depends what I'm doing.

Do you have the feeling that people are a danger to you; they're going to have a go or get at you in some way? Maybe they'll hurt you?

No, I'd fix them up.

Do you have the feeling that people are watching you or spying on you, you're under surveillance or bugged?

No, not now. I thought the insurance company was, a year or so ago, and it turns out they were.

Did it worry you?

No, not really. They want to look, go right ahead. They won't see much.

Do you have the feeling that people are plotting or conspiring against you, spreading lies or stories, or holding information back from you?

No, not really. I don't trust them but that's...

Alright, well that's not 'real paranoid' at all. That's hardly even on the horizon. Now are you a person who checks things all the time, doors, locks, keys, switches, gas taps, all that sort of thing?

Oh yeah, terrible. Four or five times.

Why?

I'm just worried about something going wrong, but mostly it's my memory now. I get in bed and ask the wife, did I check the back door? So I have to go and check it. I'm not thinking about what I'm doing.

So you're not driven to do it?

No, sometimes I say what the hell, and I just go to sleep.

Are you very fussy about cleanliness, tidiness, order, punctuality, and efficiency?

Oh, yeah, I've got it bad. Drives my wife mad. She says I'm ODC or something.

Does that get you into arguments?

Sure does. I try to be friendly about it but underneath, I'm angry. Punctuality, I can't stand being late.

I saw you were here fifteen minutes early. Do you have special ways of arranging or cleaning or organizing things; it's got to be just so, like a ritual?

Ah, mate, I'm the worst. I line things up. Everything has to be right in line. Anybody moves anything of mine, I blast them. Tools, clothes, books, furniture, you name it. Touch my car and you'll die.

What about cleaning? Do you have a special order? Or if somebody rinses the cups, do you wash them again later?

Cleaning, I'm a demon. I do most of the cleaning at home. Everything has to be done in order.

If it's not in order, would you have to start again?

No, I just don't want to forget anything.

Baby's bottles?

Ha ha, she's had about ten new ones already; I put too much chlorine in them. I've got a real phobia for dirt for her. Not me, I don't care what I eat. And washing my hands before I feed her; I'm like a doctor before an operation.

It actually makes the numbers of bugs increase. So do you count things or color code them or touch them?

I color code things, especially tools and stuff.

Do you have thoughts popping into your head all the time that you know are silly but you can't resist them?

Only about blowing up the insurers.

But you don't think they're silly at the time?

No, I know I'll never do it but it makes me feel better to think of them all hanging out the top floor, screaming, and I'll be down in the crowd, laughing. Bastards. That doesn't mean I'm crazy does it? You can't lock me up for that?

I don't lock people up, and I don't think it's crazy. Now what sort of trouble do you have physically?

I've got this hot, burning sensation deep inside my left knee and I get a clicking and pinching feeling if I do anything unusual, like climb a ladder or twist on my feet.

Where is it in the knee?

It's deep inside, in here, like somebody's put hot charcoals in there. It's bad, can wake me at night.

Is it there all the time, or does it come and go?

All the time. Sometimes it's worse but it never goes away.

Now what makes it worse.

Walking around, and climbing ladders, that's the worst.

Stairs? Have you got an elevated house?

No, ground level. Stairs are no good. Going up them, I have to pull myself up with my left hand on the banister but it still hurts. Coming down is murder. I take all my weight on my hands and actually swing my legs together.

How far can you walk on level ground, like a roadway?

Not far, about a kilometer, maybe less. But I'd pay for it that night, so I don't try. I can ride my bike a bit if I put the weight on my right leg.

Be careful about that, by favoring your left leg, you can end up with pain in your right hip.

Funny you should say that; I've said that to my wife. My right hip hurts at night when I lie down.

Can you run or jump or dig?

No way, none of them.

Twisting on your knee?

That kills me for the rest of the day.

So no dancing or mucking about?

No way.

How much can you carry?

They let me carry 20 kg for a short distance but it's too much.

And uneven loads?

Can't. Has to be balanced.

Well, at least something about you is balanced. And walking on soft sand, like the beach?

No good, I can only do about twenty meters. And my left calf cramps as well.

What about squatting or sitting cross-legged on the floor?

No, never. I have to lift the baby up on to the bed or the table to change her; can't kneel to change her nappies on the floor.

Can you drive?

I had to sell my Nissan Patrol. It was an old model with the heavy truck clutch, I just couldn't change gears in the bush. So I got that motorbike. I can change the gears on that because it's only my toes.

Yeah, well just don't come off the damned thing or you're history.

I had to sell the truck, I couldn't afford the fuel. So now we can't go bush or camping.

Anything else? What effect does this injury have on your sex life?

No good. If it's been hurting all day, that's the last thing on my mind. When we can manage, it sounds bad but it's better if the wife goes on top.

Doesn't sound bad at all. It's whatever you like.

[sheepish laugh] Well, she likes it.

Modern women. Right, now tell me how all this came about.

I was working for Consolidated doing the site work for their treatment plant at Jupiter Springs, driving a big four meter front end loader.

That's one big machine.

They're big. I had to stop to talk to some blokes about where I wanted some metal dumped and jumped down. I was looking at them and didn't see a rock about the size of a melon on the ground next to the wheel. I landed on it and went straight over, twisted my leg. I felt something tear inside and it hurt like hell.

So did you go to the first aid center?

No, that was back at the main camp, ten k's away. And I was the only one with the license for that machine, so I kept on until knock off, about three hours. After a while, it didn't hurt so much; it's got electric gear changes, so I thought it would settle down. But hell's bells, when I stopped for the day and tried to get out of the cabin, I couldn't do it. Couple of blokes had to help me and they thought I was mucking around. So I went back to camp with them and put some ice on it and had some tablets from the kit and went to bed.

You didn't see the first aid bloke?

He wasn't there, he goes back to Katherine at night and I couldn't drive. It hurt like hell all night, so the boss took me into town the next morning, he had a meeting or something. At the hospital, they said I'd twisted it so they just wrapped it up and sent me back to work.

Did they give you any tablets, or X-ray it?

Nothing. Just Panadeine. I got back to work and struggled on to the weekend, then went home. I was alright driving on the highway, as long as I didn't have to change gears.

So did you see your doctor?

He was away. He's always away.

What about the hospital?

No, they'd told me in Katherine it was just twisted, and I didn't want to wait up there for six hours with all the drunk blackfellas bumming smokes off me.

Did you go back to work?

That was my week off. We work two on, one off, twelve hour shifts for fourteen days. I stayed at home and rested it.

You didn't go back to work?

Yeah, I didn't have a medical certificate.

Well, you should have rung them and said you weren't able to climb into your machine.

And get sacked. I've never been sacked in my life.

They can't sack you for that. So how long did you last?

About four days. They brought me back to Darwin and I went to the hospital for X-rays.

What did they show?

It was fractured. Something about a plate.

Tibial plateau. What did they do?

They said it was too late to screw it; it'd have to be in plaster for three months.

Did they look inside it?

No, that was about a year later.

Did they operate then? An arthroscopy?

I've had eight operations, I think. I'm not having any more. They don't work. Everything was torn inside but they left it too long, all the tendons were frayed and torn. It just makes me sick to think of it. If I was a fucking blackfella and they did this to me, they'd have that fucking Aboriginal Legal Service holding a blow torch to their arses, believe me.

If you think you haven't been treated properly, you're entitled to go to the Health Complaints Commission.

Huh, been there, done that, fucking fat lot of use they were. They were covering up all the doctors and hospitals. They didn't give a shit about me.

You might need to see a lawyer.

They wanted $30,000 in advance. Like I've got thirty thousand to spare. I didn't get any pay for nearly three months.

Legal Aid?

Civil matter, they don't do them. They defend murderers and child molesters and help women screw their husbands for maintenance, that's all.

Right. OK, have you ever had any serious physical or mental illnesses before?

Nothing. Fit as. First and last time, believe me.

OK, tell me about your background. Where were you born and raised?

I was born in Perth but I was raised all over the place. My father was in the Navy and we moved every two or three years.

So where's he now?

He's here; actually, he's got a job with the Defense Department in the patrol boats contract section.

Oh yeah? I've heard about them.

Well, you haven't heard anything. I'll tell you another day. They drive him mad.

So what rank was he when he retired.

Chief petty officer artificer; you know what that is?

Yeah, I do a lot of the military work here. And what was he like as a person?

He's good. He was away a lot but he always tried to make up for it when he came home, took us camping and fishing. I see them every week.

Well, he lent you that money.

Yeah, but that was the worst day for me, crawling to my old man to beg for money. I've been looking after myself since fifteen.

He wouldn't mind. It's not as if you drank it. And your mother? She's here?

Yeah, she's fifty-five.

Oh, and your father, how old's he?

Ah, fifty-eight.

Does she work?

She does now but not when we were younger, she had to run the house when the old man was at sea.

And what's she like as a person?

She's great. We get on like a house on fire.

So how many brothers and sisters were there?

Just one, my little sister.

How old is she?

She's three years younger than me, so... thirty. Next month.

And where's she?

She's in Adelaide.

What's she do?

She's a radiologist.

A radiologist? Or the one who takes the pictures?

The one who takes the pictures.

Radiographer. She married or single?

Married, two kids.

And what's she like as a person?

She's OK.

Only OK?

She used to get me into trouble a lot when we were younger. She'd do something and then tell the old man I did it and I'd cop it. He wouldn't believe me; the sun shone out of her arse, that's for sure. Daddy's little darling. Still is.

And always will be. Little girls can be very spiteful, you'll find out. Now is there any family history of mental disorder in the family?

The old man had a bad spell after the Gulf War. Second one, I think. He was in Vietnam and it all got stirred up. They said it was post-trauma or something.

Vietnam? He was too young.

No, he joined at fifteen as an apprentice. So he was there when he was still nineteen. There was an explosion on their ship but he would never tell us about it.

So he's alright now?

Yeah, he takes some tablets I think.

Any other family history? Anybody drinking too much or using illegal drugs? Nobody got a criminal record?

No, only me.

Get on to that later. So where did you go to school, just local state schools?

All over the place.

How many schools in all?

About five.

That's not so bad. How old were you when you left school?

Sixteen, I think, I left in the middle of Year 11.

Passed Year 10. And what sort of marks did you get?

About average.

And how did you get on with the teachers?

Yeah, OK.

And with the other children?

No, I was good. Popular.

Were you shy, nervous, or aggressive?

I got into fights. I had no time for idiots.

What's that mean?

If the kids were mucking around on the cricket field, I'd whack 'em. Sometimes they'd get smart and try to hit back so I'd have to flatten them.

What did the teachers say?

They used to say things like, Always keep your left up, Collins, and never kick a man until he's down.

Great teachers. So you liked sport?

Loved it. I was in the NSW state schoolboys rugby team, and the cricket training squad. [New South Wales is the largest state, and those teams are highly competitive as they can lead to sports careers].

What were your main interests at school?

Well, not school. I was too active, I wanted to be working from the day I turned fourteen. Anything outdoors, that was me.

What was your home life like?

It was pretty good. I had no complaints, really. You see how some of the kids in the street lived; fuck me, you wonder how they survive.

A lot of them didn't, I see them in the prisons. Now what did you do when you left school?

Diesel fitter's apprenticeship. Four years.

What sort of marks did you get?

Yeah, good.

And where were you living?

I was with my parents for the first year; then they moved to Canberra, so I lived with my grandparents. They were cool; actually, they were really with it. They wouldn't tell my old man if I came home drunk or if they found a bit of mull in my room.

Did you stay in the trade?

For a while, then I went north and got different jobs; I don't like being bored. Sometimes I was on drilling rigs in the desert; sometimes I'd get a job on a coastal ship, you know, fun travel, and adventure. Good life. I was young and fit and the bosses loved me. I was a good worker. Try anything.

So when did you come to Darwin?

We were here in the early nineties when dad was posted here so I always had it in mind to come back; been here this time about seven years.

How many jobs have you had altogether?

Oh, heaps. I move on when I'm ready.

Why do you change so often?

Usually for something better, or for new experience. There's nothing I can't do, I've seen it all. Only thing I haven't done ever is work inside a building. Fuck that.

Have you ever been sacked?

No way, they beg me to stay. I can ring any of my old bosses and he'd have me back tomorrow. I'm a top worker. I've never been on the dole and never taken payments before. So this is why they shit me when they won't pay me now. I've earned it. I haven't been rorting the system.

But you're not a supervisor.

I have been but it doesn't suit me. I can't tell people what to do. If a bloke doesn't do his job, I'm just as likely to knee him in the balls. Anybody who has to be told what to do shouldn't be working.

Have you ever been told you're a bit difficult?

All the time. I'd be worried if somebody wasn't whinging about me somewhere.

You're a good worker?

Tops man, just tops.

OK, so what about your social life? When were you first married or de facto?

I was married at twenty-one and divorced at twenty-two.

Wow. Any children?

Two.

That was quick.

One was almost popping.

Why did that break down?

She wouldn't leave her mother. Wanted to live next door.

Do you see the children?

No, she stopped that. I pay the maintenance, I had a court order for access but I'd fly down there and knock on the door and somebody would stick their head out and say she moved three months before. It's never stopped. I couldn't pay the legal bills because she had legal aid and just moved to another state and told them she was scared of me. I never raised a finger to her; I've never hit a woman in my life. It sucks, but there you are.

How did that affect you? Do you think you were depressed then?

Hmm, a bit. I was flat for a couple of years but I always thought I could work it out. I never really gave up hope. It only really dawned on me after I had met my second wife; she said she thought the kids' mother never had any intention of letting me see them and she bet me she had another bloke all along. Turns out she was right. Women's intuition. So I never felt so abandoned as this time.

And this marriage?

We were both twenty-five. I just hope we get to thirty-five together [pauses, then eyes fill again]. I never wanted to be a bad husband or father, but it's happening. And all because of this fucking knee; that's why I'm poison on that fucking insurance company.

Do you drink?

Not much.

Any other drugs?

No, nothing. Don't do drugs, just a bit of mull when I was skiting as an apprentice.

You gamble?

Couple of times a year, a group of us go to the casino for a meal and a show, and the missus and I'll put fifty into the pokies each, but when it's gone, so are we. Doesn't interest me; I'd rather be fishing.

So would I. Any police record?

Nothing much. Few brawls.

And your general health is good? No asthma, hepatitis, anything?

Nothing.

OK, so how would you see yourself normally as a person? Normally, that means before this accident?

I was very happy, very easy-going, and active.

Easy-going except when you were smacking people in the head.

But I was very easy-going about it.

Would you say you were a nervous person?

Not at all.

Did you stand up for yourself or were you inclined to be pushed around.

Never. I'd stand up for myself.

Did that ever get you into arguments?

Sometimes, if they were silly enough.

Would you say you were easily bothered by guilt?

A bit, if I failed at anything, I'd feel very guilty about it.

And shame?

No.

And self-consciousness?

A little bit, at times. It's much worse now having this splint on my leg. And yeah, I do feel ashamed if I can't do something and I have to ask somebody. I'll just walk away and go without. People look at me and they say, You look fit enough; what's wrong; you got compensationitis? I get so fucking wild, I want to rip their heads off but I don't dare, I can't risk another injury on this knee. I'm gonna have to have a knee replacement but they won't even think about it at my age.

Not under fifty, if they can help it.

Great. Seventeen years and counting down.

Do you trust people readily enough or are you wary of people?

Sort of trusting. Sometimes.

I'll put that down as a bit wary. And you've said you're very tidy and organized. Patient or impatient?

Impatient.

You tend to follow rules?

Yes. Very much.

And you get angry if other people don't?

I'm like a pit bull.

Now are you a social person or can you get by without people?

Now?

No, I mean before. Normally, were you a social sort of person?

Yeah, I get on well with everybody.

With the odd punch in the head. Are you inclined to be jealous?

No.

But you hold grudges, I'd say.

Very much. Oh yes, nobody puts one over me.

So how do you get on with authority? Bosses, managers, police, government?

Good. Very good. They trust me totally.

How did you rate your temper?

Out of what?

Mild, moderate, severe, off the planet?

Yeah, pretty quick. But I get over it quickly, few minutes and it's all forgotten.

Except for his head.

You got it.

OK, how do you rate your intellect?

Good. I'm pretty cluey.

And how did you rate your self-esteem?

Heaps.

So now you'd say you're nervous and irritable and not very social. You don't trust people and you're not able to enjoy yourself. You feel guilty all the time over failing, your grudges are off the gauge, and your self esteem is what?

Shithouse.

Alright, nearly finished. What do you think this trouble is all about? What would you say is wrong with you?

Well the doc said it's a chemical imbalance of the brain.

No no, not what anybody told you; what would you say is wrong yourself?

I've dropped my bundle. I dunno. I was the strongest, fittest, happiest bloke around; everybody loved me, and now look at me! It's this fucking crying, look; it just gets me and I can't stop it. So does this mean I'm depressed? That's a brain disease, isn't it? It says so on all those ads on TV. See your doctor, get some tablets, go to the funny farm, shock your brain. Not me, no fucking way!

Well, what's caused it?

Work. Must be, couldn't be anything else. My knee. I'm an invalid. I'll never run down a hill with my daughter, never carry her on my back... Oh Jesus, I can't... [collapses in convulsive, agonized crying] What's the point? What's the fucking point? If I was a fucking racehorse, they'd take me out and shoot me. Maybe they'd all be better off that way. My baby, my baby...

And what would you like done?

[fights the tears down] I've got to get better. I've got to get back on the road. I'm 33; I can't lie down and die now? But I'm not going to hospital; you're not locking me up.

But what sort of treatment do you want?

I dunno mate; you're the specialist. I gotta do what you say, I suppose.

We'll talk about it in a moment. Now why did your doctor say you had major depression?

He gave me one of them question things, Beck or Peck...

Beck Depression Inventory.

That'd be it. I got the top score, it said I got extreme major depression and I need to go to hospital as an emergency.

But you don't want to go?

No fucking way.

When did he say chemical imbalance of the brain?

That's what he said. He gave me this pack of tablets to start and I looked up their website on the internet and it was all about brain chemicals or some shit. And side effects? I threw 'em out. I don't know. I'm not a doctor. I just do as I'm told.

Well you do sometimes. Alright. All that talk about chemicals in the brain is a theory, and in my opinion, it's not a very good theory.

[with a big grin, he reaches across the table to shake hands] Now you're talking my language, doc. So whaddawe gonna do.

OK, this is what we'll do. [see after]

Mental state examination

The mental state showed a fit man of a bit above average height with a stocky muscular build but carrying some excess weight. He was dressed in clean, faded work clothes, and had a surgical support and lateral splint on his left knee. There were no visible tattoos but he had two ear studs on the left. There were no visible scars or jewelry. He walked with a slight limp on the left. At first, his manner was loud and almost bumptious and he was clearly attempting to control the direction of the interview, but this changed abruptly when he began crying. He wept painfully several times during the interview but was attempting to control his distress by a cheery attitude. At first, he was wary, but he soon settled. He was not hostile or overtly suspicious. There were no signs of a psychotic disorder and nothing to indicate an organic impairment of brain function. He was at least of bright normal intellectual ability, if not higher, but was educated below his potential.

He was commenced on specific treatment for an anxiety state and given a small dose of a benzodiazepine to help sleep. At first review, five days later, he had no side effects from the medication. Mentally, he was transformed. He was much calmer, smiling, and cheerful, and reported a substantial improvement at home. There had been no temper outbursts; he was sleeping better and he was able to spend more time with his family. He felt he had more energy and was able to assist more around the house.

He said: "I've realized now I've been trying to pretend my knee isn't there. I've been trying to do everything I used to be able to do but it was killing me."

It probably hasn't been doing your knee a lot of good, either. You've got to look after it. It's damaged inside, you've got no cartilage to absorb the impacts, so you have to minimize the impacts. We're going to get you some proper shoes, for a start. And if you're going to ride that bike, you need reinforced racing boots. I don't care whether they're hot; they're not as hot as the surgeon's knife. And you have to keep reminding yourself, you're not doing this for yourself; you're doing it for your family and you'll do whatever it takes. Is that right?

You're only saying that to scare me, doc. It does. Things will be different from now on.

In the three months since, his improvement has continued. The anxiety is controlled and he has been able to reduce the medication. He does not need drugs to sleep. Using regular ibuprofen and ice packs, he rarely needs codeine for pain. He continues with physiotherapy aimed at strengthening the quadriceps, which had shown some atrophy. However, the main thrust of management has been to get him to change his self-perception from somebody who gained his daily sense of achievement and self-approval from a high level of skilled physical activity, to accepting that he will never be able to do all the things he once did (fishing, camping, shooting, building, servicing his own cars, etc), to working with his brains in an indoor setting. Every week, he is told to say to himself fifty times a day: Brains beats brawn. He will need retraining at some stage but he is not sure what he will do. The first step will be a tertiary bridging course but the insurer will not pay for that. His back payments have been settled and he has repaid his debts to his family.

9.3: Death before Dishonor

What is the point of this history? The point is that Sean Collins had every possible symptom of Major Depressive Disorder, most of them at a dangerous level; yet he has been managed successfully as an out-patient, averaging one visit per week of up to half an hour, with no antidepressants and, for almost the whole of the three months, no psychotropic drugs whatsoever. He was not admitted to hospital and certainly was not given the ECT the depression questionnaire had suggested was needed as an emergency. He has been at work practically the whole time and his family life has improved dramatically. Yes, he is a success. And yes, there are also patients who are not successful, but he's not one of them. If you want to see unsuccessful patients, you should hang around one of the big mental hospitals or large clinics in teaching hospitals. There, any time, any day, you will see failed patients by the score.

Anybody who is familiar with this type of case would know that conventional treatment would almost certainly not have resulted in this type of improvement. Practically any hospital or clinic in the country would have admitted him for in-patient treatment. Because he would have refused to take the drugs, he may have been detained and treated as an involuntary patient, which would certainly have meant incarceration in a security (locked) ward. He would not have tolerated this. He would have been given antipsychotic drugs by injection, meaning powerful side effects, his physical strength and appearance would have declined further and he would probably then have been given ECT.

So what has this to do with my claim that 'Observable mental events are caused by hidden mental events'? We can go through this step by step.

The Beck Depression Inventory picks out certain symptoms which its authors believe are the core or diagnostic symptoms of depression. The more of these symptoms you have, the worse you are. The symptoms were selected because patients who had already been diagnosed as depressed ticked most of them, so if you tick most of them, you are more likely to be like a depressed person than you are like a non-depressed person. These have been correlated with the DSM-IV-TR so that a person with a high score on the BDI is very likely to meet the criteria for Major Depressive Disorder. All nicely circular. All these approaches do is tell you what the person is like on the surface: they pick out surface manifestations of deeper disturbances but they say nothing about what is going on underneath to cause those manifestations. This case, which to me is absolutely routine, shows that there were lots of things going on underneath the surface and that, when they were corrected, the surface manifestations corrected themselves. In this respect, the biocognitive model of psychiatry is no different from the biological: what you see is not the cause of what you see. The cause lies deeper. The biological approach says the cause is chemical/genetic; my approach is that the cause is lower-level mental events.

The long version of the BDI asks twenty-one questions whereas this man's version had only seven questions. Can a matter as complicated as a psychiatric diagnosis be made on seven questions? I don't think so, especially when the diagnosis is then used as the justification for a specific form of treatment. By this means, psychiatry is dumbed down (sorry about this expression, but it is almost onomatopoeic) to the point where, soon, it will not need psychiatrists. Put the questionnaire on cereal boxes for people to fill in when they have finished doing the crossword at breakfast, write your name and medicare number on the form, and drop it in the box at your local pharmacy on the way to work. That way, you can simply pick up the prescription on the way home and cut out the middle man (the awful psychiatrist who would only put you on drugs anyway). A score of over ten on the short form demands action, and the action is a prescription. Too bad about your broken leg and your broken heart, just take more of the blue tablets and pay as you go out.

This man had a personality, and the conflict between his changed circumstances and his personal drive was breeding the distress that was amounting to depression. Pain led to fear of failure; fear of failure led to shame and humiliation; shame and humiliation led to anger at those he believed were deliberately not helping him; anger spilled over his family, increasing his shame and guilt, leading him to isolate himself and fear more outbursts of rage, until he began to believe he was going to lose everything. How do I know? Because I heard in his voice the mortal fear of loss when he cried out "My baby, my baby." He had already lost two children; with the loss of his health and his source of self-esteem, the thought of losing his wife and baby was more than he could countenance. Terror took over his life, convincing him he was going mad. The so-called depression was guilt over his failure as a husband, father, provider, and worker, all caused by his badly mismanaged fractured knee, the growing sense of uselessness in terms of his previous self-perception and his inability to see a way out of his mess. For him, the mental hospital was looming closer but he knew that he would rather die than go there. It was a matter of shame: "Death before dishonor" is not a fairy story. Remember the millions of men in World War I who, faced with certain death on the battlefield or dishonor in their mates' eyes, scrambled up the trenches and began walking into the walls of hot steel from the machine guns. He did not want to die; he wanted to be with his child as she grew; but he could not live as a failure. Conflict.

The treatment was a pushover. I would say that 75% of it was effected in the first appointment. Simply taking the history in that way, asking all the questions the BDI didn't ask, brought him to an awareness of the complex pressures on him at that point in his life. Once he knew them, or had an inkling of what they were, he was smart enough to start to see a way out. He realized he had to shift his self-perception from 'strong and capable' to 'smart and capable in a different sort of way'. With his broad industrial experience, he was in a good position to find a suitable new career. Instead of sitting alone at the back of the house, feeling cut off from his family, punching his head in vexation at being unable to will his leg to heal; he was able to start studying, which his wife supported strongly. He was taken out of the physical job and given a desk in the store where he became responsible for ordering and tracking goods on computer. He still drove a forklift truck because he liked to but he did not climb ladders or carry anything.

His proudest moment was when he brought his infant daughter to his appointment by himself. His wife was working and he was baby-sitting for the day. She trusted him again to care for the baby properly. I do not believe that large doses of powerful psychotropic drugs, with or without ECT, could ever have done that.

At this point, the chorus of biochemical believers will come to life: "Ah yes," they will intone with mournful joy, "but everybody knows that life events can cause depression. How does your one-off case prove that his condition wasn't a chemical imbalance of the brain? Remember, doctor, anecdotes never amount to a general truth."

This is certainly true. Inductive evidence amounts to very little unless the numbers are there, but there are two parts to their objection. The first part is the question of causation of his mental disorder, and the second concerns treatment. I say that treatment is dictated by causation; so the argument here devolves onto causation. The biochemists say that, for no particular reason, this man's brain chemistry just decided to start to play up, but to do so in a particular pattern that mimicked the grief reaction. Now, by definition, the grief reaction is not a mental disorder, even though its features are exactly the same to the word as those of Major Depression. His disorder was supposed to be genetic but there was no family history of depression whatsoever, and he had never been depressed except for a time after he lost contact with his first two children. So, coincidental upon suffering a series of huge losses in his life, losses which were magnified by their significance in his personality make-up, we are asked to suppose that he developed a syndrome of loss which had nothing to do with the losses he was experiencing and the further losses which tortured him and made him think death would be preferable? If this is what the biological psychiatrists believe, then I don't think they have any understanding of the nature of causation in human affairs.

Well, on that claim, I am on very safe ground: They freely state that they don't. They don't believe in psychological causation. What do they believe in? Oh, don't ask, that's irrelevant, beside the point, not a matter of their science. They have defined causation out of their science, just because they do not have a formal model of mind in which to base their biological model of mental disorder. If there is no model of mind, there is no model of mental causation, and thus their approach drifts further into incoherence. Their concept of mental disorder has no ontology; it does not nest in a structured system of beliefs which, together, say "This is how the world is." They do not know how a person decides to raise his right arm; moreover, they do not care. They do not talk about it in their journals or at their conferences, nor is it included in their training programs. Young psychiatrists are not examined in it just because it does not exist in their world. All that exists is the belief that mental disorder is a genetically-determined biochemical disturbance of neuronal function. Worse still, a disorder is only a disorder when the committee votes for it. Grief is not a disorder; homosexuality was but is no longer; internet pornography addiction wasn't but is about to become one. A belief that floats free of any ontological attachments is not science; it is ideology. Thus you see the inestimable advantage of not actually having an ontology: you can do what you like.

9.4: Questions from Medical Students (edited)

Ladies and gentlemen, and others, that is the end of my formal presentation, so if you have questions, we can discuss the concepts informally. I'm not so concerned with the actual management of the case as with the theory behind the management. Yes, doctor?

I'd like to thank you so much for a most fascinating and stimulating...

My dear young lady, you don't have to be polite to me. I'm not a professor, so you can be as rude as you like. This is your big chance.

Well, I did enjoy your talk but I was a bit lost on the way you use the term 'causation'. You seem to jump from physical to psychological and back again, it's hard to follow... I mean...

You mean it's hard to follow. That's fine, I'll do better next time. The mind-brain complex has different levels of function, and therefore, it has different levels of causation. The biocognitive model splits the functional mind itself in two parts: the experiential, like what you see before you now, and the informational, which is where all the unseen action takes place. The experiential realm is a causative dead-end; it exists but doesn't do anything that we know of. The informational realm, what Chalmers calls the psychological mind, is the busy part, where information is manipulated and then directed to its effector organs. It's a bit like the CPU in your laptops, but you must be very careful of the computer model. Now, if I lift my arm like this, something took place in my head to make it happen. Part of that something was activity in the motor cortex and other motor centers in the midbrain and cerebellum, but a critical part was in the informational realm, where I actually made the decision to do it. Something caused the arm to lift, but introspection doesn't tell us what it was. We accept that the something was an executive event, which means it had to take place in the mental sphere, not the physical, just because molecules don't make decisions; only minds do. Ultimately, minds derive from molecules but they are not part of the physical realm, although they can interact with it.

The mind operates in its own realm, generated by the physical activity of the brain but governed by the laws of its logic, whatever they are. Now that's a fascinating topic but we can't go there. But we have to be careful not to start an infinite regress, like I lift my arm because I had an urge to do so; and I had an urge to do so because I had an urge to have an urge to do so, etc. How do we stop an infinite regress in a computational system? Dennett has given the clue, based in Turing's work. We have two lesser inputs which interact and produce an output which amounts to the decision. It's like chemistry. How do you make an explosive? You mix two non-explosive chemicals together. So in this model, we are looking for the hidden imperatives that interact to produce the observable behavior. In Sean Collins' case, he had an intense drive to avoid failure, so he had always channeled that through his physical strength. When his physical health collapsed, his fear of failure could no longer be channeled. It built up and up until his anxiety exploded. It mainly came out as rage, which is what men do, which in turn reinforced his sense of guilt and failure.

So your question leads straight to a critically important aspect of biocognitive theory which is entirely novel in the history of psychiatry, the notion of the self-reinforcing pathological state. Fear builds up, it feeds on itself, amplifying and spreading to affect more and more of the patient's life; then it drives him to the realization that his life is ruined because of the fear. One day, he thinks he can never get better, so he gives up on life itself. In turn, this activates his grief response, and we call that depression. But if we ask him: "Why are you depressed?" often he doesn't know. He does not recall giving up on life itself. All he knows is that he does not see a life ahead. One thing leads to another. We have to find the causes, which lie in the mental realm. The brain is the mechanism or agency but the mind itself contains its own causes. Remember

Schopenhauer's maxim: Nothing happens without sufficient reason. The psychiatrist's job is to find it, not smother it with drugs.

Yes sir?

If you don't like the biological approach, what's your model of depression?

This is a very good question. I would really need to devote a whole lecture to it, with lots of slides and diagrams. You must think of the mind as a series of modules working in concert, not as an entity. It is not a single, uniform thing, and any sense we have of having "a mind", as compared to lots of little mindlets, is an artifact. It's the same sense that an orchestra isn't a single thing; it consists of clusters of instruments all working in harmony, and each cluster is composed of single entities with a role to play that adds to the total outcome. OK, so one major module of the mind is the informational module, which is itself composed of many subparts, and they in turn of many, many sub-subparts. It takes information in from the peripheral senses, compares them with instructions coded in memory, then jumbles them together in a computational space until one bit of information and that we call our decision. This is not magic. Machines do it all the time; even turnstiles do it. But we're not just machines; we have other modules called emotions.

Now, it happens from time to time, by means we can't even begin to comprehend, that certain inputs result in an output called "Loss." Just as we recognize a chocolate ice cream or we recognize threats, so we recognize losses. This output activates certain pathways in the lower brain which impinge on what we loosely call the pleasure centers. You've all seen those experiments where rats have electrodes implanted in their brains and they sit happily pressing the switch all day. I presume something like that is involved in normal human life. We have modules subserving our emotional experience. A signal from the computational mind activates them, and we feel pleasure. However, they are doubly innervated. A signal from another tract which is only activated in conditions of loss will cause a long-lasting inhibition of just those neurons. Because of this blockade, we are unable to activate our own pleasure centers from within, and this we call depression. We lose the capacity to enjoy anything, nothing looks good, or sounds good or feels good, because it can no longer activate the pleasure centers. I presume this is where drugs and ECT work, in that they can partially reverse the blockade. There are, of course, very good models of this type of learning, because that is what it is, chemically-mediated neuronal learning, and Kandel has had a lot to say about them. You should also be aware of the work of Aleksandr Luria on cerebral inhibition; he actually started the whole field nearly seventy years ago but his work was unknown in the West almost until he died. Karl Pribram was influential in introducing him, before he went off into some sort of fantasy land.

So gradually, over the months, the inhibition fades and the depression lifts, as we say. That's my model: depression is actually a long-lasting cellular inhibition in critical centers devoted to the experience of pleasure. Those centers are rendered incapable of responding to daily inputs but this is the crucial point: the input that rendered them insensitive was itself psychologically determined. They were switched off by an instruction coming from a higher center, not by an impulse coming from within their own cellular mechanisms. The genes that were activated to produce the inhibiting proteins that constituted the blockade were not activated by mindless biochemical factors. They were activated by psychological factors, travelling as volleys of impulses in ordinary neurons. I have described this mechanism in another book. It is not magic. Of course, if the centers are repeatedly inhibited, then we get a picture of chronic depression. If life experiences are repeatedly negative and hurtful, the person never seems to come out of one depressive phase before sinking into another. Can you give us an example of that? Yes, you sir. Your question, you get first right of response.

Um, I suppose… failing your exams over and over.

Is that one a bit close to home, is it? And why would you fail? Not you, of course, but any student? Give me an example of why a student should repeatedly fail. He should not, according to Skinner. Failing is so aversive that he should be warned off it by one experience. Well, don't be shy; I can think of lots of reasons but they are psychological. Think of personalities. Yes, you. Drinking, of course. He drinks, so he fails. He feels bad for failing, so he drinks more. And fails again. Which group of students are likely to start drinking early? Come on, don't be shy… there, I gave it away. You're right, young lady, shy students. They drink so they can socialize. And my clinical work shows that unsuspected chronic anxiety states are the most powerful cause of recurrent depression. Why are they unsuspected? Yeah, you.

Because we aren't taught to ask about anxiety. We ask about depression; then we stop asking questions and prescribe antidepressants or ECT.

You're right. Modern institutional psychiatry is obsessed with depression. They want to see it as a biological disease; so they don't ask about psychological causes. That's what I said earlier. If your model of mental disorder consists of one sentence floating in ontological space like a party balloon, it is never wrong. It's also never right, but if you can get enough people to say what a wonderful model it is, there is no dissent. And if the institution of psychiatry actually represses criticism of itself, it can never correct itself. Criticism is the foundry of progress. No criticism, no progress. Alright, we're running out of time. One more question. You sir, right up the back, with your bloody great feet on the desk. You've got a question. Speak up, boy; I saw you grinning and nudging the others. OK, everybody, big round of applause. What's your name?

Jake.

OK, Jake, shoot.

This long term inhibition you talk about, would that be an epigenetic effect?

That is not quite the question I thought you would have but you've put your finger right on it. Is everybody familiar with epigenetics? Take the example of insulin resistance in type II diabetes. The relationship with obesity is now thought to be causative. The plasma of the obese has all the nasties you would expect from pigging out on hamburgers all day, like salt and sugar and long-chain fatty acids, but it also has high levels of cytokines. If you take a culture of murine somatic myocytes and flood them with salt, sugar, fatty acids and cytokines, something happens. The myocytes develop insulin resistance. The mechanism appears to be that the genes which begin the process of building and activating mitochondria are methylated. Blocked, in other words. So the myocytes have fewer and smaller mitochondria, meaning...? You tell them, Jake.

Glucose can't be metabolized. It builds up. So you would have high plasma glucose with insulin resistance. Type II diabetes.

Absolutely correct. So the environment has an epigenetic effect which becomes a diseased state. In order to treat type II diabetes effectively, we need to reverse the epigenetic blockade. Isn't that fascinating? Now the blockade I'm talking about in depression is different. It is a normal blockade. It is not, most definitely NOT, pathological. It is the normal state of affairs for those neurons. They receive a particular instruction that they are hard-wired to receive, so they switch themselves off. That has to be by gene activation, it couldn't be any other way. After the signal, the neurons produce a protein which blocks transmission in just that group of neurons and no others. It may be pre-synaptic, as in lowered production of neurotransmitter; it may be post-synaptic, say from reduction in the numbers or sensitivity of receptors; it doesn't actually matter at this stage. But it does mean that signals are blocked for months on end. Gradually, the blockade diminishes and the person starts to feel things again. We would say, his depression lifts. I presume drugs and ECT somehow reverse the blockade but not very well. Does that seem reasonable, young man?

Sounds OK. So you're saying depression is a normal state, not like NIDDM?

Correct. Look at chimps and baboons. What happens to a young male who challenges the alpha male and gets walloped?

Gotcha. It protects him.

Absolutely. But it is a psychologically determined state. It is not random. It is not a diseased state in the sense of sick neurons, like a confusional state in renal failure or hypoxia means sick neurons. Depression may be a pain in the arse but is has a function. It is the neurons doing their job to protect their owner from his own folly. They're saying to him, Hold on there, junior, get back in your box or you'll lose more than a bit of hair. You have to see that this hypothetical blockade is the brain doing what it is designed to do. The blockade is a physical state of the neurons but it is activated by a psychological instruction, a thought. I don't mean that in the sense that you may have the thought, "Ohmigod, this is a boring lecture", or "I'd rather be sailing", but it is a thought process or mental event in the sense that getting a joke is a thought process or mental event, or putting your foot on the brakes when you see a red light is a thought process or mental event. So depression has a role in the psychic economy, if you wish; but sometimes, it gets out of hand. If we accidentally flick the switch and activate a happiness blockade, then we're in trouble. Chronic anxiety will do that. Any more questions?

He's got one.

Is he a friend of yours, Jake?

Sure is.

Sir, I see the role of depression in that sort of loss, but what about grief? Why would that result in depression?

You two lads can see me afterwards for a job. I can give you a suggestion, but can you answer your own question? Think of chimps and baboons, because that's how our emotions evolved.

I think... Yeah, if you're a baboon and you lose your mate in a fight, it wouldn't be a good idea to try and mount the first baboon chick you see. You'd need to be in a depressed state for a while until you worked out which chicks were available.

You're so sensitive, young man, you could almost be a baboon yourself...

He is. You should see him on Saturday nights. [laughter]

I'll pass. If you're a baboon, then losing your baboon friends means you have to keep a very low profile, say if you've been excluded from the troop or you got lost. I see grief as the price we pay for being able to form social bonds. But it is a normal state of the brain. It is not pathology; it is not a disease. It may not be desirable but it has a job to do. Jake, you're...?

Gotcha. Actually, you were right. I did have another question. I just wondered what treatment depressed psychiatrists get?

They get psychotherapy, whaddayer reckon? They find the best and most sensitive psychotherapist in town, and they sit there and talk about their deprived childhoods.

10 Locking the Revolving Door

10.1: Introduction

In order to save space in the remaining histories, I won't repeat the questions as they are always exactly the same as the past two chapters. Instead, I will give the history in the form of a normal case report with headings, paraphrasing my notes so that the history reads as prose. From time to time, I will quote the patients' own statements verbatim so they can speak for themselves. It is important that we don't try to speak for them as our objective language necessarily smoothes and homogenizes their experiences.

Kerry Palmer was 46 years of age and had been in Darwin three months when she was first referred for treatment. About a year after her mother died, she moved to Darwin to join her much older, single male cousin as she had no other relatives. For many years, she had been receiving an invalid pension for Bipolar Disorder, so she was not required to look for work. However, she wanted to work and had no trouble finding jobs but was rarely able to keep them for more than a few months. When she arrived here with her dog, she knew nobody other than her cousin but she soon joined AA as she had previously been a member.

Following a number of admissions to hospital in her twenties and thirties, she had been prescribed large doses of a variety of psychotropic drugs which she had taken religiously for many years. When seen, she was taking:

- Venlafaxine 375 mg per day;
- Diazepam 20-40 mg per day
- Sodium valproate 800 mg per day.

She arrived about fifteen minutes early for her appointment and was clearly in an agitated state as she went in and out to her car several times and appeared to be on the verge of driving away. When she entered the office, she was practically distraught.

10.2: The History: Life's Little Ups and Downs

Presenting Complaints

(Barely able to talk): "I've got mood swings and bipolar and a long history of taking antidepressants and I need to see a psychiatrist and a psychologist." In general, she said, she was feeling terrible all the time. Her sleep was erratic. She went to bed at any time of night, depending on her mood. Usually, she got to sleep fairly quickly but, most nights, she woke after a few hours and some nights, had no sleep at all: "Thinking is my problem, my mind never stops." Her appetite was "dreadful" and she had lost about 7 kg in four months. She had little energy but she was constantly active, always on the move, and did various exercises when she had no housework or gardening to do. She said she had no interest in her normal activities and her motivation to do things was "zero." Socially, she actively avoided people and often did not go to AA meetings as she felt unable to mix. She had no sexual interest at all.

She described her memory as "shocking" and her concentration was also poor. She had great difficulty making decisions and put them off where possible as she feared making mistakes. She had trouble thinking clearly as she became flustered and agitated under the slightest pressure and lost the train of her thoughts. The thought content was dominated by worrying and feeling angry at herself for having made such a mess of her life. There were no disturbances of perception.

She described her mood as "very despondent and useless". She felt low and miserable most of the time, often feeling "pretty bad and sometimes overwhelming". By this, she meant she was sick of life itself and often had the feeling that death would be a relief but she did not have active suicidal ideas. She wasn't sure why she was unhappy but felt it was probably because she had failed in life.

She had frequent bouts of feeling tense and agitated, during which she felt irritable and unsettled. With these bouts, her heart raced and her stomach churned, and she felt shaky and sweaty, mainly in her hands. She was short of breath, had a dry mouth, and was light-headed and unsteady on her feet. She felt tight in the throat and often clenched her jaw until the muscles ached. She had trouble speaking clearly during these bouts as she tended to stumble over her words. With these bouts, she felt angry and frightened but it varied a lot from day to day.

She was having two or three bouts a day, each lasting from five minutes to several hours. On a bad day, the bouts of agitation tended to run together, lasting the whole day until she went to bed. They were caused by any sort of delay or minor upset in her routine, by having to mix with people, by appointments or interviews, and by dealing with aggressive people. Because of the agitation, she tended to stay home when possible but, when the cousin's friends visited, she would either take her dog to the beach or stay in her room.

On questioning, she had an extensive list of fears, mainly social in nature. She was easily startled by sudden noises, including thunder, and was very frightened of lightning (for background, Darwin has more lighting strikes than any other city in the world), but not by animals. She was frightened of crowds, queues, public speaking, and public transport, so she avoided them unless absolutely necessary. She was very fearful of threats or criticism, disputes or arguments, even if they did not involve her, and confrontation or saying no to people. She greatly feared letting people down, causing trouble, or giving offence and was especially frightened of humiliation or disapproval. She feared making mistakes or failing at anything, to the extent that she would simply walk away from tasks or duties (this was a big factor in her leaving jobs). One of the main fears that kept her awake at night was the idea that she would slip back into a serious mental illness and be committed to hospital again. She was very frightened of all groups of aggressive people, including drunks and teenage gangs.

From time to time, she had a sense of danger from people but no other paranoid symptoms (sense of persecution, surveillance, or conspiracy).

She was fastidiously fussy about cleanliness, tidiness, order, and punctuality, which often got her into arguments with people: "I'm a bit of a control freak like that." She had to check and recheck doors, locks, keys, switches, and gas taps as she constantly doubted her memory and couldn't be sure she had done it. She was tortured by the idea that, if she left a switch on, the house would burn down and she would be blamed. She had quite a number of minor rituals about cleaning and tidying or organizing things and hated anybody moving her possessions, but did not attempt to organize other people's belongings. She described repetitive thoughts but these were mainly ruminating on the same worries, day in, day out, until another one took over. There were no true obsessions or compulsions.

Physically, she had some low back pain but was generally fit and could work whenever she found a suitable job.

Recent History

At first, she said she developed mental problems in her mid-thirties, but it was pointed out that she was granted the invalid pension at age 27. She then recalled being admitted to hospital in her early twenties but she had been drinking heavily for some years before that. She couldn't recall any particular incident as the cause of her mental trouble. Over the years, she had been admitted to a number of hospitals in several cities, mostly following overdoses of drugs and alcohol or in states of intense agitation.

Personal Background

She was born in Sydney but spent her childhood on a remote cattle station in North Queensland. When she was aged ten, her father was killed in a mustering accident so she moved back to Sydney with her mother. He had been the area manager of a large cattle company but she had very little recall of him, except that he drank a lot. There had never been a step-father. Her mother died at the age of 79, a year before Kerry moved to Darwin. After they moved back to the city, the mother had part-time or casual work in shops but lived a very withdrawn life. She had little contact with her own relatives and none with the husband's family. She was described as "very quiet, closed and smothering", and she also drank quite heavily. Kerry was an only child. As far as she knew, she had only the one cousin on her mother's side and had never met any of her father's relatives. Her maternal grandparents lived in Perth (on the other side of the country) so she had met them only once before they died, soon after she started high school.

While they lived on the cattle station, her mother supervised her schooling via radio. When they moved back to Sydney, she attended a Catholic girls' school but she hated the strict religious atmosphere. Her mother would not let her go to a state school because she did not want her mixing with boys, and actively discouraged her making friends in their street. By the time she left school, she had never been to a birthday party and had never spoken to a boy except one or two who worked at the same place as her mother. However, the mother watched her constantly to prevent these meetings. She passed Year 10 at school, but her marks were never good. She did not get on well with the teachers as she was frightened of the nuns. She did not get on well with the other girls as she was very shy and nervous and was unable to mix. She did not play sport as her mother wanted her home immediately after school finished, and would not let her go out on weekends. She never belonged to any youth clubs or groups, even those at the local church. Her home life was "very controlled" but she did not argue much with her mother: "I never thought of it. If I argued with her, what else was there for me?"

On leaving school, she attended a secretarial course for twelve months but began drinking, which quickly led to arguments with her mother. On finishing her course, she soon found work in an office but was becoming increasingly unsettled and never stayed long in jobs. However, she was easily able to get work and gradually gained responsibility, to the point where she was managing stores in shopping centers and malls. She then began working in security and stayed in this type of work until she stopped work after she was given the pension. She could always get work with security firms and went back to it whenever she was well enough. Socially, she had a brief relationship with a sailor at nineteen, became pregnant, lost the pregnancy, then began a lesbian relationship with an aggressive and domineering older woman who drank heavily. Over the next eight years, her own drinking became a real problem and she was convicted of disorderly conduct several times for fighting in hotels and bars. She began using amphetamines because she felt more in control.

Her first admissions to hospital were during this stage of her life. She was diagnosed as having Bipolar Disorder and was prescribed large doses of psychotropic drugs while detained in hospital and then under community treatment orders. At the age of twenty-nine, she took a serious overdose after her lesbian partner left her; then went back to live with her mother in a distant suburb of Sydney. For the next few years, she was very withdrawn but was drinking steadily and arguing constantly with her mother over her irreligious life. At the age of thirty-four, she met a man who came to work on her mother's house and soon moved in with him.

She reduced her drinking and was generally more settled during this time but still was unable to mix with people unless she had been drinking. She stopped using amphetamines and had no further trouble with the police. After several years, they were married, but they separated after another six years because of her mental disturbance. She went back to living with her mother but stopped drinking and led a secluded life until her mother died when she was about forty-five. Although very distressed, she was not admitted to hospital. In desperation, she contacted her cousin who offered her accommodation.

Self-Assessment

When asked to describe herself, she quickly replied: "I'm always a very confident and active person and I really like myself." When it was pointed out that she had been intensely agitated when she entered the interview room, she became embarrassed: "Well, you said normally, and I was normally confident before I was bipolar. Yeah, OK, so it was twenty-five years ago. I dunno; I'm just a mess. That's what bipolar does to you."

On direct questioning, she agreed she was very nervous and intensely bothered by guilt, shame, and self-consciousness. She was unable to assert herself with people but always resented being pushed around. She was fanatically tidy, followed rules rigidly unless she was having "mood swings", and expected other people to follow rules as well. If they didn't, she became angry, but mostly kept it to herself. She was inclined to over-trust people but also had trouble mixing, so she avoided company where possible. She was jealous and held grudges for long periods (she still resented the sailor from twenty-five years before). At first, she said she got on well with authority but then agreed it was because she was very polite and cooperative and never spoke out. She felt she had a bad temper but she tried to keep it to herself as she always feared getting into trouble. She felt her intellect was "pretty good" but her self-esteem was "low, real low".

Mental State Examination

The mental state showed a rather chubby woman of about her stated age and a little below average height, dressed in tight denim shorts and a black singlet. She had short blond hair with two old professional tattoos and some chunky silver jewelry. She had two large, Indian-style shoulder bags stuffed full of documents and was carrying several files in her arms. When called to the office, she was sitting in the waiting room, rifling through the files and bags, with loose papers on her knees. Clearly intensely agitated, she clutched her possessions in an untidy bundle and entered the room, trembling and barely able to walk. As she dropped into her chair, her files slipped to the floor and she tried to pick them up but dropped her bags, which spilled around her feet. Told not to worry about them, she sat slumped in her chair, one hand over her eyes, and began blubbering that she didn't want to go to hospital. When told it didn't appear necessary, she began panting with relief and gradually settled. She spoke rapidly in a common accent but with an exaggerated courtesy, clearly at pains to appear polite. After half an hour, she was still agitated and tremulous but was a lot more settled. She was unhappy but not despairing or suicidal. She was not hostile or suspicious. There were no signs of a psychotic disorder, and nothing to indicate an organic impairment of brain function. She was probably of bright normal intellectual ability but educated well below her potential.

Further Information

Her messy files contained her psychiatric records going back to her first admissions, over twenty years before. This was from a large mental hospital with university affiliations. The first discharge summary consisted of a page of detail such as her address and next of kin, with a one-line diagnosis of Bipolar Disorder. More recent discharge summaries had more medical detail but most started with a statement such as "This well-known patient presented in a depressive state six months after discharge from a manic attack." There was no description of her condition at any stage, and nothing to indicate a full history had ever been taken. She had been prescribed large doses of drugs including chlorpromazine, thioridazine, amitriptyline, imipramine, phenelzine, lithium, carbamazepine, valproate, and, more recently, olanzapine and quetiapine. She had attended various programs run by psychologists as well as drug and alcohol centers. She had copies of all the documents from the various hearings she had attended, relating to her detention orders, but none of them gave more than the skimpiest details of her condition. In the main, they simply repeated that she had been in hospital before and was not taking her drugs or had taken too many.

Management

She was commenced on specific treatment for her very obvious anxiety state and all other medication was slowly reduced. The valproate was discontinued after about two months but it was just over a year before the venlafaxine stopped. She had suffered bad withdrawal symptoms from it in the past and was fearful of stopping it suddenly. She is still taking diazepam 2 mg, morning and evening, and is reluctant to reduce the dose further, although she forgets it from time to time.

Early in her management, she was referred to a support group called GROW, which has a similar type of program to AA. GROW runs activity programs for people with chronic mental disorders so she attended these until, after about a year, she felt she wanted to find work again. She started working twelve hours per weekend in the storage area of a small franchise firm but, after several weeks, was weepy and distressed as she felt it was too demanding. She displayed typical anticipatory anxiety about mistakes she might make. After recognizing the problem and developing suitable plans to forestall reasonable errors, she settled and continued with the job, gradually increasing her hours until she was working three eight-hour shifts, from Friday to Sunday. One weekend, a staff member was sick, so she offered to work in the front of the store. This went well and she was given a bonus by the manager, which pleased her enormously as it was the first bonus she had received since her early twenties. Gradually, she increased her time until she was working twenty-four hours a week, at which point her pension payments ceased.

Over the next few months, she continued working in the front of the store, dealing with the general public, including over the Christmas period. When the position of deputy manager became vacant, she was invited to apply for it by the manager but there were several other applicants and she was not successful. As a result, she became distressed and weepy, complaining that the job was too much for her and she should resume her pension. This was managed in her ordinary visits and the "crisis" passed without further complication. A few months later, the manager took leave, so Kerry was promoted to act as deputy manager for a month. She worked full-time for this period and continued full-time when she went back to her normal post. She has now worked longer in this job than any job since the age of eighteen, and will soon break that record.

Socially, she met a number of her cousin's friends and has formed a relationship with one of them. This man drinks very little but is quite happy to go to AA meetings with her. She has now bought a small car and is considering moving to the friend's apartment on a permanent basis.

10.3: Conclusion: When Up and Down is Not Bipolar

The discharge summaries from her previous hospital admissions gave her diagnosis as Bipolar Disorder. When she was drinking and fighting with the lesbian friend, she was sometimes given the diagnosis of Borderline Personality Disorder. At no stage was her severely anxious personality recognized or treated; yet, as soon as the proper diagnosis was made and appropriate treatment instituted, her condition began a steady improvement. After more than twenty years, she is no longer receiving a pension but is working full-time and is fully self-supporting. She is seen only once every three weeks for a short visit (cost $37.50) and her monthly medication costs are about $15.00, down from something like $350.00. On any measure, her management has been successful, but only because she is no longer treated as a case of Bipolar Disorder. Even though she met all the criteria, the diagnosis was incorrect.

The expression 'bipolar disorder' is a surface diagnosis and does not give any indication as to the actual causes of the recurrent bouts of depression and agitation. In fact, her problem was severe anxiety. She drank and used illegal drugs because they calmed her. Whenever she was not anxious, she was active and outgoing but, as she tried to do more, she became increasingly anxious that she would fail. Before long, she had to drink to control her agitation, which led to further trouble and always culminated in a depressive episode. Anxiety states mimic the bipolar syndrome, but they are a separate disorder and require precisely targeted treatment; otherwise there is no improvement. Generic "anti-bipolar" treatment (long-term antidepressants and so-called 'mood stabilizers') does not tackle the underlying problem. Essentially, it converts the anxious patient into a heavily sedated patient with an untreated anxiety state. The natural history of untreated anxiety states is that they get worse with the passage of time.

For a conventional, biologically-oriented psychiatrist, the notion of an "underlying cause of the bipolar syndrome" is a solecism. To them, there is no bipolar syndrome; there is only Bipolar Disorder: the symptoms both define and constitute the disorder. At the same time, the symptoms are irrelevant as they are mere artifacts of a biochemical lesion. That the biochemical lesion is also unknown is a bagatelle: as an act of faith, it exists, and will eventually be revealed by neuroscience. This is absurd. Firstly, it is not possible to nominate and to define or describe something in a single illocutionary act ("What's that patient go?" "Bipolar disorder." "I see, and what's Bipolar Disorder?" "It's what he's got."). Second, there is the classic error of promissory materialism. When he described the manic-depressive syndrome, Emil Kräpelin was quite sure that a biological cause would soon be found. 120 years later, we are still waiting for it. That might be plausible but for the third objection, which is that, if it turns out that the cause of the manic-depressive syndrome is actually psychological, not biological, then the biological psychiatrists will never know they are wrong. If, in science, a researcher is unable in principle to say whether he is right or wrong, then he should stop his research project as it can never yield reliable results. We return to the challenge I set the biological psychiatrists some years ago: what is the evidence that will show your research project is wrong? If they cannot answer that, then they should close up their shop.

In a case like this, the problem is that the DSM-IV project is so convinced that its surface diagnosis accurately charts an underlying biochemical disorder that they stop asking questions. They do not ask their patients the full range of anxiety symptoms. Thus, they can never know whether their patients have a primary anxiety disorder with secondary depressive reaction, or whether they have the "genuine" bipolar state, whatever that turns out to be. Anybody who makes a diagnosis is saying not only that the patient has this condition, but he is also saying the patient doesn't have any other conditions. Unless the patient is systematically questioned about all the psychiatric syndromes, diagnosis becomes a Procrustean exercise of responding to the obvious while ignoring the subtle. If our police departments do that sort of thing, we are outraged, but it seems to be all the rage in psychiatry these days.

<table>
<tr><td>

11
</td><td>

The Case of
A Pain in the Back
</td></tr>
</table>

11.1: Introduction

Alexander McBride is a 36-y/o Scotsman who was referred in late 2008 for management of back pain and a chronic mental disorder. He arrived in Darwin in September that year, looking for work. Two days after he arrived, while waiting to cross the road to his car, he was knocked down by a reversing truck. He was taken to hospital by ambulance and remained there for nearly two weeks with a minor spinal fracture, broken ribs and a pneumothorax. While in hospital, his car, with practically all his belongings in it, was stolen and wrecked. He was discharged from hospital but had very little money, so he was given a bed in a homeless men's shelter. On his second day there, he was pushed by a mentally-disturbed man and fell to the ground but was unable to get to his feet. He was taken back to hospital with severe sciatica and was discharged after two days with narcotic analgesics. He went back to the shelter but it closed for six hours each day. As he was unable to sit in a nearby park in the pre-monsoonal heat, he had to walk 2 km to the public library which was air-conditioned. He was very worried as he could only stay in the shelter a maximum of three months, and he had already been there two months.

When he was referred, he had no money and very few possessions. He had found that his interstate car insurance was not valid in the Northern Territory and his claim for damages from the public Motor Vehicle Insurance Trust was delayed as there were no witnesses to the accident and the hospital had not submitted his reports. Pending approval of his MVIT claim, he was being provided benefits by the Social Security Department on a fortnightly basis. This meant that, each two weeks, he had to go to the DSS office, about 12 km away, and submit all his forms again. As he was not an Australian citizen, he had to complete extra forms with certified copies of his passport and various other documents, all of which either cost money or had to be approved in different offices around the city. He had used his last possessions, his laptop and a digital camera, as security on a loan for $200, on which he was paying an astounding $50 a month interest.

Several weeks before his appointment, the narcotic drugs were stopped abruptly on the basis that he had had too much. He had been given paracetamol but this caused gastritis, so he was not taking anything for pain. He was still taking drugs prescribed by a hospital psychiatrist, including an antidepressant (mirtazepine 30 mg at night) and small doses of diazepam as a muscle relaxant. He was on the waiting list for spinal surgery but had been told it would be at least a year.

The day he was seen was extremely hot and humid, with no breeze at all. To reach the appointment, he had travelled for over two hours, including two buses and walking nearly a kilometer. He was soaked by sweat and in considerable pain when he arrived. He explained that he had left a small town in Victoria, some 4000 km away, in a state of intense agitation with no clear idea of where he was going. This followed the final breakdown in a relationship with a much younger woman with whom he had a child of eighteen months. He had met the woman in a mental hospital where they had been in-patients together. He had no relatives in Australia and knew nobody in Darwin.

11.2: The History: Taken Aback

Presenting Complaints

Close to tears, he said he was feeling "depressed and hopeless and close to suicide". He immediately added that he did not want to go to hospital as it had never achieved anything and he would lose his place in the shelter. He said he was barely able to sleep at night, even when he had been taking narcotics, but, without them, he was getting no more than two hours of broken sleep a night. He was waking from nightmares, but then the pain stopped him from going back to sleep. The bad dreams mostly related to his failed relationship and his childhood. His appetite was poor and he had lost 5 kg since discharge from hospital. He had very little energy and his activity was limited to walking to his appointments. He had no interest in what was going on around him and felt unable to do anything beyond holding his life together. Socially, he did not want to mix. He was frightened of the men in the shelter and spent a lot of his time there sitting near the supervisor's office for protection. From time to time, he was able to talk to the mother of his child and to the child herself, but it was becoming clear that the child had no idea who he was. He had no sexual interest at all.

He said his memory was patchy and he had trouble concentrating as he was highly distractible when around people but, when alone, his mind drifted back to the past. He felt he could not make decisions and delayed them or asked for help where possible. He had trouble thinking clearly as he became flustered under any sort of pressure, even if it was as simple as trying to decide when to call his child because of the time zones. His thought content was totally dominated by his problems and he could not think of anything else. Asked about disturbances of perception, he said he often found himself conducting arguments in his head but these were never resolved. He knew the "voices" were his own thoughts, even when they were critical of him, but he felt unable to stop them.

He described his mood as hopeless and useless. He was feeling low and miserable most of the time. This was "pretty bad", meaning he was sick of things as they were and often sick of life itself. He had often had the feeling that it would have been better if the truck had killed him and had had vague suicidal ideas, but had no urge to act on them. The unhappiness was due to the separation from his child and his injuries and losses since he arrived in Darwin. He never felt good except briefly while he heard his daughter's voice but that didn't last and seemed to leave him feeling worse.

He described frequent bouts of agitation during which he was physically agitated and mentally irritable. He was shaky, sweaty (especially on his palms), his heart raced, and his stomach churned to the point he thought he would vomit. At its worst, he was unable to eat and would often have cramping abdominal discomfort and the urge to defecate. He felt short of breath, his mouth was dry and he felt light-headed and unsteady on his feet so he would usually try to lie down. In addition, his throat felt tight and he was unable to speak or swallow properly. Mostly, he would stumble over his speech unless he was enraged and started swearing.

During these bouts, he felt frightened and a bit irritable and had to get away from whatever was troubling him. At the time, he was having two or three bouts a day, each lasting up to several hours; so he was disabled for a large part of each day. They were brought on by "everything". On questioning, he was frightened of heights, electricity, and water. He was unable to put his head underwater and would not go on the ocean. He feared darkness, dirt, disorder and contamination, and washed his hands frequently each day. He was fearful of dogs, lizards, snakes, spiders, geckoes, and maggots; but most of his fears were social in nature. These included public speaking, standing in queues, interviews, tests and exams, and threats or criticism. He was very fearful of conflict or disputes of any sort and went out of his way to keep the peace. He feared humiliation and disapproval, letting people down or causing any sort of trouble, making mistakes and failing at anything. He had always been scared of hospitals and dentists but this was worse since his accident. He was very frightened of all aggressive people but especially the aboriginals who hung around the shelter and demanded money from him. He had never felt comfortable near any sort of authority.

When he was near people, he had the feeling that they were looking at him or talking behind his back. He felt all people judged him and he had to make sure he did not give offence. He had a strong sense of danger from people, that they would hurt him or assail him in some way, not just physically but also by humiliating him. Sometimes, he had the feeling he was being watched or followed and he felt several of the men in the shelter were spreading stories about him. For example, he was sure that one of them had told the supervisor he was selling his narcotics, and this had been conveyed to the hospital: "They've got the wrong idea of me, I'm weak."

He had always been very fussy about cleanliness, tidiness, order, punctuality, and efficiency. This had caused a lot of arguments with his former partner, who was untidy, disorganized, and had no concept of time. He had repeated intrusive thoughts of being in danger or impending trouble, but there were no true obsessive-compulsive features.

Physically, he had constant low back pain, starting deep in the midline and spreading sideways, especially on the right. The pain drove deep into his right buttock and thence down the back of the right leg to the ankle. It was an intense, boring pain which was often so bad that it stopped him from moving. At different times, he had deep, crushing pains in his thigh or scalding sensations around the knee and calf. His right foot felt weak and he tended to stumble when going up stairs. He had to grip the banister tightly when going down stairs, especially at night, and avoided walking on wet or slippery surfaces. He could not carry more than a few kilos and did not believe he could operate power tools etc. Since the accident, he had had no sexual function at all but his interest had long gone, anyway. He was not incontinent.

Recent History

He had been in Australia about five years and had recently been granted permanent residency on the basis of his de facto relationship, just before it ended. Some years before, he had been admitted to a rural mental hospital in what he said was a psychotic state. He described intense agitation associated with paranoid ideas about people in his boarding house making fun of him. He had become depressed and weepy, and was given the diagnosis Bipolar Disorder. He was discharged from hospital on fluoxetine, quetiapine, and sodium valproate. While an inpatient, he met a woman of about half his age and moved to stay with her after they were discharged. The relationship was tempestuous and he was admitted to hospital twice more after taking overdoses. After the baby was born, he was very happy for a time, but then discovered his partner was having an affair with a biker who was plying her with amphetamines. She became violent toward him and assaulted him a number of times but, when questioned by the police, he denied the assaults. He was readmitted once more before suddenly fleeing the town in a state of overwhelming agitation. He wanted to keep in contact with his child but did not want the mother to know where he was in case her boyfriend had contacts with the bikie crowd in Darwin.

Personal Background

Alex was born in Aberdeen, Scotland, and raised in a small town further north. His parents separated when he was fifteen after which he lived with his mother until he went to university. His father, a retired forensic pathologist, was then aged 62. The father, who drank heavily, was highly demanding and critical and had no friends. He loathed religion and communists and had been treated for depression for years. He was described as "an angry, angry man" and Alex had always been terrified of him. The father hit him for every minor transgression until he was nearly fifteen. His mother was then 60 and was still working as a nurse. He described her as "very calm and serene" and he had always got on very well with her, except that he felt she had done nothing to protect him from the father's temper outbursts: "She just didn't hear what was going on, but she was very nice afterwards." She was very involved in the local church. He kept in regular contact with her. He was the second of three siblings. He had a 38-yo married sister who was working as a teacher in England. He described her as "OK, but very judgmental" and was not close to her. He had a 33-yo brother who was the head chef in a luxury resort but he was "just like our father, the same volatile temper". They were not close. Apart from his mother, half a world away, and his infant daughter, who did not recognize his voice, he had no affectionate relationships in the world.

He attended the local government schools to the age of twelve, then a local church college for the rest of his schooling, finishing at 18. His marks at school were "very high" and he got on well with the teachers, although he was frightened of most of them. He did not get on with the other boys: "I was no good, a classic nerd. I was terribly shy and nervous. I was bullied and teased because I was too scared to hit back. If I'd ever been in a fight at school, my father would have killed me." In primary school, he had suffered minor bowel incontinence. For the rest of his schooling, he was terrified of having to change for sport in case his underwear was stained so he managed to avoid sport by cultivating incompetence. His only interests at school were reading and computers. He had one or two friends who were almost as bad as he was, but never visited them after school and never had any friends visit his home. His home life was miserable and his schooling was a nightmare. Toward the end of their marriage, his parents argued constantly.

On leaving school, he moved to Aberdeen to study computer engineering. He lived with an elderly relative and, for the first time, started to enjoy himself. With a friend, he joined the Army Reserve combat engineers and found he could keep up with the other men. However, over the next two years, he became increasingly shy and withdrawn as he did not drink and could not mix with girls. He graduated with mediocre marks and was not offered a higher course. For a time, he toyed with the idea of transferring to the regular Army but the idea of combat in the Gulf terrified him, so he resigned. He found work with a small local engineering company in the oil industry and started studying a diploma part-time. The company was involved in developing self-controlled underwater vehicles and also had military connections, so he was fairly happy for several years. He completed his diploma and enrolled for a higher degree, working full-time and studying at an advanced level part-time, which meant that he had no social life at all. As the company was struggling, he guaranteed a sizeable loan for the owners. However, not long after, the company declared bankruptcy and he had to surrender all his assets to repay the loan. The industry was in a downturn so he found a similar job in the off-shore gas industry in Victoria and moved to Australia. For a year, he was reasonably happy; then he lost his job and became very depressed. He was first admitted to hospital in this state, and met the young woman. Because of his mental state, he lost his clearance with the company and was forced to find work as a fruit packer and casual laborer.

Socially, he was almost totally inept. He had never been much of a drinker, did not use any illegal drugs, and had no police record. He had never had a girlfriend until he met the mother of his child in the mental hospital, and had no sexual experience: "She had to show me what to do; I was terrified." She appeared to take control of him. The relationship was poor as she was using drugs throughout and was incapable of holding a job more than a day or two. She became physically violent, which terrified him as the neighbors sometimes called the police, who invariably treated him as the offender. After the baby was born, he worked as a taxi driver so he could come home at different times if she called him. He was largely responsible for the baby's care as the mother often went out without telling him where she was going. He knew she was using drugs and was hanging around with the town's couple of elderly bikies but he was too scared to do anything. Her behavior deteriorated and he became increasingly distressed. She began threatening to report him to the police as a child molester until, in a state of intense agitation, he loaded his belongings in his car and disappeared into the night.

Self-Assessment

Tearfully, he said: "I try to be a good person. I'm helpful and I always avoid trouble." He saw himself as very nervous and incapable of asserting himself. He was intensely troubled by guilt, shame and self-consciousness. He was over-trusting of people, which often led him into trouble, but he was not jealous and did not hold grudges. He was tidy, organized, excessively patient, and fearful of authority. He always followed rules as he was too scared to do otherwise. He saw his temper as very mild, his intellect as "very high" and his self-esteem as "abysmal, the worst."

Mental State Examination

The mental state showed a thin and well-presented man of about his stated age, dressed in clean but sweaty casual clothing and wearing a spinal brace. He had no visible tattoos, studs, scars, or jewelry. His movements were careful and considered and he lowered himself gingerly into his chair using the arm-rests. He spoke softly in a gentle, quavering voice and was often close to tears. His answers to questions were full and he appeared keen to talk. He was anxious and tremulous throughout the interview. He was very unhappy with a strong sense of guilt and worthlessness. There were vague suicidal ideas and he was using the child as his justification for resisting these ideas: "I've got to live for her. Her mother is too disturbed. I'm all she's got." He was not hostile or suspicious. There were no signs of a psychotic disorder and nothing to indicate an organic impairment of brain function. He was clearly of superior intellect.

Management

He was prescribed narcotic analgesics, the antidepressant was doubled, and he was commenced on specific treatment for his life-long anxiety state. When reviewed a week later, he was much improved. He was sleeping four to five hours a night, had better pain control by day, and was much less agitated: "I can deal with things at last. I can talk to people without panicking and running away." Over the next few weeks, he contacted his mother to see if he could borrow some money but she had none so, with great trepidation, he called his father. As expected, his father flew into a rage and refused, so he hung up. He was pleased with this as, before, he would not have been able to ring or, if he had, would not have been able to speak or hang up. The men's shelter found him a place in a charity hostel in the city which gave him a single room for the same price and he did not have to leave by day. He recovered his computer and was able to do some jobs for the hostel, showing them how to network their own computers.

Unfortunately, his run of bad luck continued. His social security payments were stopped so he lodged an appeal and presented it himself. He was successful but the department immediately lodged a further appeal although his payments continued with the requirement that he look for work. This meant attending an employment agency that were paid a fee by the government if he attended, not otherwise; so they would not accept that he was not able to get out of bed some days. A call to the hospital showed that, for unknown reasons, he was not on the surgery waiting list, which meant he had to start the process again, getting appointments, waiting, more X-rays, review, a trial of physiotherapy, etc. Physiotherapy was not successful as he had to catch two buses from the city and was in more pain when he got home than when he started. However, because he stopped attending, his name came off the waiting list again, which meant half a dozen phone calls to the hospital, who couldn't find any record of him, then sent him to the rehabilitation clinic. This clinic decided he needed to go to the pain clinic before they would consider treatment. After a two-month wait, he attended the clinic at 1:00 pm. He was seen by a physiotherapist, an occupational therapist, and a psychologist for an hour—each, consecutively. At 4:45 pm, in tears of pain and agitation, he hobbled out and caught a taxi home. A week later, still in a lot of pain, he slipped on the stairs at the hostel while going down to collect his mail. He fell heavily, landing sideways with one buttock on the step. When he finally got his mail, it was a letter from the hospital saying that, as he had failed to complete his assessment, his appointment at the rehabilitation clinic had been cancelled. Quite often, people enduring this sort of difficulty become very paranoid, especially when they have been injured at work. In a sense, it was fortunate that his entire life experience had been the same so he was not especially troubled: "Same shit, different country."

After nearly two years, he appears to be no closer to surgery but, mentally, he is better than he ever has been. Despite the trouble he has had, he has not been in hospital, has not taken overdoses, and his only psychotropic drug is the antidepressant.

11.3: Life Experiences vs. Chemical Imbalances

Once again, this case demonstrates the conflict between the idea that the symptoms say it all vs. symptoms being only the clue to what is actually happening in the person. Discharge summaries from his admissions to the hospital in Victoria were skimpy. They focused on his mood disturbance (meaning his complaints of depression) without ever explaining why he was unhappy. Even though the summaries had a space for a diagnosis on each of the DSM-IV axes, they were rarely filled in and nobody appears to have suspected his severely anxious personality. Because it was never suspected, it was never treated. Because it was never treated, he kept getting depressed.

Depression has to be seen as a reaction to life events. It is not a "black dog" that comes snapping around your heels just because it can smell a defect in your genes. It is not a black cloud that randomly catches in your hat as you come home from work. It has a cause. Everything has a cause; nothing is without a reasonable cause.

Every human comes equipped with the cerebral machinery to experience emotions, and one of them is sadness. The grief state appears to be the price we pay for being able to form social bonds. If we were not able to form bonds, we may still be here but we would be more like ants than the creatures we suppose ourselves to be. Be that as it may, our emotions are rational. Emotions don't just fire off randomly otherwise we would all be dead. They have to be appropriate and precisely-directed responses to life events in order to maximize our chances of survival. They have to make sense in the overall context of our lives.

The biological psychiatrist will object: "Ah yes," he will say, "but that's the whole point. Mental illness doesn't make sense in the context of the patient's life, that's why we call it mental disorder and not mental order." This might be true if the biological psychiatrist could show that he has thoroughly explored the patient's life and, sad to say, the depression or anxiety or suspicion is unrelated to the totality of his experience, but that never happens. Biological psychiatrists are the people who claim that mental distress is unrelated to normality, and they are also the people who don't take psychiatric histories. Why don't they take histories, teasing out the many threads that go to make up the patient's life? They won't say, but we already know the answer: they don't take histories because they believe the history has no bearing on the mental disorder just because the disorder is genetic, not psychological. *Petitio principii*: thus, they beg the question. They assume the truth of that which requires proof, namely, that life events are irrelevant. By assuming that life events are irrelevant, they ignore them, which means they never find life events that could make sense of the patient's disorder. Because they have an absence of proof, they take this as proof of absence.

Let's go back to Alex McBride's miserable life with a tyrannical father and a fatalist mother. I would say that the father had a severe personality disorder, with high interpersonal anxiety, low self-esteem and high mistrust. He was bitter, controlling, and self-righteous, all of which are facets of the paranoid personality. This led to a miserable life and self-treatment with alcohol (a powerful anti-anxiety drug). Eventually, he was given antidepressants but he had to take them all his life because his personality was so awful that being sober would inevitably lead to depression. The mother was simply weak. She was frightened of her husband's temper and wandered around the house in a detached ("serene") manner, ignoring the ructions or disappearing into church when it got too bad. Young Alex talked to her but couldn't rely on her. He told her he was having a miserable time but she simply patted him on the head and told him to trust in the Lord and play more with his little friends. Eventually, he stopped telling her but she didn't notice. By the time he reached university, he was socially crippled. What does this mean?

Alex was an anxious personality, meaning he habitually responded to neutral events in the environment as though they were a threat. His burglar alarm was set too fine, you could say; it was set so that it went off with the slightest disturbance in the neighborhood. He spent his life in a state of high alarm, startled by every change in the breeze, panicking over every frown on the teacher's face. If anything was delayed or didn't quite fit, he reacted as though he had discovered a cancer eating his vitals. For him, there was no such thing as "Dinnae fash ye'self, laddie". Everything was about to blow up in his face; everything was a catastrophe in the making. That's what anxious personality means. I fully appreciate that DSM-IV does not recognize an anxious personality; it assigns excessive anxiety to the formal mental illnesses, but that begs the question of what causes anxiety.

Biological psychiatry (of which DSM-IV is the roadmap) argues that an anxious person (often known as "the worried well") has a biochemical disturbance of the brain which is manifest as excessive and inappropriate anxiety. To my simplistic way of thinking, this doesn't make a lot of sense. Why should a person (say, a 21-y/o Army private I saw yesterday) have a single "chemical imbalance of the brain" which makes him frightened of cockroaches and nothing else? What claims are we making of the wiring of the brain to say that one insect of many thousands should provoke such widespread terror as the harmless cockroach? It can't even bite. I have never seen anybody with a phobia of mosquitoes.

Let's look at some of the "chemical imbalances of the brain" (true phobias) I have seen over the years:
- Doll's eyes. That is correct. A woman was mortally afraid of the doll's eyes that close when you tip the doll over.
- Clusters of little round objects, like grapes, bubbles in the bath, small boiled sweets (candy) in a plastic bag, or collections of washers.

- Rust on boats. Not rust on cars, not woodworm in timber boats, not water, not pirates, but streaks of rust on steel boats.
- Rubber ducks. Nobody believes this one but it is absolutely true.
- Ants, but not snakes or spiders.
- Pythons, but not poisonous snakes.
- Tree frogs (harmless) but not cane toads (poisonous).
- Toenail clippings.
- Earthworms, but not snakes or anything else.

Conceptually, we cannot account for these aberrations without invoking a mentalist explanation. The notion that we can distinguish between poisonous snakes and pythons at the level of our DNA is utterly implausible; yet this is what biological psychiatry entails.

In my view, the mentalist account of phobias is the more economical. It simply says that the individual person is accidentally switching on his fear circuits without knowing that that is what he is doing. This is not implausible, just because none of us knows how we switch on our fear circuits anyway. The decision to respond fearfully to an event is not taken consciously. The decision is made for us silently and at high speed, in the psychological or computational realm of the mind, and is active before we are even aware of it. It has to be; otherwise it wouldn't save our bacon. The whole point of the fear response is to save lives, meaning it has to be very fast, very sensitive, and very powerful; otherwise we would ignore it. We would keep looking for mushrooms while the bull is pawing the ground. So for an anxious person, we are making no further claim than this: his life experiences have taught him to react fearfully to events that most people see as harmless. We are not making any claims on his genes or his biochemistry; it is simply a matter of ordinary learning which has gone a bit further than normal. If I burn a cake, I am not claiming there was something wrong with the recipe, or the ingredients, or the oven. I am simply saying I took the normal process of cooking a cake a bit far. Same goes for anxiety.

In Alex's case, the claim is not that he had a genetic defect of some kind but that he had learned to see the world as a very dangerous place, where anything that went wrong would result in an explosion, where he would be blamed and he would be unable to defend himself. So why didn't he just get over it, let it go, and move on, as they say these days? If I put some new horses in the paddock near the railway line, they will snort and run away the first time a train roars past. A few days later, they won't even lift their heads from the grass. Why didn't his fear responses extinguish, to lapse into behaviorese? Why didn't he learn that he could talk to girls at university and so break down his terrible loneliness? His fear responses, including his vast social phobia, did not extinguish because they were constantly being negatively reinforced, but internally, not by the external environment.

A person with a fear of frogs will always say: "I know it's silly; I know they can't hurt me; but I am terrified of frogs." Every time she goes near a frog, she will feel a jolt of fear, so next time, she doesn't go near them.

Nobody sees the fear but she knows it is there. A while later, she starts to avoid places where she thinks frogs are likely to be, but this is not a fully conscious matter. The computational mind does that for us; we are only apprised of its decisions. Why should I say that humans don't sit down and work out where frogs are likely to be? Because chimps work out where the fruit is likely to be without having round table conferences. There is a large lagoon not far from our house where the egrets have worked out frogs that are likely to be. Their decision was not conscious in any normal sense of the word, yet it is definitely a decision (they never look for frogs in trees) and it is very effective. It has kept them alive for untold millennia. Unfortunately, the mechanism isn't perfect. Cane toads (*Bufo marinus*) have invaded the lagoon and the birds are dying. Because they die rather than just feel squeamish, they can't learn not to eat toadlets.

Alex's fear of speaking to girls was wholly internal, wholly cognitive. He had the belief: "If I try to talk to that girl, I will surely blush and stammer and sweat and look a complete idiot." This is not to say he had this thought in his mind at all times, just as I don't have in mind the thought: If I punch that wall, it will hurt my hand. It was simply there, a part of his general belief system of the world and of his place in it. He did not think: "The professor will shout and rant if I am late, and I will surely blush and stammer and sweat and look a complete idiot; so I'd better not go to the lecture." His computational mind took this belief about authority figures into account when he looked at his watch; it calculated his likely response and fed him the result in the form of an expectation, so he turned and went home, humiliated. Next time he was running late, he remembered not just his expectation of the professor's temper but also his humiliation, so he pulled back earlier. We don't know every bit of information we take into account when we make a decision. The decision is made and the anxiety response activated before we are fully aware of what is happening. It has to be that way. If it were not, the saber-toothed tigers would have finished us off long ago.

This point reminds me of the work of the neurophysiologist, Benjamin Libet. He found that, on the basis of cerebral physiology, people were acting on decisions before they were conscious of having made the decision. Dennett makes a lot of this in his Consciousness Explained. I cannot see why anybody has the slightest problem with this. We all do it all the time. Daily, we make a million decisions and put them into effect without giving them anything like conscious attention. Even while I am typing these words, I am not giving my fingers any attention at all; they just do their job. I ride my pushbike and my legs just keep going round and round. I talk to you, and the words just keep coming. Decisions are fast and essentially pre-conscious. If they were not, we would move like sloths. This point is of central importance in understanding the anxiety states.

The difference between the fear response of humans and of, say, white rats, is that we can imagine a bad outcome before it happens. We activate our fear responses on the expectation of a threat. Well, says a Skinnerian, so do white rats. They can be conditioned to react as though a threat was about to engulf them. True, but humans take it one step further. If the threat we expect just is our own fear response, then we are trapped in a vicious circle of steadily intensifying fear. However, we don't have to think about this in any ordinary sense of the term "think about it". The decision is made for us at the computational level of mind, very fast, outside introspection, and very effectively. It has to be this way. Anything else would take too long.

Fear is the only truly recursive human emotion: it reinforces itself. It is also the most powerful. It can override every other drive or impulse. It inhibits humor immediately, can override the need for food, for shelter, water, sleep, warmth, or cool, anger, misery and, of course, sex. For what seem like very sensible reasons, fear is completely inhibitory of sexual arousal. So it didn't matter how much Alex wanted to meet one of the young ladies in his class at university; his fear of humiliation crushed his sexual drive before it had even begun to push him toward her. He feared humiliation but he was only humiliated when he was fearful.

A detailed assessment of this man's personality shows why he was depressed. He was highly intelligent and a pleasant and considerate person. He didn't break laws and had always supported himself to the best of his ability. He was not violent and did not drink or use drugs; yet his life was torture. Whatever he tried failed because of his high levels of anxiety—in which fear of failure figured very strongly. As a result, he withdrew and became increasingly unhappy. The historical causes of his anxiety were crystal clear. He grew up in a household with rigidly enforced and excessively strict rules, where punishment was swift and brutal. There were so many rules that he never really knew which one he had broken; until you know all the rules, punishment seems random. In fact, he was more scared of his father's ferocious rages than he was of the actual beltings. At the first sign of anger, he froze with fear; once the belting actually started, he knew it wouldn't last long and he would be sent to his room. Once his childhood history was clear, his adult personality fell into place. Successful treatment of his anxiety resulted in a huge improvement in his performance, and thence in his self-esteem.

Orthodox psychiatry sees depression as a primary disorder in its own right. The biocognitive model of psychiatry says this is wrong. Depression is a reaction to life events. Some of those events are outside, some are inside. Some are in the present, some are in the past. And, confusingly, some of them are in the future. If we believe that life is bad and can never get better, then we have to give up on it. We have to take all our hopes and plans and drop them, one by one, until there is nothing left. Giving up induces that particular reaction called the grief reaction which is not unique to humans. People do not give up on life for laughs; it is forced upon them. If we come across a healthy, intelligent, good-looking, educated, pleasant young man with no terrible secrets or moral conflict who is depressed, we have to explain why he is depressed. It is not good enough simply to say, "Oh yes, he's feeling low and miserable, but that's what depression is." Everything, including depression, has a cause. Our job is to find the cause. An unrecognized anxiety state is by far the commonest cause of unexplained depression. Anxiety is a devastating problem; it wrecks young lives and forces the sufferer to abandon all his hopes for the future. Anxiety is not "comorbid" with depression; it is causative. Depression is the secondary or reactive emotion. To treat chronic or recurrent depression, treat the anxiety.

Why do people not recognize their anxiety as the primary problem? I think there are many reasons for this. Firstly, people often say: "I know I'm anxious, but isn't it normal? I thought everybody felt this way but they just controlled it better." This is why they see their anxiety as a moral failing: "Everybody has it, so all it takes is a bit of will-power and it will be brought under control. I have not brought my anxiety under control, therefore I have failed. If I had tried harder, I would now be as bright and cheerful as everybody else; I am not cheerful, therefore I didn't try. I didn't try, therefore my failure is moral." Men in particular do not want to admit they are anxious. They have had years of training from people who are not anxious who take their own good fortune as a sign of their moral superiority. In fact, it is very largely luck.

Second, psychiatry is obsessed with depression. It would be a very interesting topic for a PhD in the history of psychiatry to trace this peculiar preoccupation from its origin to the present. Third, and closely associated to this, the drug industry applies remorseless pressure to the medical profession, who are mostly only too pleased to be pressured, to find depression and treat it—with drugs. Why would we prescribe antidepressants if depression is a secondary disorder? We would treat the causative problem and leave the antidepressants for the really severe cases. Fourth, I suspect many psychiatrists can't be bothered with anxiety. Anxious people whinge and whine and carry on over nothing and can't be reassured. It is easier to hand them to the psychologists who, many years ago, made a grab for anxiety because they thought they had a theory (behaviorism) that explained it. They never had, of course, but they more or less deserve each other. Finally, of course, biological psychiatry demands that each disorder be seen as primary, an entity in its own right. Because depression is such a common condition, it would shatter the biological project in psychiatry if it were found to be secondary. Patients like this, of course; far better to tell your family "The doctor says I've got a chemical imbalance of the brain" than to admit "I'm a moral failure".

We could almost say there is a conspiracy between psychiatrists and their patients to pretend that anxiety doesn't exist. That's a tragedy, because it condemns a lot of people to lives of despair.

12 | A Case of Somatization

12.1: Introduction

Sally Jones, a 28-y/o mother, was initially referred for a second opinion only. She was being treated by another psychiatrist but her mother was concerned she wasn't getting any better. Sally lived in an isolated fishing village about 70 km from Darwin while her mother lived on a small farm some 20 km closer to town. The road to Sally's home was little more than a track in places and was regularly washed out during the monsoon season. Whenever there was a cyclone warning, she packed her five children into an ancient four wheel drive wagon (SUV) and drove to her mother's home to shelter until the storms had passed (her parents had survived Cyclone Tracy, which wiped Darwin out in 1974). Her partner, the father of her five children, had a fishing license which meant that, during the season, he was away for a week at a time. Outside the fishing season, he found work in the area as fencing contractor so he often stayed away overnight rather than drive the long distances home. Even when he was home, he worked long hours on their own property, repairing their home, building sheds and fences or checking the water supply and the small power generator.

Sally's mother had been a patient of mine some years ago, after she was assaulted at work. She made a reasonable recovery and went back to a different job but several times had mentioned that she was concerned about her daughter. She felt Sally had always been a nervous girl but she seemed to be getting worse. Every week or two, she would get a call from her eldest grandson saying his mother was having a turn and had to go to hospital. Sometimes, Greg, her partner, would take her but if he was busy or had been drinking, he refused and it would fall to the grandmother to drive along the rutted road in the inky night to collect her, drive back to town, take her to hospital and wait the five or six hours until she was seen. If Greg wasn't home, all the children had to be bundled into the car with their bedding and left with the grandfather.

When my former patient, the grandmother, rang to ask whether it would be possible for me to see her daughter, I asked what the trouble could be that would cause so much inconvenience. "It's terrible," the weeping lady said, "she's got this awful mental disease but there's no treatment for it. We have to rush her into the hospital but they can't do anything for her. They just settle her down and we take her home but I'm scared what will happen. And they said it's genetic, something to do with the chemicals of the brain. I'm terrified for those children."

"That's no good," I agreed, "but I wouldn't have thought you'd have a genetic disease in your family. I'd be interested to see her. Has anybody given you a diagnosis?"

"It's called Somatization," she replied.

Sally arrived on a pleasant, sunny morning about two weeks later. Her mother had brought her because her own vehicle had broken down again. Grandmother and children drove away to the shops for the morning, so Sally had some peace and quiet. "This is lovely," she said brightly, looking around the office. "I haven't been by myself for years. I always have children or my parents or Greg's family. They'll come and stay for a week or two; our place is always a madhouse."

She was then aged twenty-eight but would have passed for sixteen. She was thin and slightly built, a little below average height, with long blond hair, tight teenage clothes (embroidered denim shorts, a flowery singlet, and chunky sandals) and a lot of Indian tribal silver jewelry. She had a couple of small professional tattoos on her bare shoulders and was carrying a large shoulder bag stuffed full of baby things. With her cheery and effervescent manner and her almost flat chest, she looked like a skinny teenager on an outing to the beach. Two days before, she had spent the night in the hospital. High on her thin left upper arm, next to the tattooed bluebirds, were two small round fading bruises, like finger marks.

Within a few minutes, it was clear that, despite her bubbly exterior, Sally was well-practiced in the dark art of appearing to cooperate with an interview but revealing nothing.

12.2: The History: I'm Fine, Can I Go Now?

"I don't really think I need to be here," she said with a disarming smile, "it's just for my mother, you know how nervous she gets. The hospital is looking after me, I'm sure everything will be fine." At present, she said, she is feeling "fine." She sleeps as well as can be expected, their home consists of three transportable units arranged in a U-shape with an awning over the center. Each unit is nine meters by three, the middle one has the kitchen and laundry, and each of their other two units has two bedrooms on either side of a bathroom, so they have plenty of room, she certainly isn't complaining, their neighbors about 400 m away have only one unit and their children sleep under canvas in the dry season. Her partner got their units from the old Andromeda mine when it closed, they had an amazing time transporting them down their wiggly old road from the mine but everybody helped and it was wonderful how the children did their bit; one of the boys found a python in the laundry and he's looked after it ever since, it wanders around the place and...

What time do you go to bed?

Me? Oh, I just go to bed when the children have gone down, you know; we don't worry too much about time out there. I get plenty of sleep; I'm not complaining.

So what happens when you spend the night in the hospital? Do you get enough sleep then?

Oh, that's not so much as everybody makes out; they're all fussing over nothing. I'm fine, really, they're so lovely to me at the hospital; I've got my favorite nurses in the Emergency Department and the girls at the desk all know me; we have such a fun time; I really don't think anybody needs to worry... So what time do we finish; should I ring mum to come back and pick me up now? The baby, she frets if I'm not around, you...

What time do you get up?

Oh, the children get me up; you know what they're like. They have to catch the school bus at the corner, that's about two miles away. I drive them in the wet but this time of year, they ride their bikes and leave them at the bus stop. Gosh, that's an interesting picture on your wall; I just love dolphins; did you take that yourself?

No. So when you wake up, how do you feel?

Oh, I feel great. I've got heaps of energy; nobody believes it when they look at me; they think a strong wind would blow me away, but I eat. We grow our own veggies and we've got chickens; they sleep in the trees but the pythons still get a few; and we've always got a couple of pigs wandering around the place; gosh but they...

The interview progressed like this. It seemed they lived a feral existence on about five hectares (12.5 ac) of land on the edge of a beach. They had their own power supply and their water came from a bore well. Their block was littered with old vehicles, boats her partner was working on, tractors and other discarded farming equipment he collected on his jobs, and piles of second-hand steel and timber that he used to build the various sheds and shelters he needed. In addition to the money he earned, she received social security benefits for the children of about $300 a week, and they also received money from a number of federal aboriginal development agencies, such as the Education Trust, the Homelands Development Agency (which had paid all the costs for their home including the power and the water supply) and a number of others she couldn't remember. "And don't write this down," she giggled, "but we hardly pay any tax, so it's better than it looks."

A quick calculation indicated they were getting through the better part of $50,000 a year. "Oh," she laughed brightly, "it's heaps more than that. But you wouldn't guess it, looking at us. I mean, I get my clothes from those lovely ladies at the Salvation Army. They just give them to me; I think they feel sorry for us. But it's a wonderful life for the children; they've got the bush and the beach. They can swim 'cause the water's clear and we can see the crocodiles if they come too close. But we know all the crocs there; they're like friends."

She said her appetite was good and she ate regularly. She had never weighed much, and her weight was steady. She was always on the move, never sat around moping or worrying; there was always something to do and if she got bored, she would just take the children to the beach and play with them. She had plenty of interest in things, too much interest, and was always keen to get things done. Her problem was not enough hours in the day. Socially, she got on fabulously well with everybody; it was her nature, and she had no sexual interest at all.

She said her memory and concentration were both "fine". She had no trouble making decisions although Greg made all the big decisions but she looked after the children and that was fine. She could think clearly except when she was having one of her turns and her thoughts were mostly on what was happening at the time or what she had to do for the children and the house.

So no particular worries that keep coming back?

Oh, no, I don't have any worries.

There were no disturbances of perception.

She described her mood as "fine, no worries", and said she never got to feeling down in the dumps or miserable.

Have you ever felt low and miserable in your life, depressed for any length of time?

[long pause as she twists her mouth in thought] No, I'd say no, never been depressed. I'm just not that sort of person. That's why it was so hard for me to understand what was happening to mum; she just slipped down into...

Do you ever feel the opposite of depressed; you feel fantastic, full of energy, and on top of the world for no good reason?

I always feel good; I mean, I've got a great life. I've got enough energy but I wouldn't say it's too much; I sleep if I'm tired; when the older ones are at school, I try to lie down with the baby after lunch and get a kip, you know how...

Do people ever comment on how much energy you've got?

Everybody loves my energy; they all say they wish they had it too; they're always saying they don't know how I do it but I tell them...

Further detailed questioning did not reveal any suggestion that her buoyant mood was anything but normal for her.

Do you ever feel tense and jittery, as though you're starting to lose control?

Oh no, never. I've never lost control in my life.

Do you ever have a sense that you're in danger; you feel frightened for no good reason?

No, never. I'm not in danger. I mean, we've got snakes living under our dongas (units) but I know where they are and I don't worry about them.

So going to the hospital in the middle of the night doesn't worry you?

Nope. I'm fine; I'm used to it. I know that road like the back of my hand.

I see. So why do you go to the hospital?

I'm having one of my attacks. I'm not worried about it anymore, I used to be but I know what it is now. If Greg's not there, I call the children and we all jump in the car. But now we've got the satellite phone; I just call mum and she drives out. It's only twenty minutes; I can wait.

So what condition are you in when you call her?

She was fine, she insisted, after they called her mother, she lay on her bed and talked to the children and played games with them, so they wouldn't be worried. At the hospital, the nurses just put her on the ECG and gave her oxygen and made her move her arms and legs every fifteen minutes until the doctor arrived.

I see. So what does an attack consist of?

Oh, it's a somatization attack; you'd know more about that than I do. I've seen everybody in the hospital, Dr K (cardiologist), Dr L (neurologist), Dr M (gastroenterologist), Dr N (gynecologist) and Dr O, the rheumatologist, everybody. I've had heaps of tests and X-rays, CAT scans , MRI scans, nuclear medicine; you name it, I've had it. And then...

Just go back to how you are when you decide you need to go to hospital. What are you actually experiencing?

Well, I was just getting to that. And then after I'd been going there for years, they finally decided they had to ask a psychiatrist to see me. It wasn't that they didn't believe me; it was just that I had them stumped. It was that Dr P, actually, she's Professor P now; they promoted her. She'd be younger than you, wouldn't she? She's absolutely brilliant but it even took her a while; then she worked out what it was. Somatization. It was amazing; my mum looked it up on the internet and I've got every one of the symptoms. And do you know, one day, they put me up in front of the medical students as a difficult case. It was in that new lecture theater near the Red Cross; the nurses took me down; they were wonderful; they said not to worry; it wouldn't...

Just a minute. Before you went inside that lecture theater, how were you? What sort of condition were you in?

Well, it's funny you should ask that because, believe it or not, I had one of my attacks. A real somatization attack, just in time for those lovely students to see it. They would never have seen anything like that in another hospital, they were all amazed. So I was really pleased I could help them; I'm like that; my mum says I'd help the devil if his tail got stuck in the lift to hell. Not that I'm going to hell of course.

OK, now what did the medical students see?

See? What do you mean?

You said the medical students saw a genuine somatization attack. What did they write in their notes that they were seeing?

Oh, I don't know; you'd have to ask them.

But you were there, what condition were you in?

I was in my usual condition. I don't know what they saw; I was having an attack.

Did they video the lecture?

Yes, they did actually; funny you should ask that. They said...

Right, now what did the video show you were doing?

I don't know. I never saw it.

What was the difference between the way you were then and the way you are now?

I don't know; like I said, I never...

Well, were you on a couch or on a chair?

They had me on one of those trolley things with wheels.

Were you lying there calmly, watching the students or looking away?

Sort of lying there. Like in an attack.

Were your eyes open?

Sort of open. They roll back.

I see. And what were your hands doing?

Well, isn't that amazing you should ask that. They go all funny.

Like this? [demonstrate carpopedal spasm]

How did you know that? That's amazing; you've got it exactly.

And what do you breathe like?

I'm breathing. Yeah, I breathe but they give me oxygen.

Well, do you breathe normally like you're breathing now? Or do you struggle to get your breath?

Yes, that's it; it's a struggle.

Do you have to force your breath in and out?

Gosh, you're even better at this than Prof. P. It took her ages to work this out but you've seen it in ten minutes.

So do you have to force your breath in and out or does it go easily like now?

Yes.

Yes what?

I don't know. What was the question?

Do you have to force your breath in and out or does it go easily like now?

Um, I'm not... Force it, I'd say. A bit.

Now what about your heart?

My heart? Oh, they have me on the ECG monitor.

Yes, but what's it doing?

I don't know; I can't see the ECG and even if I could, I wouldn't...

You can tell what your heart is doing. Does it seem to be beating faster, like racing, or beating very forcefully, up in your throat?

[laughs] That's amazing. It seems to be right up in my throat, pounding, thump thump... My eldest boy, he looks after me in my attacks; he sits there and counts my heart, he says...

Right. And what rate does it go?

I don't know; he counts it, not me.

But what does he count up to?

In a minute?

In a minute.

A hundred and fifty, sometimes more. We laugh about it now that I know what it is; it doesn't worry me.

Right. So your heart's beating very fast, you're short of breath, your hands and feet go into spasm and your eyes roll back. So what is your stomach doing in all of this?

[Her phone rings and she jumps and answers it loudly and cheerfully, clearly talking to one of the children, then hangs up] Look, doctor, I'm really sorry but I'm going to have to go. That was the children; I told them to ring me if they were worried. I'm terribly sorry but they're not having a good time; mum's not handling them; she's going to bring them back.

What? Can you get your mother on the phone now?

I don't think so; they're heading for the car now.

Well, ring her.

I don't think it's necessary. She knows how to handle them; they're her grandchildren after all; she had five of her own and we've all got big families; it's like a family tradition; my nana did...

Can you just ring your mother or I will. I've got her number out there.

I'm sure it won't be necessary. The children will be fine; they just want to make sure... well, if you insist but I really don't see why... Mum? It's the doctor; he just wants to talk to you. No, I'm fine, it's just that... You come on over now, I'll be waiting outside.

Just sit there until I talk to your mother. Yes, Mrs. A? Dr. McLaren here; I'm fine. What's happening? Why do you want to come back now?

[Mother] I don't but the children do. They're very upset.

Why?

Well, it's not clear; they're all shouting and crying.

Yes, but why are they shouting and crying?

[Sally] Oh my god, are my children shouting and crying? Give me the phone, quickly; I've got to talk to her...

Sit down there. Mrs. A, why are the children upset?

[Mother] I can't... Jimmy, stop that and tell me why you're upset.... He says they have to see their mother and take her home.

Why?

Jimmy, stop that. Why do you want to see her?... He says they have to take her home.

I heard you but why did he say that?

[Sally] Doctor, I'm going to go now; just tell my mum I'll be waiting outside. I don't want anybody to be upset.

Mrs. A, this is ridiculous. Find out from the boy what he's talking about.

[Mother] Jimmy, what's the problem?... He says you're going to lock her up.

What? Who set this up?

[Sally] Doctor, I'll be going now; thank you so much, it's been so helpful...

Sit down in that chair now. Mrs. A, tell the children to stay there; she will be there in exactly 40 minutes. She is not going to be locked up; whoever told them that is lying.

[Mother] I'm sorry, doctor, but she told them that herself.

I know she told them that herself; and I know why she told them. Sally, sit in that chair now and don't leave this office.

[trembling and panting, she sits in the chair as though it may be electrified and begins to weep] My children, I've got to... they need me...

They don't need you at all. You scared them. Your mother can look after them [phone rings]. If that's the children, you tell them you're fine and you'll see them in half an hour.

[weeping] Hullo darling? Yes, mummy's fine. You stay with nana, I'll see you in half an hour. No, I'm fine... No, no....

Is he asking whether you'll be locked up?

Umm, I don't, like I...

Gimme the phone. Yeah, g'day boy, how's it goin? No, she's fine; that doesn't happen anymore. We don't have a lock-up here; you can have a look when you pick her up. Half an hour, no, make it 45, we've wasted a lot of time on phone calls. You go to MacDonald's; she'll meet you there in 45 or an hour. Bye. There's your phone, Ms Jones, turn it off. Put it on the desk where I can see it and no more texts to your children telling them you're going to be locked up.

[She takes the phone and slowly switches it off] I didn't... I mean, it's not necessary... Professor P looks after me, the hospital [people] are wonderful...

Yeah, well, we'll see. So... Where are we? So what does your stomach do when you're having an attack? What's your stomach doing right now?

It's... I mean, it's full of butterflies.

Could you eat like this?

No way, I'd vomit.

And your heart? Give me your wrist. Wow, that's easy 170. Stand up.

I can't. I'll faint. I'm all weak.

Hold your hand out in front, like this [she does so and her hand is trembling violently]. And your palms? Are they sweaty? Yerk, have a tissue and wipe your hands. Now... Just sit up straight. You're not in any danger. You're not going to the hospital. This is a typical panic attack; I wouldn't waste their time. I'm going to give you a plastic bag to breathe into; breathe in and out until you feel better. We've got a diagnosis. And a cause.

[starts up fearfully] What do you mean?

Don't worry; we'll get to that shortly.

The process of sorting out the triggers to her very obvious panic attacks was a little easier as she was unable to discern the direction of the questions, so she seemed to be answering them honestly (see Chaps 8 and 9 for the list of questions). While this was going on, she stopped crying and went back to her bright self. She was not afraid of the natural world. Even moving her son's pet python from the kitchen chairs to serve breakfast did not worry her. However, the human world terrified her. She could not go near a crowd alone or stand in a queue without her family around her. She feared appointments and interviews, tests and exams of any sort, threats, criticism and arguments, or disputes with anybody. She was very frightened of loneliness, humiliation, and disapproval, and especially of letting people down, causing trouble, or giving offence. She feared making mistakes or failing at anything, to the extent that she would not try but would move the task to somebody else. She feared illness, death, and mental illness, and was morbidly fearful of being sent to the psychiatry ward or locked up. She feared all aggressive people and voiced a powerful need to keep them happy at all times; otherwise she felt their temper outbursts were her fault.

When she was out, she had the strong feeling that people were looking at her and talking behind her back, judging her, and making unpleasant comparisons. She did not feel in physical danger from people, only their disapproval. She often felt she was under surveillance and sometimes had the idea that their new phone was bugged. She did not describe a sense of conspiracy.

She was a fastidiously fussy person, constantly preoccupied with cleanliness, tidiness, order, and punctuality with many cleaning rituals but these didn't bother her, and her family thought they were simply amusing. There were no true obsessive-compulsive features.

Recent History

At first, she said her symptoms had begun a year or two before; then she admitted she had been a nervous child: "All my life, I suppose. My brothers used to frighten me with snakes but I got over it." Over the past couple of years, she had begun having her "attacks" and had to go to hospital. The first one, she said, caused great concern among the hospital staff who thought she had had a stroke as she was lying rigid on the bed and could not move her limbs. She had a number of blood tests and scans which showed nothing. Gradually, as she attended more frequently, the hospital began to take her appearances less seriously. From being given priority in the Emergency Center, she was left more and more to the nurses so that, by the time she was seen by a medical officer, hours later, she had largely settled and was ready to go home.

Personal Background

Now, tell me about your personal background. Where were you born and raised?

Oh, you already know all of that; there's nothing much there. [in fact, there was a great deal there but it was important to see how she viewed it]

No, I see so many patients... [true, but has nothing to do with the fact that her family history was known in some detail] So how old is your father now?

Ah, he's coming up to 56 yrs.

And what sort of work does he do?

He's a farmer and he also drives trucks.

What's he like as a person?

Oh, he's fine. We get on so well, I'm his pet, really [bright laugh]. Daddy's girl, you know how it is.

So you get on well? How old's your mother?

She's two years younger; 54 now.

And she still works, I see. What's she like as a person?

She's great. She's the greatest mum in the world; we get along just so well, you wouldn't believe.

She had a number of brothers and sisters but their story is not relevant. She attended the local state schools to the age of fifteen, passing only Year 8 with poor marks. She got on "really well" with the teachers and "fine" with the other children and still has friends from her schooldays. She was not shy, nervous, or aggressive at school, or "maybe just a teensy bit shy at times, nobody ever hurt me, I was fine." She didn't play much sport as they lived too far out of town but she had "heaps" of interests and activities, especially horses. She had her own pony throughout most of her schooling and there are still horses on her parents' property where she takes her children because they want to learn to ride, too. Unfortunately, there are no horses at their home as her partner is away a lot and she couldn't look after horses as well as everything else. She also liked fishing and other outdoor activities as well as cooking, and her home life was "wonderful". On leaving school, she worked in a local store and service station until she became pregnant at the age of seventeen to her first boyfriend. After the baby was born, they lived with her parents until they were given their own property through the Aboriginal lands trust. They were not married but she used his name as it was easier. She said she rarely drank alcohol, used no illegal drugs, did not gamble ("Where would I gamble out there?"), and had no police record. Her general health had always been good until she developed "her" somatization disorder.

Self-Assessment

Asked to describe herself, she hesitated, then smiled brightly: "I try to be a good person. I'm helpful and friendly; I always try to keep the peace." She said she does not see herself as a nervous person but has always been bothered by guilt, shame, and self-consciousness. She is unassertive, over-trusting of people and enjoys company. She is not jealous, does not hold grudges, and gets on well with authority. She is fairly tidy and organized and follows rules. She sees her temper as "yep, no," by which she meant "not really, no, never." Her intellect is "not real flash" and her self-esteem is... [no answer].

And your self-esteem? How would you rate your self-esteem?

Umm, sort of... Like, it could be... I dunno.

But you must have some idea. Give yourself a score, low, average, high, superman. What is it?

Well, maybe... you know, like... No. None. Bugger all.

Mental State Examination

Her appearance and behavior have been described above. Initially, her general behavior was bright and cheery with no evidence of anxiety, depression, hostility, or suspicion. However, this changed abruptly and she became intensely agitated and weepy, although she forced this down in short time. There were no signs of a psychotic disorder and nothing to indicate an organic impairment of brain function. She was of average intellectual ability.

Management

She was told that the somatization problem was actually due to a hidden anxiety state and it would continue to cause her problems until she was given the precise treatment she needed. This could be done as an out-patient if she wished; she did not need to be admitted to hospital and she could not be detained in any event so she did not have to worry about it. She was free to go to join her mother and children at the shops but if she wanted to talk the matter over further, she would have to make another appointment.

Oh, so you're not going to give me tablets?

No, you came here for an opinion and that's what you've got. You need specific treatment or this problem will slowly get worse.

So is it a chemical imbalance of the brain, like they said?

There's no evidence for that. You're an anxious person. Something upsets you; you get into a panic and you get over it; like you did this morning. Think about it, talk it over at home, and come back if you like. See you later.

Several weeks later, after a couple more midnight trips to the hospital, she came back. Her mother was keen on her trying treatment if it meant they didn't need to go to hospital so much as it was exhausting her. She was given specific treatment for an anxiety state and showed a rapid improvement. Over the next few months, she stopped going to hospital and became more revealing of her home life. Her relationship with the partner was poor. He had a large family who were always arguing and she could never keep up with who was on their side or the other. She was frightened of his sister who had been in prison several times for assault. Her partner was a very difficult man. He worked non-stop but had periodic bouts when he became bitterly angry at everybody and suspicious and wouldn't talk to anybody. During these times, he became "insanely" jealous of her and demanded to know who she had been calling on the phone or where she had been when she was ten minutes late coming home from the store (a 30 km drive). One week, he would be friends with their neighbors, then the next he would stamp around the place, saying he ought to blow the man away. He had over twenty firearms, and she knew he had others hidden around the place or stored with his friends.

His moods could change from moment to moment, from laughing to blind, screaming fury. He drank heavily and smoked marihuana constantly. She brewed their beer but if it wasn't to his liking, he would hurl the bottle at the wall over her head. She lived in fear of him but, more particularly, for her children. She knew his father had argued with his children one by one and forced them out of the house on to the streets where they had all met one grief or another. She did not want this to happen to hers. However, she did not want to leave her partner, partly because she knew he would not survive without her, partly because she felt she owed him for all his hard work, and partly because she was terrified of his temper. He knew the country back to front and she would never be able to hide from him.

In fact, none of this was new to her. Her own father was an equally difficult man, who had worked hard during his younger years and had the same bouts of hostile suspicion. Over the years, he had become more and more withdrawn, with longer periods in which he refused to leave the property and wouldn't talk to anybody who visited. He had argued violently with both her brothers, one of whom lived alone in a hut at the back of her parents' property and was steadily drinking himself to death. The other had been in and out of prison and used amphetamines constantly. Her father and her partner hated each other and she struggled to keep them apart. At the same time, she wanted her children to have good relationships with all their relatives, even though the relatives could not be on the same property together. Often, her father would order her off his property and not speak to her for months, which caused her enormous distress but she could not tell her partner because he would either laugh or threaten to go down and blow her father away. She never took this as a figure of speech.

After about two tortuous years, her position is improving. Eighteen months after her first interview, she described the problems at home: "He's constantly at me; he drills me; he wants to know everything I do or everybody I ever talk to, so I don't talk to anyone. I would never talk to a man, not his relatives, not anyone. Especially not his relatives. He believes all his family have sex together and he thinks I would, too. He's so jealous; he's completely nuts over it. He's threatened me with knives and guns. Once he pointed a loaded rifle where the children were sleeping to try to make me admit I'd been sleeping with his brother. As soon as he starts freaking out about something, I panic and I have to get away. He's schizo and bipolar, I know it, but if I leave, he'll go completely mad and he'll come after me. The police would never stop him. Do you remember that case where the policeman was shot? He knew all about it; he knew that man and he said they'd never get him like that; he'd take out the whole police force before they found him."

12.3: How to Look and Not See

In classic Freudian theory, the subject cannot become conscious of repressed material just because it is kept at bay by powerful psychic defenses which are themselves unconscious. The patient or, because it is a general theory, the ordinary person, cannot analyze himself nor can he become aware of his hidden impulses except by accident. Freud used the example of a person with torticollis (wry neck) who cannot see something next to him because his head is forcefully turned away by matters which are outside his power to control. However, one of Freud's earliest collaborators, Wilhelm Stekel, disagreed and took sides with the apostate Alfred Adler, whom Freudians loathed passionately. Stekel's view was that it is not the case that people cannot know; rather, they choose not to know because full acknowledgement of their problems would overwhelm them. Therefore, they choose to live in a restricted little fantasy world rather than face the horror which waits just outside the circle of light. Instead of the Freudian notion of a torticollis, he used the concept of a scotoma, or blind spot. People look at something but don't see it because they choose not to; they blot it out and go on with their lives as though it didn't exist. But inside, somewhere, somehow, they know. In 1940, at the age of 72, Stekel committed suicide in Britain. Had he survived the war, he would certainly have been interested in the huge numbers of his countrymen who "looked but did not see" what was happening in their country during World War II.

In the case of Sally Jones, there is not the slightest doubt that she knew all along exactly what the problem was, but she could not bring herself to admit it, even to herself. Acknowledging that the father of her children was seriously disturbed and dangerous would have forced her to do something about it, but she couldn't. Whatever plan she thought of, there was a block. Behind it all was her intense reluctance to admit what her father had always said, that Greg Jones was a total loser, so she should get his brat out of her and keep the hell away from him. As his behavior became more and more bizarre and threatening, her anxiety rose until she was unable to control it. The panic bouts were a warning that she was attempting to live in intolerable circumstances and she should do something about it. She did. She went to hospital. This got her out of the firing line, got the children off the property, and took her to a place where she felt safe and valued. After a few hours calming down in hospital, her guilt got the better of her, and she rushed home again. All fairly normal and explicable in a dumb, human sort of way, but what was the hospital's part in maintaining her sick role?

Normally, it would be about ninety minutes from the time she left home to the time she was wheeled through the hospital doors. From there, she would either be seen by nurses who were convinced she was in some sort of life-threatening crisis and treated her as dangerously ill, or she was put in a quiet corner until people had time to see her. Either way, she felt reassured that she was having a nasty physical turn and the nice hospital staff would put it right. By the time she was seen by one of the busy emergency medical officers, it might be six or eight hours since the explosion with her partner. She would be feeling more like normal and the guilt would be starting to bite. They would satisfy themselves that she wasn't in danger and let her go. However, she kept coming back, so they referred her elsewhere. Elsewhere didn't find anything so, after a long time, somebody wondered if there might be psychological factors affecting her presentations and referred her for a psychiatric assessment.

The psychiatric assessments were, as the records showed, superficial. She was seen by a nurse who gave her several questionnaires to complete. She was then seen by a trainee psychiatrist who couldn't work out what was happening, mainly because trainees are nice young people who aren't yet acquainted with the wiles of Homo sapiens. The diagnosis of Somatization Disorder appears to have crept in somewhere between her seeing the nurses and the psychiatrist, i.e. nobody was responsible for it. It just appeared one day and stuck. Psychiatric labels are very sticky. Essentially, the psychiatrist had been told beforehand it was probably a case of Somatization Disorder, and stamped his approval. At no stage did anyone take a history of her social circumstances although, to be fair, nobody at the hospital would have pushed her hard enough to get through her wall of denial. Their interest lay in the surface manifestations of her behavior, not the underlying causes. This is because modern psychiatry does not recognize underlying causes. It doesn't recognize underlying causes, so it doesn't look for them. When it does see them, it has no means of incorporating the information into its theory: where does "mad husband" fit with "chemical imbalance of the brain"? As Thomas Kuhn noted many times, observations which don't fit with the theory are discarded. Sally Jones, it must not be forgotten, was a "lovely girl", an ideal patient—cheerful, grateful, and uncomplaining. Only a curmudgeon would think she was a liar.

A diagnosis of anxiety is a positive diagnosis; it is not the diagnosis left in the box when everything else has been excluded. I am forever saying to the real doctors: "You should have asked for a psychiatric opinion at the beginning of your investigations, not at the end. An opinion costs less than an MRI scan. Why don't you use it as part of your diagnostic work-up?" One day, I'll get an answer.

In about 1930, Wilhelm Stekel said: "After thirty years experience of analysis, I no longer believe in the overwhelming significance of the unconscious." Psychoanalysis, he said, required "the skill of a physician, a detective, and a diplomat rolled into one." The clue in this case was that, over the years, she had made perhaps a hundred nocturnal dashes to the hospital. Her children were well and truly used to them. They had stayed with their grandmother dozens of times while their mother was in hospital. Yet the one day she went to see a psychiatrist away from the hospital, they panicked and demanded she leave and go home with them. It was a set-up, the detective in me said, and it was. In her charming, friendly way, she had warned the children that she was only going to the appointment to keep their nana happy, that she didn't need to see another psychiatrist as she had a real professor to look after her at the hospital, and psychiatrists were nasty people who locked patients up so she would only be a few minutes and then they could all go home.

Just in case the little dears had missed the point (and I have never known children to miss a point they want to see), she had asked their father to give them his opinion on the value of psychiatrists. That was all the children needed to be terrified. She needed them to be terrified as it was the only way she could decently get out of the appointment. She needed to get out of the appointment as she didn't dare tell the truth. She couldn't have one of her usual turns in the office because there would be a doctor on the spot, so she arranged for the children to have a turn instead. It's clever. It's also very common. People get away with it because the institution of modern psychiatry is so dumb. It has been 'dumbed down' by the DSM committees who seem to think that psychiatry is so easy that it can be farmed out. Sure, bad psychiatry is dead easy.

The good news is that Sally has at last accepted there is a problem and that it can only be managed one way. Things are now better although there is a long way to go. I will admit that knowing her family background before she arrived was very helpful; it allowed me to see immediately that she was lying. Also, I knew Greg's family and they are every bit as bad as she says. He is a tortured man himself. It comes from his father. I haven't seen Greg yet, but I expect to, one day. I hope it's before he commits suicide and before the Jones family madness gets handed on to his children.

Having said that, I wonder how people practice psychiatry in big cities? It wouldn't be anywhere near as interesting as having "local knowledge". Now that's an interesting point. I wonder if the DSM Committee opted for a 'dumbed down' psychiatry just because they have no experience of a psychiatry with local knowledge, and they couldn't make theirs work.

A last point: it has been brought to my attention that it is not currently fashionable for psychiatrists to speak about patients 'lying'. These psychiatrists are in denial. Sadly, fashion is not my strong suit. Even though 'denial' sounds so cute, so yummy, it cannot be defined without incorporating the central elements of the definition of 'lying'. I think it is the psychiatrists who are in denial.

13

A Case of Personality Disorder or Mental Illness?

13.1: Introduction

The Procrustean tendencies of modern psychiatric are nowhere more powerful than in the personality disorders. In Humanizing Madness, I argued that the system of classification of these difficult conditions is based upon several major misunderstandings. The first one is the question of whether categories of personality actually exist, or should we be looking at personality as a dimensional construct. The debate roars on and DSM-V is likely to move in this direction, but only because nobody can actually make the categorical system work. My prediction is that DSM-V will not make any real progress. Just as trouble in the remote American subprime housing market eventually triggered the global financial collapse, so the collapse of the whole DSM project could well start in the personality disorders, the one field that nobody in psychiatry sees as important.

The second problem with personality disorders arises because of a misuse of the principles of cluster analysis. When we group a population into clumps or clusters, we try to make the clusters internally uniform. We do this by writing a list of criteria that each member of the cluster must meet in order to be included in that category. We can call these the inclusion criteria. DSM-IV has done this, and a quick look at the section on personality disorders shows how each category of disorder has its different criteria. However, that's not enough. We also need to make the clusters externally distinct, and the way this is done is to use exclusion criteria. That is, we need to specify criteria which would disqualify each member of the population from all clusters except the one he should be in. The whole purpose is to distance each cluster from its neighbors, to minimize overlap. Of course, if the clusters were genuine categories, there would be no overlap but we will overlook the overlap because everybody else does.

Unfortunately, DSM-IV couldn't do that, just because there are no categories of personality disorder. All personality traits are distributed throughout the entire population. It doesn't matter what personality factor is chosen, we all show it to some extent or another. So if you believe there are just three personality traits (such as Eysenck's Introversion-Extraversion, Neuroticism, and Psychoticism), then you can neatly classify everybody on a three-dimensional array. If you believe there are five (usually named Openness, Conscientiousness, Extraversion, Agreeableness, Neuroticism, or OCEAN), then people will distribute in a five-dimensional matrix, but the important point is that everybody will get a score on every factor. It is impossible not to score because they are measures of what people do while running their lives.

A fairly obvious trait such as Agreeableness measures your tendency to deal with people in a pleasant, cooperative and compassionate manner rather than in a suspicious, antagonistic, and unforgiving way. Your score may be zero, it may be one hundred, but that just is your score on that factor. So for this reason, DSM-IV didn't have exclusion criteria. It couldn't say that, for example, the paranoid personality will show high paranoid thinking and all the other disorders must show none because all humans show paranoid thinking. Instead, the committee rewrote all the inclusion criteria in such a way that they read as totally different. They seem to be describing categories of personality which are completely removed from each other, whereas they are not. All too often, the inclusion criteria for one disorder are just rehashes of the criteria for another. I have shown this in more detail in Chapter 7 of Humanizing Madness. Thus, personality diagnosis using DSM-IV becomes little more than an exercise in assigning people according to one's prejudices:

Because there are no exclusion criteria in personality diagnosis, people can be categorized by whatever strikes the interviewer as most obvious. Anxious psychiatrists may well over-rate aggression, particularly in big men who don't speak much English; conspiratorially-minded interviewers will not condemn someone who sees a plot at every turn, while grandiose psychiatrists are hardly likely to damn their adoring clientele as "dependent". There is nothing to stop this happening. The lack of exclusion criteria affords too much potential for the circumstances of the patient's presentation and the interviewer's bias to prejudice the diagnostic process.

The third problem to mention is the inability of the DSM process to "look beneath the surface" of the clinical presentation to find out what is generating the overt behavior. To a biological psychiatrist, this is just dumb: peering beneath the surface means looking at an fMRI or PET scan, or going straight to the genome, because that is where "overt behavior" is generated. For them, the idea of peering beneath the surface in the hope of finding causative psychological factors is irrational, on a par with peeking under the bark of a tree to find its tree sprite. The failure of conventional psychiatry to inquire after the psychological causes of overtly disordered behavior is the primary cause of the failure of modern psychiatry to engage with the hugely important field of personality disorder.

There was a line in the 1965 film Cat Ballou when the heroine comes across her drunken gunslinger, Kid Shelleen (really). "Your eyes look terrible," she snapped. He stared up at her mournfully: "Lady," he slurred, "you should see them from my side." Psychiatrists just don't get personality disorder, and it's not just because they don't have a model of personality; it's because they don't look. They don't know where to look. In order to understand personality disorder, you have to see the world through the subject's eyes. Very often, it isn't pretty, as this case shows.

13.2. The History: How to Make a Psychopath

Kevin Johnson was 34 yrs old when he was referred for urgent assessment by his general practitioner. He was due in court the following day and had already been seen by the forensic service that diagnosed an aggressive psychopathic personality. He had not been offered treatment. He saw his GP because he felt he was likely to kill himself or somebody else before he got to court. Two months previously, he had separated from his girlfriend after she found a policeman as a boyfriend. Kevin had been outraged by this and threw some of her belongings into a storm drain. She obtained a domestic violence order against him but he was due in court for breaching this order several times by threatening her over the phone. He expected to be sent to prison. At the time, he was living in a room in a house owned by an alcoholic friend. There were four men there, all of whom drank heavily. He had been working as a driver for about six months but had just lost his job due to arguing with other drivers. He was taking no medication.

Presenting Complaints

He said: "I'm a mess. I'm angry and violent and unhappy." He was barely able to sleep unless he was very drunk. He had no appetite at all and was drinking but not eating. He had lost a few kilos in the preceding two months. He had no energy at all and his only activity was walking to the liquor store to buy alcohol. He had no interest and no motivation to do anything except when he was enraged and wanted to strangle someone. Socially, he actively avoided people except for the other men in his house when they were all drinking. If he was sober, he had to stay in his room. He had no sexual interest at all.

He said his memory was patchy, which had been causing problems at work as he was forgetting deliveries. His concentration wasn't good and his mind tended to wander unless he had set jobs to do. He was having trouble thinking clearly as his mind was "scrambled" whenever he became angry, which was most of the time. He was not able to make decisions, or he made wild, impulsive decisions which usually got him into more difficulties. The thought content was dominated by thoughts of gaining revenge on the ex-girlfriend and her new boyfriend who, he said, were constantly taunting him in one way or another. There were no disturbances of perception.

He described his mood as "terrible", by which he meant he was feeling low and miserable all the time. He said this was "real bad, I want to die." This time, it was due to the separation but he had felt suicidal on and off for most of his life. In addition to the court appearance, he was about

$50,000 in debt, a large part of which was expenses run up by the former girlfriend. His car had been seized and he had lost practically all of his possessions. Since he had lost his job, he had been drinking on the last of his credit card but he knew he could not pay it back. He had never felt good in his life except for when he was using drugs, and that was never for long.

He described bouts of intense agitation during which he was unable to settle. By this point of the interview (barely ten minutes), he was becoming increasingly agitated. He was shaking and sweating and was close to tears so the interview was stopped for a few minutes to give him diazepam 5 mg, and let him outside for a cigarette (I cannot remember the last time I stopped an interview to tranquillize a patient). When he came back, he said the bouts of agitation caused intense shaking which he could only control by lashing out at somebody. During these bouts, he was sweaty, his heart raced, his stomach churned to the point that he could not eat and he was short of breath. He had a dry mouth, was tight in his throat, and stumbled over his speech. He felt light-headed and unsteady on his feet unless he got into a fight, when he would feel crystal clear in the head and acutely focused. In addition, the agitation caused numbness and tingling in his fingers and creepy sensations all over his skin and scalp.

During these bouts, he was intensely angry and wanted to smash anything within reach or get into fights. He would smash things (including twelve phones), punch walls, and kick doors. If men had annoyed him, he would try to pick a fight with them but he would never hit women. In his arguments with the former girlfriend, he would become so enraged that he would bang his head against the wall until he was bleeding. These bouts were caused by any sort of upset with people or minor friction, seeing the police and anybody threatening him or criticizing him. It was difficult to be clear how often he had these bouts. For the past few months, he had been agitated more or less all day unless he was drinking, which calmed him although he could still get into blazing arguments with people when drunk. He could not remember a time when he did not suffer the same sort of agitation although it was definitely getting worse as he got older.

On direct questioning, he had a lengthy list of social fears. He had to avoid crowds as they agitated him immediately. He could not stand in a queue with people behind him. He was completely unable to speak in public which had caused him a lot of trouble in court as people assumed he was simply being difficult. He disliked appointments and interviews and would not apply for unemployment benefits because of the delays and interviews he had to endure. This meant that, if he walked off a job because of arguments, he had to get another very quickly. He was unable to travel on aircraft, partly because of being confined and because he could not sit close to another person. He was immensely agitated by any sort of threat or criticism, even if he felt someone was looking at him in an aggressive or taunting manner. Arguments tipped him into blind rage in a few seconds and, if he heard raised voices, he always made sure he got right away until it had settled. He was very frightened of loneliness, which was why the separation bothered him so much. He was incapable of saying no to people, and was forever giving away his money, which he then resented and became very angry when they didn't pay him back. He feared disapproval and humiliation, making mistakes or failing at anything and mental illness.

When he was on the streets, he had a very strong feeling of people looking at him, talking behind his back, and judging him. He had a very strong sense of danger directed at him by anybody who came too close and would never let anybody stand behind him. He felt police were always watching him and could not stay anywhere near them, which caused problems in his driving job as he would not stop if he saw a police car parked near his destination. He had a very strong sense of people plotting and conspiring against him, particularly the ex-girlfriend and her new police friends.

He was extremely fussy about cleanliness, tidiness, order, punctuality, and efficiency, and was easily angered by delays or disorder. He loathed government inefficiency and prided himself on being a neat and efficient worker: "I'm a real perfectionist; I really have this urge to tidy your desk" (my desk is almost bare of objects). He was highly ritualistic in the way he wanted things ordered and organized and in cleaning things. When he was sober, he had his belongings neatly arranged in stacks that did not touch each other. Everything was organized by color and he had a habit of counting things in threes and touching doorjambs as he went past. If anybody moved his things, he became very angry. He could not sleep if he knew his belongings were not in their proper order. All of this caused conflict with people around him but he could not stop it and did not feel the need.

He had been this way all his life. He had been seen by psychiatrists and other mental health services in hospitals and prisons in three states but had never been treated: "Nobody wants to help me. Nobody has ever asked me so many questions. They reckon there's nothing wrong with me so I tell 'em to get f...d and walk out."

Personal Background

At first, he did not want to talk about his family background but began doing so in an accelerating flood of words (perhaps under the influence of the diazepam). He was born and raised in an isolated timber town in the south-west of Western Australia (not far from where I went to school). He did not know anything about his mother. She had apparently left his father when he was still a baby, and he was raised by his father and the paternal grandparents. He did not know how old his father was as he had had no contact with him since the age of sixteen. He said the father was a paranoid schizophrenic who had been in hospital a number of times during his childhood so he often stayed with the grandparents on a small farm just out of town. His father was exceptionally violent: "He bashed me all the time, never stopped. He was real crazy and very scary; he always threatened to kill me and he tried a couple of times." He said his father hit him with anything that came to hand, including an ax handle. He also burned him on the arms with cigarettes, and pointed to some faint circular scars on his upper arms. Over the years, the father had any number of drunken or violent girlfriends coming and going, all of whom Kevin hated like poison. Whenever he stayed on the grandparents' farm, he had to sleep in the same room as an uncle who drank heavily and who used him sexually until the age of fourteen. There was no violence but he shuddered as he recounted it. He had one older paternal half-sister but he hardly knew her. During his childhood, he never had any contact with welfare services: "They didn't care. I was a real shit of a kid; why did they care who was flogging me and f....g me?" He thought this was perhaps because his grandparents were well-respected in the area.

He attended local state schools but was expelled at twelve for drinking and attacking a teacher. He often truanted but was never reported because he knew how many days he could stay away. He hated school and all the teachers, and his marks were very poor. He was intensely shy and nervous but he covered this with aggression and bravado. He did not get on well with other children who were frightened of him and because he was often dirty and had nits. His only friends were one or two similarly disturbed boys, often part-aboriginals from broken families. He showed real talent at football but could not stay on the teams because he was too aggressive. When he left school, he could barely read and write although he had improved a lot with lessons in a remand home and in prison.

When he left school, he simply avoided contact with officials by getting casual work on neighborhood farms. This suited him because he never had to stay long. He lived mostly with his grandparents during this time, but he was drinking regularly and started smoking marihuana. He had no friends in town and started to move further afield. At fifteen, he was put in a remand home for stealing cars and growing marihuana but he quite enjoyed it because he was able to go to school and, compared with the aboriginal boys, he could read quite well, so he improved quickly. When he was released, he refused to go back to his home town but found a job with a delivery firm in the city, travelling with the drivers and also learning to drive forklift trucks. At nineteen, he was imprisoned for two years for armed robbery. He said the robbery was stupid and unplanned; he and some friends were drunk and one of them dared the others to rob a drive-in alcohol store. They were arrested by police within ten minutes. By that stage, he had a number of other charges, mainly fighting when drunk and resisting arrest etc.

On his release, he moved around getting work, then went interstate where he led much the same sort of unsettled life. He wandered on the edge of two cultures, the mainstream culture of work and families, but he was also unacceptable to the true criminal culture because of his violent and unpredictable temper. He never had any trouble getting jobs but could not hold them because he became too suspicious of the other men or argued with the managers. Throughout this, he was drinking heavily as well as using drugs, including methamphetamine, heroin, and flunitrazepam. He stopped using drugs abruptly at the age of twenty-eight and had reduced his drinking but still drank heavily when he became too agitated. Over the years, he had had "lots" of girlfriends but he usually left after a few months because of drinking, dishonesty, and temper: "I lie about everything. I can't stop it. I can't tell anybody the truth about myself."

Are you telling the truth now?

Yeah, I am actually. Do you believe me?

I believe you, but I can see why a lot of people wouldn't.

Mostly, I don't say anything. I can see they hate me so I just play dumb and let them hate me. It saves me trouble.

Self-Assessment

He said: "I'm not a very nice person." He saw himself as intensely nervous and overwhelmed by guilt, shame, and self-consciousness but he always hid this. He was extremely assertive in dealing with people and frequently got into arguments or fights because of it. He was fanatically tidy and organized but often became so distressed that he would not shower for days on end. He was very impatient, ferociously jealous, and held grudges passionately. Except for safety rules at work, he did not follow rules. The rest he ignored as he saw fit but he had no urge to break rules or laws for their own sake. He was not very social and saw himself as "a bit of a loner" except that he feared loneliness. He saw his temper as "… ten out of ten, the worst; it's shocking and even scares me." He felt his intellect was "not real good" but he was good with machines and sorting out problems if he could be patient long enough. His self-esteem was "no good, real bad".

Mental State Examination

The mental state showed a big, solidly-built man of about his stated age, dressed in clean but faded casual clothing. He had many tattoos and smelled of sweat and tobacco. He was profoundly agitated and was barely able to sit. He was weepy and constantly jiggled his legs or rubbed his face and hair. His talk was jerky and strangled and at times, he could barely speak. He expressed intense worthlessness but no self-hatred. He was enraged by the world but not hostile or overtly suspicious of the interviewer. He was not suicidal at the time but had been three weeks before. There were no psychotic features and nothing to indicate an organic impairment of brain function. He was of average intellectual ability.

Recent History

He had not been in Darwin very long when he met his recent girlfriend. He was working at the time and was making good money but she was completely irresponsible and spent everything he earned. She drank every day and gambled so he began using a credit card to take her to the casino. She had a voracious sexual appetite and he was happy to try to satisfy her but she was also highly flirtatious, which infuriated him. Before long, they were having ferocious arguments and the police were called. He was removed from her flat several times but, within a few hours, she would be ringing him to come back. He began drinking more and more and lost his job, found another and lost that too. She had a minor accident in her car while drunk and told the insurance company he had taken it without her permission so the insurers refused to pay. This led to terrible arguments and he was arrested after he smashed the windows of her car. She bailed him out, took him home, had sex, then called the police while he was sleeping and told them he had raped her.

After two days of absolute terror in the police station, part of which was a withdrawal state, he was abruptly released and told not to go near her. However, all his belongings were in her flat, so he went around to collect them. When he arrived at the flat, he found his possessions dumped near the rubbish bins and an expensive car parked in her parking lot. He collected what was left of his things, scratched obscenities in the car's paintwork, and left, with no money and nowhere to go. Unfortunately, the car was the prized possession of a married policeman who was visiting the lady in question. Next morning, he saw his car, realized the dumped clothes were gone, rang the lock-up, and put two and two together.

That day, Kevin found a room in a house with a group of hard-drinking men he had met at work and spent the next few days hopelessly drunk while the police searched the city for him. A week later, he was arrested while walking back from the local shops. When told he would be charged with damaging a policeman's car, he laughed and called their bluff. He was released with a number of new charges and went back to his room. Over the next few weeks, the woman called him a dozen times and began taunting him. When he retaliated in kind, she recorded his ranting and applied for a restraining order. This was soon breached as she kept calling him and he kept responding. He was arrested again and charged with various offences such as threatening homicide, etc. He continued drinking and became suicidal but somehow managed to get himself up to find a job. A few weeks later, he went to the hospital for help but, after waiting six hours, he walked out. He went to a general practitioner to get something to help him sleep and was referred for psychiatric assessment. By that stage, he was distraught.

At the first interview, he was commenced on treatment to stabilize his anxiety and his paranoid thinking. At the second appointment, he reported that he had not been able to get his tablets as he had been arrested and charged with stealing $58,000 from a former employer. While in the lock-up, he had punched a wall and fractured two fingers. On his release, he was driven to the hospital where a cast was fitted. He then walked 15 km to the employer's business and demanded to know why he had been charged with theft. After a confused and angry meeting, during which he threatened to kill everybody involved with the matter, he was told the problem had been sorted out (the money was not missing after all) but that nobody had remembered to tell the police after they had been given his name as a suspect. He was due in court the next day on a variety of charges relating to the ex-girlfriend.

At the next appointment, he said he had found a job but, while getting out of the cabin of the truck, his foot rolled on some gravel and he fell, dislocating his left hip. By the time he reached hospital, it had reduced spontaneously, so he was discharged home with morphine tablets for his considerable pain. Unfortunately, one of his flatmates had stolen them; so he belted the man, breaking his jaw and hurting his own hand. Bizarrely, when he collected his mail from the post office, there was a letter from his ex-girlfriend's lawyer claiming some $20,000 damages for a cancelled wedding. He explained that she had insisted on marriage, even though he was very dubious, but she put if off after he was hit by a car. The problems multiplied. He lodged a claim for worker's compensation for his hip injury but this was rejected on the basis he had not revealed his injured hand when he signed on (he had signed his forms in front of the manager with his hand in plaster). As he was unable to work, he applied for social security benefits, but his claim was rejected as he had been injured at work. He had no money for a lawyer and could not get legal aid to represent him on his many charges as he was still officially employed, even though he had not been paid for his day's work. He was unable to eat or sleep and was trying not to drink. Crying, he said: "Sometimes I wish I was never born. Why does this happen to me? I can't fight any more; they can do what they like to me."

He kept his appointments fairly reliably over the next few weeks but nothing improved. At one stage, it seemed he was developing osteomyelitis in one of the fractured fingers but this settled slowly after the plaster was removed. He got back to work but was hit by a forklift truck and injured his hand again. In a rage, he punched the driver with his injured hand and was dismissed on the spot; so, clutching his injured hand, he kicked the manager and left. The various charges were brought to court but were repeatedly adjourned, which made it impossible for him to leave town to get work. He was finally granted unemployment benefits but these were terminated after he missed a rehabilitation appointment due to being in court. He then disappeared for several months and, when he was next seen, said he had been in prison but his medication was not provided as the medical service would not contact a private psychiatrist for details of his treatment. On his side, he refused to see the prison mental health service as they had previously labeled him a psychopath and had declined to treat him. The guerilla warfare with the police, his former girlfriend, and his many enemies continued and he was due in court on Christmas Eve to face 97 charges. He was last seen just before he went to court. He was not drinking and not using drugs. He was working as a tire fitter but was very unhappy. He was continuing with specific treatment for the anxiety and was keen to do so as the side effects were minimal. With the medication, he could think clearly and had lost some weight.

One morning, about a year later, he walked into my office. He had just been released from prison and wanted to leave the Territory but he needed some medication as he had not been given any during his sentence. I gave him the prescription and talked to him for a while; then he left. Six months later, a request was received from the coroner's office in another state asking for information. After he had been arrested for kicking in the doors of a police car, Kevin Johnson had hanged himself.

The orthodox psychiatrist will shrug and say "Yes? That's what psycho-paths do."

13.3: When is a Psychopath?

I served my medical apprenticeship on the neurosurgery wards and on the burns unit of a major teaching hospital. Patients died. Very often, they were young and healthy. One night, they went out to a party and, a few hours later, their shattered parents signed consent for their organs to be removed for grafting. I remember one young man, a farmer's son of twenty, who was brought into the burns unit with over 90 percent of his body affected. His name was Kelly. He had been burning firebreaks using a knapsack spray of diesel when it ignited, turning him into a ball of fire. The only parts of him that were not burned were his feet, where his socks had protected him, and the area of his underpants. In desperation, the senior surgeon agreed to try homografts, using skin from a cadaver. The other resident and I went down to the mortuary and peeled the skin from a young man of thirty who had committed suicide. The only room available for our macabre operation was the relatives' viewing room, which was tastefully set up as a tiny chapel. Under a backlit cross, in muted light, we wielded the heavy, old-fashioned silver dermatomes and flayed him. My colleague was a devout Christian. To my astonishment, he began talking of how the dead man had betrayed his family by killing himself and he would burn in hell for ever. The whole thing was grotesque. We were first year residents; he was twenty-six, I was just twenty-three. I think he was doing that to comfort himself.

We took the precious skin upstairs and placed it on Kelly's swollen, blackened body. To our surprise, over the next few days, the grafts took and his blood chemistry started to stabilize. His kidneys began to work again and his blood oxygen levels improved. I was on duty on the Friday and, when I went home on the Saturday morning, Jack lifted his hand and waved faintly to me (he couldn't talk as he had a tracheotomy). Next morning, when I came in, I pushed open the door to the unit. As always, I glanced at the patient board to check the names. Kelly's was not there. A nurse came out: "Kelly died last night," she said, and began to cry.

The next day, eleven days since the boy's ghastly accident, I went back to the mortuary to see his autopsy. The cadaver skin had indeed taken and could not be pulled off. The pathologist was delighted with this remarkable experiment and took dozens of specimens. However, every internal organ was pale and enlarged. His liver was large and floppy and the pathologist poked his finger straight into it. The adrenal glands looked like a pair of squashed strawberries that had been left in the rain. The fact that the grafts had taken said that his entire immune system had failed. Under the terrible assault of his injury, his body had simply given up the ghost.

Kelly's death affected me more than I wanted to admit. I come from a farming family and had often enough helped with the burning off, using a mixture of sump oil and kerosene. His people were just ordinary farmers; I am sure they never once imagined that their beautiful son would be lying on the pathologist's slab while curious, masked and gowned people poked casually among his tortured remains. Why has his short, sad life come back to me after nearly forty years? I think it is because medicine is a tough game. It isn't glamorous, it isn't clean, and it's never pretty: don't ever believe Hollywood. Every day, every minute, lives are wrecked, people die, and mostly the wrong people. And psychiatry is the least pretty, least glamorous of all. It's the orphan specialty, the one that nobody wants to know. Governments don't care about psychiatry; there are no votes in madness. A government can't win an election by being nice to crazies but it sure can lose one by not being tough enough. And the worst part of psychiatry is personality disorder. In the orphan specialty, personality disorder is the orphan diagnosis, the bit that everybody wishes would just go away.

When you look at the types of patients I see, my suicide rate is mercifully low. Just over 60% of my patients are male, which is the reverse of the normal figures for private psychiatrists in this country. Most of them are young, the average age being about 33 yrs, and are struggling to pay their bills. Many of them come from shattered families or have their own broken families, and most of them have failed at school in one way or another. About half of them have criminal records, often with serious drug and alcohol problems. A lot of them have bad teeth and quite a few of them stink. Very often, the question is not how they survive, but why they would ever bother. Even then, a suicide is a blow. A suicide is just as bad as the immolation of a farmer's handsome son. There's no difference.

Modern psychiatry doesn't care about personality disorder. The great psychiatrists are not interested in psychopaths and certainly don't want any of them wandering into their tastefully furnished, discreetly-muted clinics. In fact, they dislike them so much that orthodox psychiatry has activated a program to eradicate personality disorder.

I have not conducted a multi-center, multi-authored double-blind survey on a government grant but it is clear that modern psychiatry is no longer diagnosing personality disorder (if you would like me to, please send the grant). The symptoms and behaviors which would once have earned a person a label as a hysterical personality or a psychopathic personality are now manipulated and shoved through that all-purpose blender called DSM-IV to emerge as a ticket to a genetic illness. In a welfare state, such as Australia, this is very helpful because it means the person is no longer expected to fend for himself but will be given an invalid pension for life for his new mental disorder. Better still, his relatives can extract a caregiver's benefit from having him in the house, he can see a psychologist for regular chats; he will have an endless supply of drugs he can trade and a ticket out of jail for a wide range of offences. Because psychiatry doesn't have a model of personality disorder, much less an effective means of treating it, the institution has agreed to solve the problem by reclassifying all people with abnormal personalities as mentally-ill, most commonly as Bipolar Disorder and Adult ADHD.

For psychiatry, this has any number of benefits, starting with the enormous sums of money that are made available for "research" in Bipolar

Disorder and ADD/ADHD (there is practically none for personality disorder). In practice, it means that obstreperous people can be heavily sedated to the point where their relatives stop complaining to the government. It means that wealthy people with objectionable personalities are not sent away but are drawn into the system and fed on drugs while their hip pockets are mined using the very latest sophisticated techniques. Insurance companies can be fooled into paying for lengthy and totally unnecessary admissions to expensive clinics. Large numbers of people with perfectly healthy brains can be sent for expensive scans and EEGs so the radiology department can keep buying machines it doesn't actually need. Drug companies can make sizeable fortunes manufacturing drugs that were not needed thirty years ago before the diseases were invented, or by finding dubious uses for old drugs. Psychologists and social workers can build empires based on counseling the families of the afflicted. School teachers can insist that their difficult students be sedated under threat of expulsion, and the school has to employ a nurse to dish out the drugs and a counselor to help the afflicted adjust to their genetic illnesses. Philandering politicians and televangelists can hold tearful confessions on daytime television revealing that they have been grappling with mental illness for years when everybody else thought they were grappling with a blonde.

When you look at it from this point of view, you might wonder why anybody would take exception to one of the outstandingly successful growth industries of the late twentieth century, the medicalization of personality disorder. I take exception, not just because it is poor science, or because it is likely to be the next major scandal for psychiatry, but because it ruins people's lives.

The problem is very simple: DSM-IV licenses misdiagnosis of personality disorder because it is so poorly and ambiguously worded that it has all the subtlety of doing neurosurgery with a claw hammer. Psychiatrists start taking a history but, as soon as they have found enough symptoms to pull the diagnosis they want from their manual, they stop. Just to preserve appearances, they will ask a few peremptory questions about the person's background but they don't believe there is any point to the exercise. Their theory says that mental disorder is biochemical, so all talk of early life experiences is necessarily besides the point. In fact, they think personality is so unimportant that they dump it on Axis II, along with intellectual handicap, even though personality is always prior to mental disorder. The critical reader might wonder whether this was in fact deliberate, to stop people thinking that personality was somehow causative of the mental disorder but I doubt it. My view is that it merely represented blind prejudice at work. The DSM committee didn't for a moment consider that personality might somehow determine the mental disorder just because they didn't believe it. Even if it had occurred to them, they would have dismissed it as it didn't fit with their conception of mental disorder as the surface manifestations of underlying biochemical lesions.

But why does this lead to psychiatrists consistently failing to recognize personality disorder, classifying it instead as an illness they can treat with their drugs? Exactly. Why should they do themselves out of a job? If they started a program of taking reliable histories and correctly assigning people according to the causes of their conditions, who knows where it would end? Look at the following history:

13.4: How Not to Have a Personality Disorder

Barry Martin, a 42-y/o single man, fled to Darwin from Adelaide, in South Australia, after he had sustained a head injury in a bashing. He said he could not go back to Adelaide as he was too frightened of further trouble. He had been in hospital for several weeks with a "small blood clot" but he hadn't had any operations. Soon after he reached Darwin, he told a GP he was taking stimulant medication and wanted a script for methylphenidate 30 mg bd (Ritalin LA). He was living in a men's shelter and was receiving an invalid pension for "ADHD and bipolar" which was granted many years before. When asked if he had any letters from the hospital, he pulled a sweaty and dog-eared letter from Royal Adelaide Hospital from his pocket. It was dated a few months before and confirmed that he had been admitted with a small extradural hematoma which resolved without surgery. The letter said he had been bashed with a baseball bat. I pointed out that it was a sign of a drug dealer, at which his bubbling prattle abruptly stopped for a few moments.

On questioning, it was learnt that he was sleeping about six hours a night in the dormitory and was feeling reasonably active and interested. With a laugh, he said he could never get on with people as everybody thought he was an idiot. His memory hadn't been so good since he was hit on the head but he was able to concentrate and could think clearly. There were no disturbances of perception.

He was not suffering any bouts of unhappiness and hadn't done so for "ages"; he couldn't remember the last time. He had never experienced a bout of elevated mood but was always bright and happy. However, he agreed he had frequent bouts of intense agitation with many somatic symptoms of anxiety. Most days, he had four or more, lasting up to half an hour each, and he felt very frightened during them. They were caused by any minor upsets or friction with people. He had a long list of true phobias, mostly social in nature (i.e. intense fear with active avoidance). He had strong feelings of persecution, of conspiracy, and of being under surveillance. He was a fussy and ritualistic person, which often got him into arguments. He had been this way all his life and was first commenced on amphetamines at about age six.

Barry's family background in a small town near Adelaide was very disturbed. His father was a bad-tempered and violent alcoholic with a criminal record and, after a very stormy marriage, the parents separated when he was eleven. At first, he lived with his father but there was too much drinking and violence, so he went back to his mother and rarely saw his father again. He had one full brother who was an alcoholic and two maternal half-brothers who were both disturbed and had psychiatric histories. Their father, Barry's stepfather, was a pleasant person but he cut contact when Barry started going to prison.

Barry said he did not do well at school as he was "too fast for everybody, hard to handle". He was constantly in trouble for talking and playing up and he often truanted. He had no idea how many schools he attended in eight years, probably more than ten. He was small and nervous and usually hung around with the bullies if he wasn't being bullied himself. When he left school at fourteen, he could barely read or write. Since leaving school, he had never worked regularly but had been drifting around most of his life, often supporting himself by dealing in drugs. He had had three relationships and had three children but never cared for them and had lost contact with them. His last relationship was for six years with a working prostitute and he appeared to have spent most of his time drinking and brawling. He had used opiates most of his life and, for six years, was selling morphine obtained on prescription by an old man who was doctor shopping. He had a lengthy criminal record for stealing, breaking and entering, and receiving stolen goods. He had served four prison sentences totaling about four years. He was hepatitis C positive from IV drug use.

He could not describe himself. He said he was "a bit nervous" and was highly assertive which often got him into arguments. He said he was not bothered by guilt, shame or self-consciousness. He was either fastidiously tidy or very untidy, depending on his mood, and was highly impatient. He liked company because he couldn't stand being alone but was very jealous and "always" held grudges. He broke rules all the time but still tried to keep on good terms with authority. He said his temper was "real bad" but claimed his intellect and self-esteem were both good.

The mental state showed a small, skinny, and prematurely aged man with a scruffy goatee. He was wearing frayed old clothing and smelled of sweat and tobacco. There were some old tattoos on his arms and legs and recent scars to his face and arms. At first, he was bouncy and cheerful but soon became tense, edgy, and jittery although he tried to laugh it off. He kept making silly jokes until told to stop. He gave brief, dismissive answers to questions and became increasingly resentful of the questions as the interview progressed. Finally, he demanded to know why this (questioning) was necessary when he had only come for "his" drugs. Under his zany exterior, he was very guarded and wary. He was not depressed and evinced no signs of guilt or despair. There were no signs of a psychotic disorder, and nothing to indicate an organic impairment of brain function. He was of average intellectual ability.

At the end of the interview, I explained that he did not meet the criteria for stimulant prescription in the NT. He had a moderately severe, personality-based anxiety state which needed treatment. When he realized he would not be getting the stimulants, he flared into anger. All traces of humor vanished and, if he hadn't been so short, he would have been quite threatening. He refused to believe that the laws in Darwin are different from Adelaide (about 4000 km away), and began ranting about all the "useless f...g doctors in this f...g dump of a town". He wanted to know where he could get "his" drugs and kept up a barrage of demands, masked threats, and manipulation, alternating with whining pleas for sympathy. After several minutes of this, I put the prescription pad away. Suddenly, he became quite eager to learn about his new tablets and leaned chummily across the desk. After being given the prescriptions and instructions, he was taken to the reception area to make his appointment but immediately began agitating for drugs. He kept demanding of the receptionist why he had not been given the drugs and where he could get them. When he finally left (as I was coming out to eject him), he walked up and down outside the office for a long time, apparently speaking on a phone.

13.5: Mad or Bad? Mental Illness vs. Personality Disorder

The critical question arising from Barry Martin's history concerns the relationship between personality and mental disorder. The first point to remember is that biological psychiatrists are not qualified to comment on this question just because they do not recognize such a relationship. They have no theory or account of personality, and are committed to the idea that mental disorder arises from the genome, meaning there is no point at which psychological factors could intervene. Some may say this is taking too extreme a view, that they do take life events into account but they have no model for doing so and, in practice, it is little more than lip service (e.g. the spurious 'biopsychosocial model').

The second point is that a proper history looks at all symptoms, not just those that satisfy the particular psychiatrist's interests or prejudices. Barry Martin showed a pervasive disorder affecting all aspects of his life: on what authority did the psychiatrist choose just the symptoms of ADHD (then known as hyperactivity) and assign them primary value, leaving all the rest to sort themselves out? From childhood, he had had a severe, generalized anxiety disorder; anxiety causes learning disorders; so why was his anxiety not addressed? It wasn't addressed because it didn't register with the psychiatrist. Even if he had seen the boy shivering and twitching and jerking around, he would have said to himself: "Ah, yes, that's what ADHD is, that's what aberrant brain chemicals do. There is nothing further to understand, no mystery to unravel, no hidden mechanism to be uncovered. These little tablets will bring him back into the realms of normality." They didn't, because his behavior was generated by personality factors, which drugs don't touch.

The reason drugs don't touch personality factors is because drugs and personality factors belong to separate realms of discourse. They are, to paraphrase Orwell, like a sausage and a rose: their purposes hardly intersect. Drugs belong to the physical realm and personality factors are informational states encoded in that realm but functionally removed from it. True, we can give people drugs that will affect their brains to such an extent that they may not act on their particular beliefs but there will never be drugs that can compel a person to stop liking Stravinsky and chase after Eminem. Drugs cannot and never will act at the level of recoding information in the brain. They suppress symptoms but do not eliminate their causes.

Personality is the sum total of the rules, attitudes, and beliefs which constitute the core informational state of the individual. In order to make the definition workable, we restrict personality to the set of beliefs that are unique to that individual. There is no limit to the beliefs individuals can have, and no reason to believe all people have the same clusters. I may show tidy, organized behavior but my reasons for doing so may be totally different from yours. A person may show socially avoidant behavior because he is frightened of making mistakes, or he fears people ignoring him, or he fears attack, or he believes that talking to people is self-indulgent and is therefore bad or that his opinions are never worth hearing. There is no limit. We use the symptoms to work out what the hidden beliefs are, often having to cross-reference or triangulate them; then we work on them. Drugs are only used to alleviate particular symptoms to bring the person within reach of psychotherapy.

It will be fairly clear that this model makes some strong claims on the notion of morality but I can only indicate them in briefest terms here. As outlined in earlier volumes, I see humans as autonomous agents with the capacity to control their behavior. Observable behavior is generated by the high-speed interaction of a vast number of informational states, some long-standing, some derived directly from current input. In crude terms, our current sensory input percolates through a complex matrix of beliefs, attitudes, rules, dispositions, ambitions, proclivities, inclinations, hopes, dreads, inhibitions, prohibitions, and any other term that can be used to convey the sense of a predetermined response to an input. Even though this is very fast, it actually takes time and, typically, we have moved on to the next input before the last one has been processed and decisions made. Attention flickers from one sensory modality to another, which only means that one input is promoted over another. Thus, from moment to moment, as we meet different contingencies, we must compute the correct behavioral outcome. Our job, as moral agents, is to ensure in advance that all our rules and dispositions conform to the prevailing standards. The rules must be in place before the event happens; we cannot compute new responses to every contingency from first principles. The constant apprehension that our next move may be wrong is consistent with Kierkegaard's "existential anxiety".

For any input, there will be an output, even if it is "Do nothing". Every output consists of a set of behavioral instructions, including overt movement, speech, emotion, and physiological responses. If the complete set of behavioral instructions always conforms with what the society has decreed is "decent behavior", we would say that the person has a normal personality. If his behavioral output clashes with society's standards, we say he has a personality disorder. Depending on what sorts of behaviors he typically shows, we tend to categorize him (that word) because that's what humans do: abhorring chaos, we still it with a name.

The set of behavioral rules an individual can have is near-infinite; the set of all rules ever used by a human anywhere is imponderable. However, certain rules pop up all the time. Some of them are the result of living but some of them probably have a more primitive origin: we call them human nature. Fear of strangers, the tendency to form dominance hierarchies, territoriality, and even the sense of fair play are probably as close to innate as human cognition can be. Can there be free will with innate cognitive rules? There has to be, as Isaac Bashevis Singer said; we have no choice in that. The question is not the rules we are born with, but the rules we leave in place. Every person has a unique or peculiar combination of rules resulting from his life experience. These have to be seen in the setting of his intellect, his physical health, his skills and weaknesses, and many other factors. His rules constitute the totality of how he sees the world, himself, and his place in the world, and determine how he will react to it. Every input bounces through this bewildering array of instructions, some of which the individual knows, many of which he knows only dimly, while some are quite outside his awareness. Because there are so many influences acting at each point, we can only quote one or two for each decision. From this complexity arises the subtlety of human behavior in its infinite range, its nuanced power and adaptability. However, people still tend to behave in characteristic ways because of the over-riding influence of major blocks of similar rules.

All of these rules are coded into the brain in a manner which is still far beyond our current understanding of the neurosciences. Each individual's response to his life experiences constitutes his career path in life. We have very little control over the first rules we learn; that is almost entirely the product of early family life. Children do not set the tone of the family, it is set for them. The child arrives at school, day one, with a functioning set of rules and suddenly has to cope with a much larger society than the family. If he is lucky, he will be able to mesh smoothly into the playground society (and don't underestimate how complex it is) and generalize his rules to incorporate his new world. If he isn't lucky, if he has been raised in a household where parents brawl and children are walloped randomly, then school is going to be a problem. He might be bright and get a teacher who sees his potential and encourages him; or he may be unlucky and get the teacher who can't stand mouthy boys and so school becomes just another battleground, as it did for Barry Martin.

The concept of the career path is not well understood in psychiatry, mainly because we have spent all our research dollars on brain scanners which can't actually read mental rules. We need a new emphasis, one which shows how the individual relates to his environment and, in turn, the environment feeds back to him responses which govern the new rules he acquires and the old ones he modifies. The individual's career path is defined by his prior set of rules and his history of environmental contingencies (pace Skinner) insofar as they cause him to gain or change rules. Psychotherapy therefore becomes the process of bringing to full awareness the major rules that govern one's life. We use the symptoms to uncover the hidden rules or to show their full impact. Most people are at least dimly aware of their rules; very often it is just a matter of their not according them their true weightings. There is a constant dynamic interchange between the individual's set of rules and the society around him. The biggest risk we face is that, very often, our rules are self-reinforcing or self-fulfilling. Self-fulfilling rules are the basis of the anxiety states, and anxiety is very often the stone that starts the avalanche.

Let's look at the rules that were knocking around in Kevin Johnson' head when he arrived at adulthood. The first and most important was something like: "I am absolutely on my own in this world. Nobody cares whether I live or die." Next, he had a cluster of rules which added up to: "The human world is a cruel and dangerous place, it will never give me a chance and it will probably destroy me just for fun." He had no fear of the natural world but it couldn't give him much comfort as he feared loneliness: "Loneliness is too scary to think about." Other people with very similar early family backgrounds may have had comforting experiences while alone in the bush, so they will tend to retreat into solitude when the world gets too much. Kevin Johnson couldn't do that. He had to find a human for comfort but he didn't trust ordinary people. His experiences of life in small town society had taught him that ordinary people despised him, even when he no longer had nits. He was therefore driven to find company among outcasts because he knew they were less likely to turn on him and he also knew he could dominate them physically. Intuitively, he knew that most outcasts are easily frightened. At the same time, however, he was profoundly suspicious of male affection. He could not tolerate a man who looked upon him approvingly as he immediately translated that into sexual interest, and his early experiences revolted him. Thus, he gravitated back to disorganized women, but his experiences with them tended to reinforce his prejudices. In particular, the bias in judicial services in favor of women and against large tattooed men filled him with rage and amplified his sense of betrayal.

A lot of his trouble came from his intense anxiety. He had a huge list of social fears, mostly about how people saw him or how he was performing. He could not tolerate failure because he feared the sense of people looking down on him. He feared people looking down on him because, like the rest of us, he wanted to be liked, to be one of the society: he needed approval, but he had no sense of self-approval. He was therefore at the mercy of those around him for his very sense of self-worth and, as many years of bitter experience had taught him, their approval was not likely to be forthcoming. Just as the other children sneered at him and taunted him in the playground and ran to the teachers when he lashed back at them, so he was caught in the bigger playground of the adult world, where police sneered at him and taunted him, and nice people (doctors, nurses, lawyers) told him to wait his turn, there was always somebody else before him. It is an amazing thing about being a psychopath: everybody treats you psychopathically. If a human is treated badly enough long enough, he has to adopt certain attitudes as a matter of survival. It's either that or go under.

Montaigne said: "The laws of conscience... rise and proceed from custom, every man holding in inward veneration the opinions approved and customs received about him" (Essays, Lxxii) Because we can change our rules, we can change our behaviour. Morality becomes just a matter of rewriting our rules.

13.6: Conclusion: The Nature of Mind

In his Devil's Dictionary, the inestimable Ambrose Bierce defined mind as follows: "A mysterious form of matter secreted by the brain. Its chief activity consists in the endeavor to ascertain its own nature, the futility of the attempt being due to the fact that it has nothing but itself to know itself with…" I believe we have come some little way since then.

I am drawing a model of vast, perhaps incalculable, complexity. We can never know what goes on inside another person but we can make some fairly good guesses. Very often, we may not even be entirely sure what is going on inside ourselves, which is what training psychotherapy is for. If, for example, I had approached Kevin Johnson with a strong need to gain his approval, I would have triggered his homosexual anxieties and pushed him into a panic. His standard way of dealing with anxiety was to flip it into aggression, which would have been troublesome for both of us. However, he was fairly comfortable with my deliberately low-key approach. The model says that our beliefs and rules generate behaviors, including emotional behaviors. As we don't have a very large number of emotions, these are common to all humans. What counts, therefore, is not so much the emotions we generate but what we do with them. That is the difference between saying one person has a mental illness compared with his neighbor who has a personality disorder. If I quake in my boots, I have a mental illness but if I turn my fear into rage, I am a psychopath. If it stops me learning, I have ADD, but if it makes me vomit, I am somatizing. If I drink to calm it, I am a worthless drunk but if you give me medication, I am a grateful patient.

In Chapter 7, Mark Jones had much the same problems with anxiety as Kevin Johnson but his response was to freeze. He couldn't do anything so he became more and more depressed until he saw no option but to take overdoses. That was what his life had taught him. Kevin Johnson's life had taught him to come out fighting because if anybody saw him sniffing, they attacked. Such is the nature of the playground, as well as the larger playground we call life. He switched his anxiety and used it to power his rage so he survived each attack, but each incident drove him deeper into the netherworld. Mark Jones swung from states of agitation to states of despair, so he was labeled bipolar. Kevin Johnson drank and used drugs to control his agitation and got into fights in between, so he was labeled a psychopath. Another boy of the same age and in the same school, who was smaller and brighter and had delayed puberty, could not fight as Kevin had done, so he used his verbal wit to keep one jump in front of the bigger boys. Because he had to keep a constant stream of blather going, and tried to score points in class by making fun of the teachers, he fell behind but he could not admit it, so he became the class clown, was labeled ADHD, and was put on drugs. Mark coped by withdrawing into himself and daydreaming, so he was labeled ADD and was put on the same drugs.

Another insecure boy came from a moderately religious family. He resolved his anxiety by becoming more and more religious and finally withdrew from the scary world into the sedate and predictable world of religious orders. His brother went the other way, violently rejecting everything his parents said and diving into the world of psychedelic drugs and Eastern mysticism. The next boy was bigger and had earlier puberty than the class clown, so he learned early that he could kick a football further than the others, and snatch it from the other boys more often. He soon learned that he could get any amount of approval from the male teachers and his father's friends, so football became his career. At the same time, a girl who was also anxious in company learned that she could be very popular if she made herself available behind the stand after the football matches.

Another little boy, whose name we won't mention, realized fairly early that, if he wanted a life that went beyond booze, religion, football, fighting, and fornicating, he'd better pass his exams and get a scholarship, so he could get the hell out of that town, so that's what he did. Every night, he studied; every day after school and all day Saturday, he worked and saved every penny so that, on the day he left the school, he had his scholarship but nobody noticed. Everybody was too busy congratulating the footballer who had been chosen to play with a city club. Years later, when he was replaced in the team by a younger and fitter man, the fallen hero took to drinking to control the despair that came from being a footballer who couldn't hold his balls. Now that he was thirty-four, overweight, and his knees were ruined, the people who had cheered him as a high-flying twenty-year-old had found another twenty-year-old high-flyer to adore. He didn't recognize the psychiatrist he was sent to see (perhaps it was the beard, perhaps the footballer had never even noticed him all those years ago), but he came to see how he, too, had been used – and how, in a Faustian bargain, he had let himself be used.

The biocognitive model generates a hugely complex picture of recursive interactions of social cause and mental effect evolving over years in a multidimensional matrix. The dimensions are space and time, culture and experience, both public and private; emotions, intellect, fantasies and fears, health and intellect, strengths and weaknesses, both innate and acquired and, above all, luck. It was my good luck not to be born into Kevin Johnson's family.

Orthodox psychiatry does not recognize luck as an element in the development of mental disorder. Perhaps that is why so many of the great names in psychiatry think they are next to God in the pecking order. They really believe they have got to the top by virtue of their superior moral and intellectual equipment but actually, it was just that they were born in the right house on the good side of town and somebody gave them a break. This might explain why they react so bitterly to criticism. They had better get used to it: biological psychiatry has had its day. The coming generation of psychiatrists was born into a complex, cognitive world which has broken with the old securities. The notion of a recursive informational state that amplifies its own failings is second nature to them.

References

Chapter 1

1. cchrint.org/tag/charles-nemeroff/ Accessed November 27th 2009.

2. Turner EH (2004) A Taxpayer-Funded Clinical Trials Registry and Results Database. PLoS Med 1(3): e60. doi:10.1371/journal.pmed.0010060

3. McLaren N. The myth of 'eclecticism' in psychiatry. Australasian Psychiatry 1996; 4: 260-61. Revised version in: *Humanizing Madness: Psychiatry and the Cognitive Neurosciences.* Ann Arbor, MI.: Future Psychiatry Press. ISBN 978 1 932690 39 2.

4. Masson JM 1984. *The Assault on Truth: Freud's suppression of the seduction theory.* New York: Simon and Schuster.

5. Crews F. *Unauthorised Freud: doubters confront a legend.* Penguin Putnam; New York; 1998.

6. Changeux J-P 1985. *Neuronal Man: the biology of mind.* Oxford: University Press.

7. Kandel ER 2005. *Psychiatry, psychoanalysis and the new biology of mind.* Washington, DC: American Psychiatric Publishing.

8. McLaren N 2009. *Humanizing psychiatry: the biocognitive model.* 2009; Ann Arbor, MI.: Future Psychiatry Press. ISBN 978 1 615990 11 5.

9. Chalmers DJ 1996. *The Conscious Mind: in search of a fundamental theory.* Oxford: University Press.

10. Dennett DC 1991. *Consciousness explained.* London: Penguin Books (1993).

11. Dennett DC 1996. *Kinds of minds: Towards an understanding of consciousness.* London: Weidenfeld and Nicholson.

12. Dennett DC 2003. *Freedom evolves.* London: Allen Lane. Page numbers refer to the Penguin edition, London, 2004.

13. Bonner B. Zurich Minds Symposium. http://www.dailyreckoning.com.au/zurich-minds-symposium/2009/12/18/ Accessed December 29, 2009.

14. Dennett DC. http://ase.tufts.edu/cogstud/incbios/dennettd/dennettd.html. Accessed December 29, 2009.

15. Audi R (Ed.) 1995. *The Cambridge Dictionary of Philosophy.* Cambridge: University Press.

16. Dorbolo J. Intuition pumps. *Mind Mach* (2006) 16:81–86 DOI 10.1007/s11023-006-9012-8. Published online May 5, 2006.

17. Skinner BF. *Beyond Freedom and Dignity.* New York: Knopf, 1971.

18. Dennett DC 1978. *Brainstorms: Philosophical essays on mind and psychology.* Hassocks, Sussex: Harvester Press.

19. Turing AM. On computable numbers, with an application to the Entscheidungsproblem. Proceedings of the London Mathematical Society (1936 - 37) Series 2; 42:230-65. Available on line: See author entry in Wikipedia.

20. Turing AM. Computing machinery and intelligence. *Mind* 1950; 59: 433-60.

21. Luria AR. *Higher cortical functions in man.* New York: Basic Books, 1980.

22. Guze SB. Biological psychiatry: is there any other kind? *Psychological Medicine,* 1989; 19: 315-323.

Chapter 2

1. Guze SB, 1992. *Why psychiatry is a branch of medicine.* New York: Oxford University Press.

2. Searle JR 1999. *Mind, Language and Society: Doing philosophy in the real world.* London: Weidenfeld and Nicholson.

3. Searle JR 1993. The problem of consciousness. *Social Research.* 60 (1)   Spring. http://users.ecs.soton.ac.uk/harnad/Papers/Py104/searle.prob.html. Accessed Dec 30. 2009.

4. McLaren N 2007 *Humanizing Madness: Psychiatry and the Cognitive Neurosciences.* 2007; Ann Arbor, MI.: Future Psychiatry Press. ISBN 978 1 932690 39 2.

5. McKenzie BD, 1977. *Behaviourism and the limits of scientific method.* Routledge and Kegan Paul: London.

6. Popper KR, Eccles JC, 1981. *The Self and its Brain.* London: Springer.

7. Searle J, 2007. Dualism revisited. Journal of Physiology, Paris. 2007 Jul-Nov;101(4-6):169-78. Epub January 19 2008.

8. Searle 2002 Why I am not a property dualist. Initially in *Intentionality, an Essay in the Philosophy of Mind,* Cambridge University Press, Cambridge, 1983. Available at http://ist-socrates.berkeley.edu/~jsearle/articles.html Accessed December 30 2009.

9. Searle JR 1999b. The future of philosophy. Paper presented to Royal Society. Available at http://socrates.berkeley.edu/~jsearle/articles.html. Accessed January 4, 2010.

10. Searle JR 2000. Consciousness. *Annual Review of Neuroscience.* 23:557-578.

11. McLaren N 2009 *Humanizing Psychiatry: The Biocognitive Model.* 2009; Ann Arbor, MI.: Future Psychiatry Press. ISBN 978 1 615990 11 5.

12. Popper KR. *Objective Knowledge: an evolutionary approach.* Oxford: Clarendon Press, 1972.

13. Luria AR. *Higher cortical functions in man.* New York: Basic Books, 1980.

14. Stanford Encyclopaedia of Philosophy. Accessed Jan. 25 2010: http://plato.stanford.edu/entries/consciousness-intentionality/

15. Turing AM. On computable numbers, with an application to the Entscheidungsproblem. Proceedings of the London Mathematical Society (1936 - 37) Series 2; 42:230-65. Available on line: See author entry in Wikipedia.

For most of Searle's papers used in this chapter, go to his university website:

http://socrates.berkeley.edu/~jsearle/

It also says his office hours are Tuesdays and Thursdays, 4.00-5.00pm. That, surely, is a dream job.

Chapter 3

1. Bulhak, AC. 'On the simulation of postmodernism and mental debility using recursive transition networks' Dept. of Computer Sciences, Monash University, Melbourne, Vic. 1996. Available at: http://www.csse.monash.edu.au/publications/1996/tr-cs96-264.ps.gz

2. Doctorow EL. *Creationists: Selected essay, 1993-2006.* New York: Random House, 2006.

3. Medawar P. Critical notice: Teilhard de Chardin's *Phenomenon of man. Mind,* 1961; 70:99-106.

Chapter 4

1. Stumpf SE. 1993. Socrates to Sartre: a history of philosophy. 5th Edn. New York: McGraw Hill.

2. Kockelmans JJ. Phenomenology, in Audi R (Ed.) 1995. *The Cambridge Dictionary of Philosophy.* Cambridge: University Press.

3. Center for Advanced Research in Phenomenology. http://www.phenomenologycenter.org/

Accessed April 4th 2010.

4. Society for Phenomenological and Existential Philosophy http://www.spep.org/

Accessed April 4th 2010.

5. Russell B. 1989. Wisdom of the West. New York: Crescent Books.

6. Lacanian Ink, occasionally available from the site www.lacan.com.

7. Foucault M. 2006. *History of Madness.* (Ed. J Khalfa, tr. J Murphy and J Khalfa) London: Routledge.

8. Editors of *Lingua Franca.* 2000. *The Sokal Hoax: The sham that shook the academy.* Lingua Franca Books/University of Nebraska Press.

9. Gross PR, Levitt N. 1994. *Higher Superstitions: The academic left and its quarrels with science.* Baltimore: Johns Hopkins Press.

10. Sokal A, Bricmont J. 1998. *Fashionable Nonsense: Postmodern intellectuals' abuse of science.* New York: Picador.

11. Sokal A. 2008. *Beyond the Hoax: Science, philosophy and culture.* Oxford: University Press.

12. Lennon K. 1997. Feminist epistemology as local epistemology. *Proc. Aristot. Socy.* Supp.71: 37. Quoted in: Boghassian P. 2006. *Fear of Knowledge: against relativism and constructivism.* Oxford: University Press.

Chapter 5

1. Andreasen NC. 2007. DSM and the death of phenomenology in America: An example of unintended consequences. *Schizophrenia Bulletin.* 33: 108–112.

2. Mullen PE. 2007. A modest proposal for another phenomenological approach to psychopathology. *Schizophrenia Bulletin.* 33: 113–121.

3. McLaren N. 2007 *Humanizing Madness: Psychiatry and the Cognitive Neurosciences.*; Ann Arbor, Mi.: Future Psychiatry Press. ISBN 978 1 932690 39 2.

4. Crews F. 1998 *Unauthorised Freud: doubters confront a legend.* New York: Penguin Putnam.

5. Rosenhan DL. 1973. On being sane in insane places. *Science* 170;70: 250-58. See http://en.wikipedia.org/wiki/Rosenhan_experiment for a brief commentary.

6. McLaren N. 2010. Letter: Psychiatry's failure to define itself. *Australasian Psychiatry* Vol 18 (in press).

Chapter 6

1. McLaren N. (2007). *Humanizing Madness: Psychiatry and the Cognitive Neurosciences.* Ann Arbor, Mi.: Future Psychiatry Press. ISBN 978 1 932690 39 2.

2. American Psychiatric Association DSM-V Development Site (2010). Accessed May 29th 2010. http://www.dsm5.org/Pages/Default.aspx (note that the information on this site changes regularly).

3. Frances A. (2010). A few DSM-5 updates and commentaries. Accessed May 17th 2010.

http://integral-options.blogspot.com/2010/04/allen-frances-few-dsm-5-updates-and.html

See also: http://ondemand.duke.edu/video/22221/duke-doctor-allen-frances-on-p

4. Stein DJ et al. (2010). What is a Mental/Psychiatric Disorder? From DSM-IV to DSM-V. Psychological Medicine, 2010; doi:10.1017/S0033291709992261. Accessed May 17th 2010.

5. Horwitz AV, Wakefield JC. (2007). *The Loss of Sadness: how psychiatry transformed normal sorrow into Depressive Disorder.* New York: Oxford University Press. ISBN 978 0 19 531304 8.

6. Dennett DC. (1993). *Consciousness Explained.* London: Penguin Books.

7. McLaren N. (2010). Monist models of mind and biological psychiatry. *Ethical Human Psychology and Psychiatry* (in press).

8. Chalmers DJ. (1996). *The Conscious Mind: in search of a fundamental theory.* Oxford: University Press.

9. McLaren N. (2009). *Humanizing Psychiatry: The Biocognitive Model.* Ann Arbor, Mi.: Future Psychiatry Press. ISBN 978 1 615990 11 5.

10. Gottesman II, & Gould TD (2003). The Endophenotype Concept in Psychiatry: Etymology and Strategic Intentions. American Journal of Psychiatry 160:636-645.

Chapter 7.

1. Guze SB. *Why psychiatry is a branch of medicine.* New York: Oxford University Press, 1992.

2. Kandel ER. *Psychiatry, psychoanalysis and the new biology of mind.* Washington, DC: American Psychiatric Publishing, 2005.

3. Kandel ER. *In search of memory: the emergence of a new science of mind.* New York: Norton, 2006.

4. Engel GL. A unified concept of health and disease. *Perspect. Biol Med* 1960; 3:459-485.

5. Engel GL. The need for a new medical model: a challenge for biomedicine. *Science* 1977; 196:129-136.

6. Engel GL. The care of the patient: art or science? *Johns Hopkins Med J* 1977; 140:222-232.

7. Engel GL. The biopsychosocial model and the education of health professionals. *Ann NY Acad Sci* 1978; 310: 169-181.

8. Engel GL. The clinical application of the biopychosocial model. *Amer J Psychiat* 1980; 137:535-544.

9. Guze SB. Biological psychiatry: is there any other kind? *Psychol Med*, 1989; 19: 315-323.

10. Canadian Psychiatric Association. http://www.cpa-apc.org/browse/sections/0 Accessed May 2nd 2010

11. *The Canadian Journal of Psychiatry.* http://publications.cpa-apc.org/browse/sections/0 Accessed May 2nd 2010

12. Holmes J. Fitting the biopsychosocial jigsaw together (editorial). *Brit J Psychiat* 2000; 177; 93-94.

13. Wilson J. President's Letter. *Austral Psychiat* 1998; 6:83-84.

14. Royal Australian and New Zealand College of Psychiatrists, 1998. Position Statement No. 39: 'What is a psychiatrist, and what does a psychiatrist do?' RANZCP, Melbourne.

15. Engel PA, Engel AG. George L Engel 1913-1999: remembering his life and work: strengthening a father-son bond in a new time of grief. Aust N Z J Psychiatry 2002; 36: 443-448.

16. Taylor GJ. Mind-body-environment: George Engel's psychoanalytic approach to psychosomatic medicine. Aust N Z J Psychiatry 2002; 36: 449-457.

17. Singh BS. George Engel: a personal reminiscence. Aust N Z J Psychiatry 2002; 36: 467-471.

18. Smith GC, Strain JJ. George Engel's contribution to clinical psychiatry. Aust N Z J Psychiatry 2002; 36: 458-466.

19. McLaren N. A critical review of the biopsychosocial model. Aust N Z J Psychiatry 1998: 32; 86-92. Revised version:

20. Muir B. Comment on McLaren's critical review of the biopsychosocial model. Aust N Z J Psychiatry 1998: 32; 93-94.

21. Mullen PE. Comment on McLaren's critical review of the biopsychosocial model. Aust N Z J Psychiatry 1998: 32; 95-96.

22. McLaren N. The biopsychosocial model and scientific fraud. Paper presented to annual congress, RANZCP, Christchurch, May, 2004. Revised version Chapter 8 in Ref. 26: When does self-deception become culpable?

23. McLaren N. The myth of the biopsychosocial model (letter|). Aust N Z J Psychiatry 2006; 40:277-78.

24. Cantor C, Joyce PR. Evolution and psychiatry (Editorial) Aust N Z J Psychiatry 2009; 43:991-993 (Prof. Joyce is editor-in-chief of *ANZJP*).

25. McLaren N. Science and the psychiatric publishing industry. *Ethical Hum Psychol Psychiat* 2009; 11: 29-37.

26. McLaren N. *Humanizing Madness: Psychiatry and the Cognitive Neurosciences*. 2007; Ann Arbor, Mi.: Future Psychiatry Press. ISBN 978-1 932690-39-2.

27 McLaren N. *Humanizing psychiatry: The biocognitive model*. 2009; Ann Arbor, Mi.: Future Psychiatry Press. ISBN 978-1-615990-11-5.

28. McLaren N. Monist models of mind and biological psychiatry. *Ethical Hum Psychol Psychiat* 2010; 12 (in press).

29. Chomsky N. The Fate of an Honest Intellectual. *Understanding Power*, 2002. The New Press pp. 244-248

30. Kuhn TS. *The Structure of Scientific Revolutions*. 2nd Edition, 1970. Chicago, Ill: University Press (International Encyclopedia of Unified Science, Vol. 2, No. 2

31. Cloninger CR. Evolution of human brain functions: the functional structure of human consciousness. Aust N Z J Psychiatry 2009; 43: 994-1006.

32. Intuitions about combining opinions: misappreciations of the averaging principle. http://goliath.ecnext.com/coms2/gi_0199-6097958/ Intuitions-about-combining-opinions-misappreciation.html

Epilogue

"An error does not become truth by reason of multiplied propagation, nor does truth become error because nobody sees it. Truth stands, even if there be no public support. It is self-sustained."

Gandhi

In these three volumes, I have taken each of the major theories used in psychiatry in the past one hundred years and analyzed them using the standard tools of the philosophy of science. Each of them has irredeemably failed the tests, meaning psychiatry has no rational basis at all. These days, very few psychiatrists would be concerned to hear that psychoanalysis and behaviorism are not considered scientific but many are shocked to be told that the dominant biological approach lacks anything like a coherent, articulated model of mental disorder to guide daily practice, teaching, and research. Surprised, sometimes bewildered and quite often irritated, they point to the dopamine thesis for psychosis or the 5-HT model of depression as assurance that their work does have a proven rationale. This is not correct. These are not models of mental disorder but are simply instances of a larger model, the biological model. However, this has never been articulated and, if my work is correct, it never will be just because it is logically impossible.

I am not talking about 'technically improbable', such as when people used to say that heavier than air flight was impossible, because that only requires a change of technology. Nor am I talking about 'impossible in practice', such as the idea of curing world hunger. I am talking about logically impossible, such as a statement being true and also being false at one and the same time. We cannot use speech in the sense of symbolic transmission of information, and, at the same time, say that mental disorder is just a special case of brain disorder.

Other people take exception to my claims on the basis that we have an empirical practice that works, so why attack it? My work is not about whether some drugs work on some cases some of the time, but what is the exact nature of mental disorder, so that we can develop practices that work on practically all cases nearly all of the time. We need to shift from the pre-scientific stage of poking in the dark to knowing exactly what is happening in a person's head to cause his current symptoms.

Thus, my work has moved from simply criticizing the current models, because that is not difficult to do, to offering something in their place. In order to do that, I had to branch out of psychiatry into philosophy of mind, which has generated further controversy as some well-regarded philosophical work has shown itself to be full of holes. That can't be helped: my view is that if somebody doesn't want his theories criticized, then keep right away from science. Criticism of the status quo is the engine of scientific progress: no criticism, no progress. In science, only this point itself is beyond criticism.

This foray into philosophy has led to a specific theory of mind, or theory of mental order, which leads directly to a theoretical resolution of the mind-body problem. From this point, the theory of mind, which incorporates an account of language, allows the development of a rational theory of mental disorder and thence to a formal approach to treatment. This is the first time in our history that psychiatrists have been able to make this claim but the work needs to be developed further before we can be confident that it can answer the profoundly important questions of mental disorder. Thus, the ideas presented in these books must now be subjected to stringent criticism by a broader range of people and, in that respect, a hundred thousand heads are better than one.

Just for the record, I would like it known that I have never received a penny of financial assistance nor any material or intellectual support from any person, government, foundation, or educational body anywhere in the world at any stage. Moreover, I never discuss my work before it is edited for publication. Readers may feel that it would have been better if I had done so but it has always been beyond my control. It is the result of the antagonism of the psychiatric establishment to the idea that they can and should be criticized. That may at last be changing. As Oscar Wilde said, "There is only one thing worse than being talked about, and that's not being talked about."

Index

Y

Z